3D Imaging in Endodontics

Mohamed I. Fayad • Bradford R. Johnson
Editors

3D Imaging in Endodontics

A New Era in Diagnosis and Treatment

Second Edition

Springer

Editors
Mohamed I. Fayad
Department of Endodontics
University of Illinois Chicago
Chicago, IL, USA

Bradford R. Johnson
Department of Endodontics
University of Illinois Chicago
Chicago, IL, USA

ISBN 978-3-031-32757-5 ISBN 978-3-031-32755-1 (eBook)
https://doi.org/10.1007/978-3-031-32755-1

This Springer imprint is published by the registered company Springer Nature Switzerland AG
The registered company address is: Gewerbestrasse 11, 6330 Cham, Switzerland

Contents

Principles of Cone Beam Computed Tomography

1

William C. Scarfe

Abstract

Radiography is an essential diagnostic tool in clinical endodontics. Maxillofacial cone beam computed tomography (CBCT) has revolutionized diagnostic imaging providing high-resolution, limited field of view, and relatively low-dose volumetric data from which task-specific images can be reformatted for applications in endodontic diagnosis, treatment guidance, and posttreatment evaluation. Successful diagnosis using CBCT requires that clinicians understand the fundamentals of CBCT acquisition, the role of both scanning and image visualization protocols in image quality and patient dose, and adopt a methodological approach to endodontic enhanced CBCT imaging. Guidance on selection of optimal parameters for task-specific endodontic imaging and visualization will be provided.

1.1 Introduction

Radiography is an essential diagnostic tool in each of the three therapeutic stages of clinical endodontics: (1) pre-operative and diagnosis and treatment planning, (2) intra-operative assessment, and (3) post-operative monitoring. While providing valuable information, intraoral radiographs only present a two-dimensional (2D) representation of a three-dimensional (3D) dental structure and are susceptible to exposure (e.g., density and contrast) and geometric errors (e.g., unsharpness, magnification, and distortion). In addition, the complex nature of the anatomy of the teeth and adjacent structures contributes to limitations of intraoral radiography in the visualization of root canal anatomy, detection of periapical pathology, and

W. C. Scarfe (✉)
Department of Diagnosis and Oral Health, University of Louisville School of Dentistry, Louisville, KY, USA
e-mail: william.scarfe@louisville.edu

M. I. Fayad, B. R. Johnson (eds.), *3D Imaging in Endodontics*,
https://doi.org/10.1007/978-3-031-32755-1_1

assessment of the healing of periapical tissues. The introduction of maxillofacial cone beam computed tomography (CBCT) in dentistry has revolutionized diagnostic imaging in endodontics, providing high-resolution, relatively low-dose 3D images from volumetric acquisition.

Successful diagnosis using CBCT imaging in endodontics requires that clinicians understand the fundamentals of CBCT acquisition, the role of both scanning and image visualization protocols in image quality and patient dose, and adopt a methodological approach to endodontic enhanced CBCT imaging. Guidance on selection of optimal parameters for task-specific endodontic imaging and visualization will be provided.

1.2 Fundamentals of CBCT Imaging

The radiologic goal of CBCT imaging in endodontics is to consistently produce high-resolution, high-quality diagnostic images at a minimal radiation dose to the patient and efficiently interpret them. In this regard, the CBCT imaging chain is a linear process comprising two interconnecting chains, each with discrete "links." The interpretation of CBCT images is limited by the weakest link in the imaging chain.

- **CBCT Acquisition.** This is the *technical* aspect of CBCT radiography and requires an understanding of CBCT acquisition and an appreciation of the factors under the control of the clinician (operator-dependent variables).
- **Image Visualization.** This is the *technique* aspect of CBCT radiography and demands a methodological approach to the display of imaging data and interpretation of the 3D imaging volume.

CBCT imaging for endodontics is unique compared to other areas of dentistry in that it necessitates small volume acquisition, providing high-resolution cross-sectional radiographic images of a dental region of interest with the least noise, and minimal artifacts. This places high demands on both technical acquisition and the visualization skills of the clinician. This customized approach to imaging has been termed "endodontic enhanced CBCT" [1].

1.3 CBCT Image Acquisition

There are many manufacturers of CBCT units, each producing a variety of models. Models vary in design and footprint, projection geometry, exposure and technical controls, and visualization software. However, the principles of acquisition are the same and follow three sequential phases (Fig. 1.1):

- **Projection Geometry.** A rotating platform supports the synchronous single full or partial rotation of an x-ray source and a reciprocating area x-ray sensor around

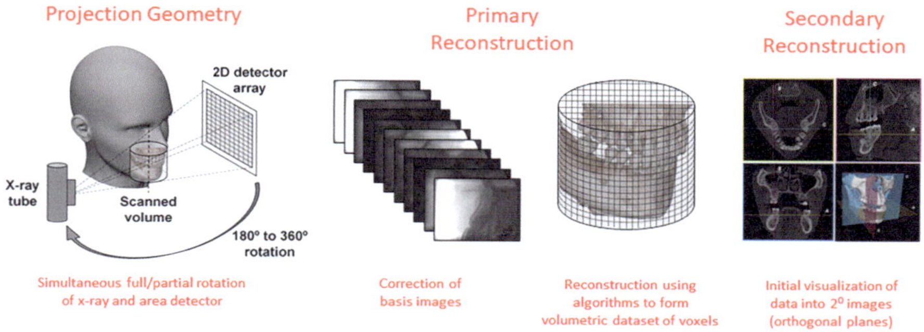

Fig. 1.1 The three phases of CBCT acquisition (from left to right): (1) geometric projection, (2) primary reconstruction, and (3) secondary reconstruction

a fixed axis of rotation (rotational arc) related to the dental region of interest (ROI). A divergent pyramidal (originally "cone-shaped") beam of ionizing radiation is collimated and directed through the middle of the ROI to provide a field of view (FOV). During the rotation, between 150 and 1000 individual single, sequential planar projection images are acquired. This series of two-dimensional (2D) *projection* or *basis images* acquired at slightly different angles forms a set referred to as the *projection data*.

- **Primary Reconstruction.** Sophisticated mathematical software algorithms process the projection data to correct for magnification, distortion, and density variances and then generate a three-dimensional (3D), usually cylindrical, *volumetric dataset* composed of cuboidal volume elements (voxels).
- **Secondary Reconstruction**. Perpendicular sectioning of the volumetric dataset to provide contiguous thin section images in three orthogonal planes (axial, coronal, and sagittal) is referred to as *secondary reconstruction*.

1.3.1 Operator-Independent Variables

Each CBCT unit operates based on a manufacturer specific, complex balance between the characteristics and geometry of the physical components of the system, and the computer hardware and software of the system. These include:

- **X-ray source and geometric configuration**. Numerous unit-specific features of the x-ray source and projection geometry of CBCT devices influence the image quality and resolution of images [2].
- **Type and response of the x-ray detector.** Most currently available dental CBCT units use coupling of a scintillator (e.g., gadolinium oxysulfide or cesium iodide) to convert x-ray photons to light photons which are then detected using a sensor array of digital elements (dexels) to produce a two-dimensional x-ray transmission image [3]. The read/write/erase ability of this detector (frame rate) together with the completeness of the trajectory arc and

the speed of the rotation determines the total number of images comprising the projection dataset and is reflected in the scan time. The scan time and therefore number of basis projections acquired differ between CBCT units and may be fixed or variable.

- **Motion of the x-ray source detector assembly**. Three rotational angle configurations are available: (1) fixed full (360°) trajectory, (2) fixed partial (ranging from approximately 200° to 240°), or (3) variable, usually with two trajectory settings, full and partial scan (180°) arc (see below). Reconstruction algorithms theoretically require data acquired from a 360° rotational scan arc; however, projection data from a reduced scan angle can be reconstructed using interpolation algorithms.
- **Type of reconstruction algorithm**. The Feldkamp, Davis, and Kress (FDK) algorithm is the most widely used for CBCT reconstruction. An alternative reconstruction method, iterative reconstruction (IR), is now available on some CBCT units. IR may be available as a pre- or post-processing option and, when applied, substantially reduces noise, motion artifacts, beam hardening and scatter artifacts compared with FBK reconstruction without sacrificing spatial resolution. Clinically the image takes longer to reconstruct and a computer with superior processing, memory, and video graphics capability is necessary.
- **Hardware and software**. Reconstruction times vary depending on the acquisition parameters (voxel size, FOV, number of projections), hardware (processing speed, data throughput from acquisition to workstation computer), and software (pre- and post-processing, reconstruction algorithm) used. Most CBCT units are provided with a single computer that performs both acquisition and display. Reconstruction times may increase, and visualization software responsiveness decrease over the operational lifetime of the CBCT unit with increasing local data storage.

The function of CBCT software is fourfold: image capture (acquisition), image processing (reconstruction, pre- and post-processing), image storage and retrieval (database), and image display (enhancement and visualization).

1.3.1.1 Recommendations for Endodontists

- **Desirable Features of a CBCT Unit.** Units with smaller x-ray tube focal spot sizes, continuous pulsed exposure, and longer source to object distance favor the production of higher-resolution images with reduced noise. Quoted values for nominal resolution are theoretical only—request data reporting actual resolution. A unit with variable scan time, providing a high number of basis projections, is highly desirable, reducing image noise. Partial scan arc systems may have reduced image quality with decreased visibility of pulp canals and increase the number of false positives when detecting vertical fractures [4]. Units that use aligned projection geometry are preferred [2]. Units with IR algorithms are desirable, especially with units using fixed exposure parameters, scan time, or partial scan arc acquisition.

- **Hardware.** Periodic archival of patient data files and use of computers with video graphics processors ensure optimal reconstruction times and software visualization responsiveness.
- **Software.** Final image quality is a complex interplay between the functions of CBCT software. Images should be initially viewed using proprietary software. Exported DICOM images imported into non-proprietary software may lose definition and clarity because of the specific features and refinements of image display software "fine-tuned" to the output of other elements in the proprietary imaging chain.

1.3.2 Operator-Dependent Variables

Unlike other extraoral dental imaging modalities (e.g., panoramic), there are two technical (Fig. 1.2) and one practical factor to consider when performing CBCT imaging for endodontics.

1.3.2.1 Scan Protocol

The choice of specific technical parameters to optimize image quality and minimize exposure for endodontic imaging is called the *imaging acquisition* or *scan protocol*. Scan protocol affects image quality and patient radiation exposure.

- **Exposure Settings.** Most dental CBCT units allow the operator to adjust the x-ray tube voltage (peak kilovoltage [kVp)], the tube current (milliamperes [mA]), or both. These can be adjusted manually or predetermined, "fixed" exposure settings be used. These settings may reflect patient type (e.g., child, adolescent, adult, large adult), scan resolution (standard or high definition), or scan mode (e.g., implants, endo) (Fig. 1.3).

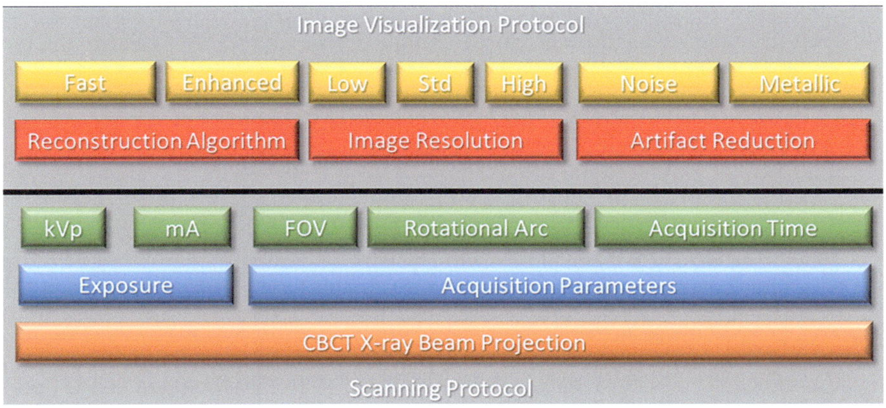

Fig. 1.2 Relationship between the two operator-dependent technical factors associated with image acquisition: (1) scanning protocol and (2) visualization protocol. Alteration of scanning factors affects dose and image quality, whereas adjustment of visualization parameters affects image quality only

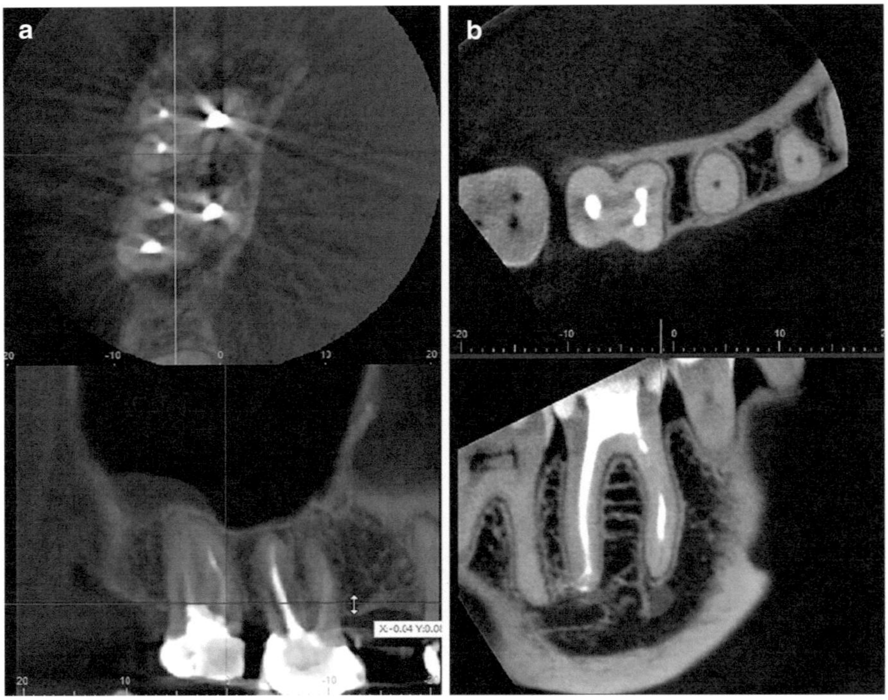

Fig. 1.3 Comparison of small FOV endodontic image quality at the same resolution between one model of CBCT taken for the maxillary right molar (90 kVp, 8 mA, 9.4 s scan time,l 270° rotation arc) (**a**) and another for the mandibular right molar (100 kVp, 5 mA, 17.9 s scan time,l 360° rotational arc) (**b**). The higher kVP, the greater number of basis images and complete rotational arc provides images with higher contrast, reduced noise, and minimal artifacts

- **mA.** mA settings are usually less than 12 mA, while some operate as high as 20 mA. Increasing mA produces overall darker images, but reduces image noise, visually observed as a "salt and pepper" inhomogeneity within a specific tissue. However, patient effective dose increases proportionately, almost in a 1:1 ratio.
- **kVp.** Most CBCT units operate in the range less than 90 kVp, with a few able to operate up to 120 kV. Higher kVp units theoretically produce images with a higher contrast-to-noise ratio, particularly at lower exposures. The effect of kVp on dose and image quality is complicated—however, increasing kVp has an even greater effect on dose than mA; with each 10 kV increase, it approximately doubles the dose [5].
- The effect of changing one or both exposure factors on image quality and dose is not straightforward and should be balanced such that adequate image quality is achieved at the lowest possible dose. Currently there is still a low level of clinical evidence on the effect of adjusting exposure settings on image quality specifically in endodontics [6, 7].

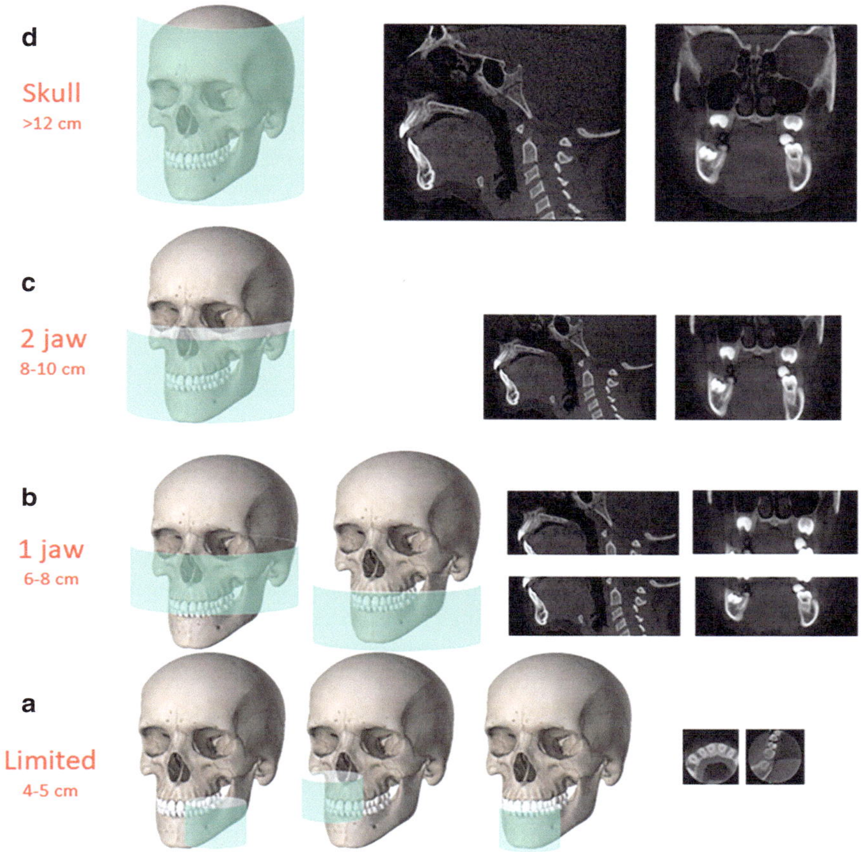

Fig. 1.4 Schematic representations of the approximate anatomical coverage provided by different fields of view of a CBCT unit. (**a**) Small or limited FOV captures a localized area of several adjacent teeth with their periapical region, (**b**) One jaw captures dentoalveolar regions of one jaw, (**c**) Two jaws capture the dentoalveolar regions of both jaws, and (**d**) large FOV captures the maxillofacial structures beyond the oral cavity and maxillary sinus floor

- **Acquisition Parameters**.
  - **FOV.** The FOV determines the extent of anatomic coverage (Fig. 1.4). It is adjusted by collimation of the x-ray beam to the ROI and must be minimized for all endodontic CBCT imaging examinations. Most FOVs are cylindrical, predefined, and reported in centimeters by a maximum vertical height and circular diameter (e.g., 4 × 4 is 4 cm vertical height and 4 cm maximum diameter). Reducing FOV improves image quality by reducing image noise by minimizing scatter radiation, as well as optimizing patient radiation dose [8]. In most units, small FOVs enable the selection of the highest spatial resolution.

- **Rotational Arc.** Units with partial scan arcs reduce scan time, minimize the potential for motion artifacts, and may provide reduced patient radiation dose. However, images from partial scan arc systems have greater noise, have lower spatial and contrast resolution, and potentially suffer from reconstruction interpolation artifacts [9]. This is offset by considerations of a proportionate reduction in patient radiation dose [10].
- **Acquisition Time.** Increasing scan time provides more information to reconstruct the image and has multiple beneficial effects on the image including greater contrast resolution, improved signal-to-noise ratio producing "smoother" images, and reduced metallic artifacts (Fig. 1.3). However, increasing scan time increases the potential for motion artifact and delivers a proportionately higher patient radiation dose.

Recommendations for Endodontics

- **Use the highest kVp setting for endodontic images.** Optimal images for endodontics require the use of the highest kVp [11], especially in patients with high-density objects such as root canal fillings and post-core restorations to reduce beam hardening artifacts (Fig. 1.3) [12–15]. This should be in combination with other dose reduction strategies (e.g., smallest FOV).
- **Adjust mA to compensate for patient size.** As endodontic images should have minimal noise, modest increases in mA from default settings provide greater noise reduction at a given dose than increasing kVp. Dental periapical diagnosis involving visualizing the periodontal ligament space and subtle changes in bone trabeculation may benefit from moderate increases in mA with larger patient sizes.
- **Use the smallest FOV for endodontic imaging, except in one clinical situation**. The FOV for an endodontic evaluation should be as small as possible and provide adequate anatomic coverage including at least 1 to 2 teeth in either side of the tooth under investigation and 1 to 2 cm beyond the apices. Practically a limited FOV scan will allow selection of the highest resolution. In addition, it reduces the effect of exomass (i.e., structures located out of the FOV and between the focal spot and image receptor) on image quality. An exception to this is in patients with invasive external root resorption, where this may be present in multiple teeth in different segments of the jaws [16]. In this circumstance, an FOV adequately covering the dentition of both jaws is highly recommended (Fig. 1.4).
- **There may be minimal difference in diagnostic accuracy between full or partial arc rotation CBCT units.** Theoretically images acquired using a full arc rotation and higher scan time produce images of optimal diagnostic quality for endodontics [17, 18]. However, this is accompanied by a substantial and proportional increase in patient radiation dose. Current evidence suggests that there is no difference in diagnostic accuracy between full and partial/half scan for numerous endodontic tasks in vitro [19] including the detection of MB2 [18], periapical bone loss [20], root fractures [21, 22], external root resorption [23], and when performing endodontic measurements [24]. However, the presence of high-density objects in the FOV (previous endodontic treatment, posts) will markedly compromise image quality in partial/half scan data.

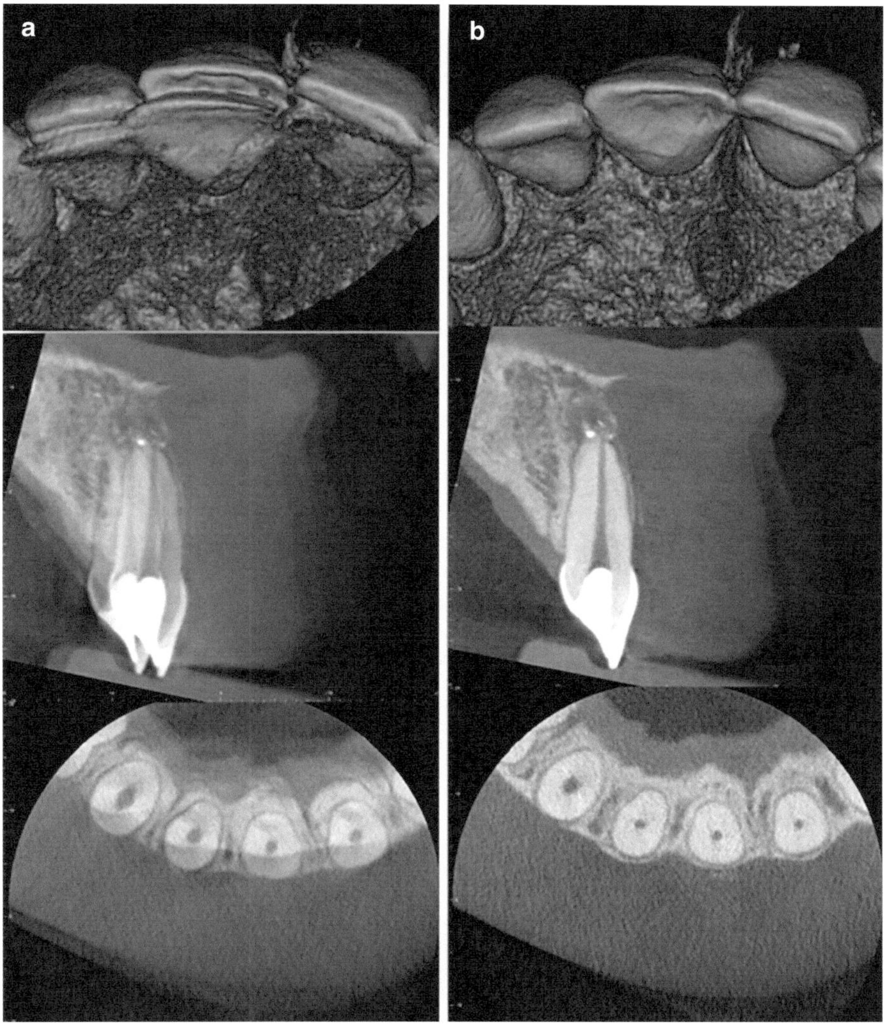

Fig. 1.5 Volumetric rendering (top), para-sagittal cross-section (middle), and axial (lower) images of the maxillary anterior region from an original (360° arc trajectory) (**a**) show marked blur attributable to motion artifact during the scan. Post-acquisition limited rotational arc reconstruction (**b**) shows excellent image quality recovered by selecting contiguous basis images from a 180° portion of the scan with minimal motion

– **Post-acquisition half scan reconstruction is extremely useful in endodontics for specific diagnostic tasks**. While only one manufacturer provides post-acquisition half scan reconstruction (Accuitomo F170 | X800; J. Morita Corp., Kyoto, Japan), this function is highly desirable in endodontics to minimize artifacts caused by patient motion and exomass, eliminating the need for a rescan (Fig. 1.5). It can also be used for follow-up imaging and is therefore a valuable dose-saving strategy.

– **The impact of the acquisition time on the accuracy of endodontic diagnostic tasks is equivocal**. While reduced acquisition time leads to decreased overall image quality and increases the presence of metallic artifacts [25], the impact of this on specific endodontic tasks is currently inadequately investigated. For the detection of VRF, reducing scan time results in reduced specificity (false positives) [21].

1.3.2.2 Image Visualization Protocol

There are three parameters that affect image quality but have no effect on patient radiation exposure.

- **Reconstruction Algorithm.** Iterative reconstruction (IR) algorithms (see above) are now provided as an option in some units. These produce images with reduced noise and artifacts and greater contrast and spatial resolution but have longer processing time.
- **Image Spatial Resolution.** Endodontics involves imaging of inherently small structures. The periodontal ligament space (e.g., acute apical periodontitis) has an average dimension of 0.2 mm and therefore demands a resolution at or below the Nyquist frequency (<0.1 mm). The smallest three-dimensional data unit on a CBCT image volume is the voxel (volume element). Voxel size depends principally on dexel dimensions. The size and spacing between dexels determine the nominal or theoretical resolution of the CBCT system, which ranges between 0.4 mm to 0.076 mm or equivalent to 1.25 to 6.5 $lp.mm^{-1}$. While often reported as the resolution of the system, it is never achieved as several other elements in the imaging chain such as reconstruction algorithms and image pre-display processing "filters" also contribute to actual spatial resolution. In general, a CBCT scan acquired with a smaller pixel size produces an image with higher spatial resolution.
- **Artifact Reduction Algorithms.** Two algorithms can be applied to the volumetric dataset prior to interpretation that may potentially improve image quality—noise and metallic artifact reduction (MAR). Both should be used with caution as they may add considerable time to the reconstruction phase and introduce other undesirable effects into the image.

Recommendations for Endodontists

– **Always use the highest resolution setting.** Most endodontic diagnostic tasks (e.g., visualization of the periodontal ligament space, lamina dura, root surface) require high-resolution (less than 0.125 mm) scan modes. These modes, especially those that are pre-set, may be linked with an accompanying longer scan time to increase the number of basis projections to reduce noise or greater exposure to increase brightness and contrast and reduce noise. This results in higher patient radiation dose and the potential for patient motion artifacts. Smaller voxel sizes, ranging from 200 um to as low as 80 um, improve the detection and, in some cases, observer inter-rater reliability of MB2 [26–29], root length measurements [30, 31], and vertical root fracture [32] (Fig. 1.6), which appear to be

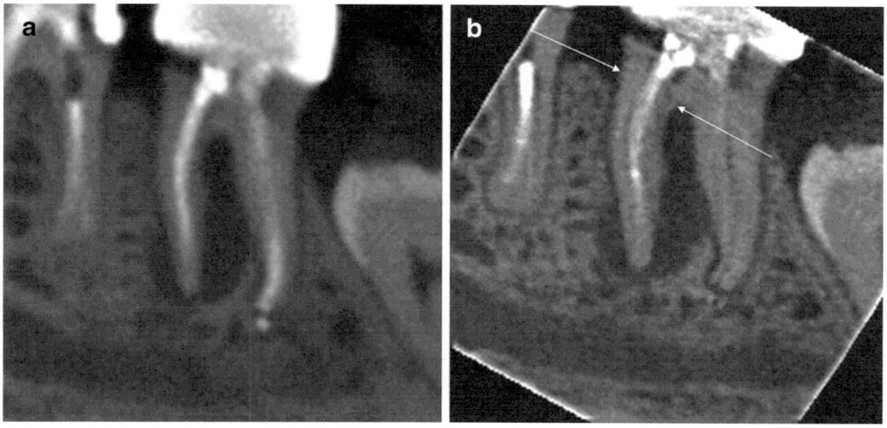

Fig. 1.6 Para-sagittal image of the left mandibular first molar at 0.25 mm (**a**) and 0.08 mm (**b**) voxel resolution. While the "J"-shaped lesion associated with the mesial root is highly suggestive of a root fracture, it is only the high-resolution image (**b**) that clearly demonstrates the location and completeness of the fracture (solid arrows)

CBCT unit dependent [33]. Scan resolutions from 0.1 mm [34] to 0.3 mm [35] voxel size may be adequate for the detection of external root resorption [36].

- **IR may improve image quality, particularly if the unit has partial scan arc.** While no specific authors have reported the effects of IR in endodontics, it has the potential to improve image quality in some CBCT units, especially those with fixed kVp or partial scan acquisition.
- **The use of MAR in endodontics shows promise in some endodontic tasks.** The application of MAR has not been reported to improve diagnostic accuracy in the detection of MB2 [37], fractured instruments [25], or furcal perforations [38]; however, it may be valuable in improving the diagnosis of VRF [39, 40], especially in the presence of intracanal posts [41], and varies on post material [42].

1.3.2.3 Patient Positioning Protocol

Irrespective of the CBCT patient configuration (standing, lying, or seated), the jaws must be firmly stabilized during the entire scan. This reduces the potential for motion during the scan, a significant source of artifact and reduced image quality [43–45]. This can be accomplished using chin rests, bite blocks, or head holders and by providing instructions to the patient to remain still during the procedure and to keep the teeth closed together or on a bite block.

Recommendations for Endodontists

- **Separate the dentition when the jaws are closed.** On units that use a chin rest for stabilization, teeth should be separated by cotton rolls or a tongue depressor such that the effects of scatter and beam hardening artifacts from high-density objects in the opposing jaw are minimized.

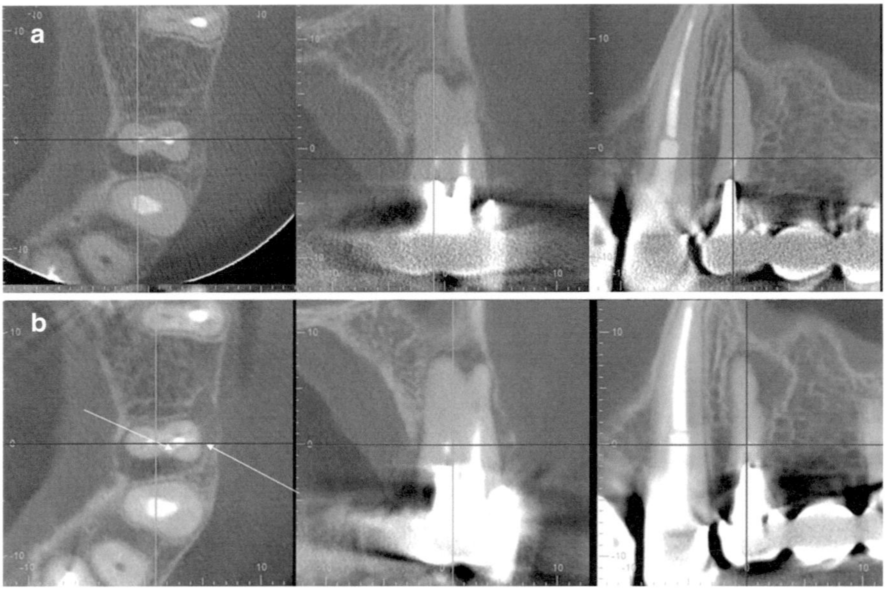

Fig. 1.7 Axial, cross-sectional, and sagittal images (left to right) of the maxillary left premolar region with labio-distal and palato-mesial alveolar defects. The initial scan (**a**) shows the extent of the lesions and incomplete obturation of the palatal canal; a second scan was performed (b) using a hard bite block pivoted on the buccal cusp and shows a complete vertical root fracture of the buccal cusp corresponding to the location of the separate alveolar defects

- **Apply occlusal force to assist in the detection of cracked teeth.** Initially cracked teeth are a diagnostic challenge as the two segments are not separated and there are minimal radiographic findings. Application of a constant occlusal force during the scan on either the labial or palatal aspect of the crown (e.g., cotton roll, bite block [e.g., Tooth Slooth]) can result in enough movement of the segments to occasionally aid identification (Fig. 1.7).
- **Ensure that the tooth under investigation is centered in the FOV**. Optimal image quality in all CBCT units is at the center of rotation. Center-scanned position has been reported to be the only position that is reliable in the detection of vertical root fractures (VRF) [46, 47] (Fig. 1.8), especially if MAR is applied [39].

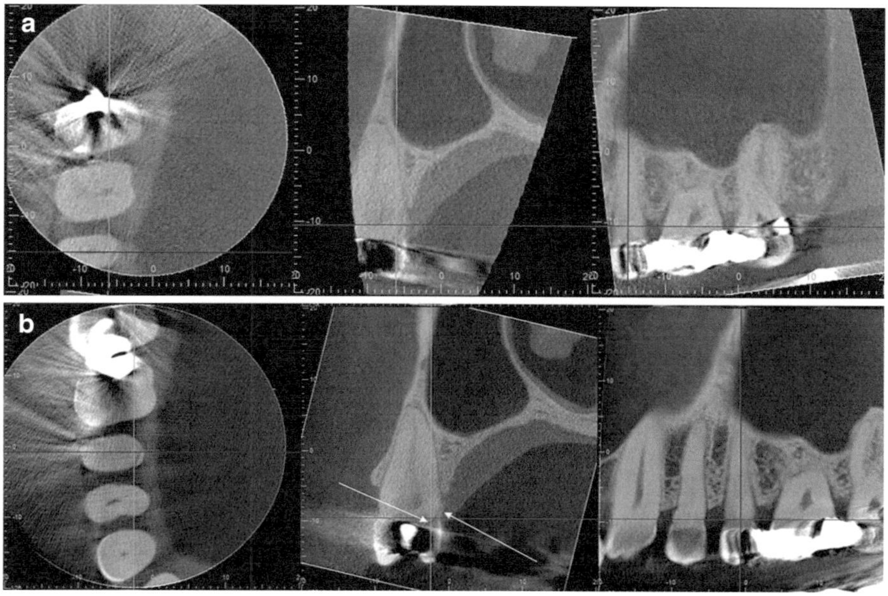

Fig. 1.8 Axial, cross-sectional, and sagittal images (left to right) of the maxillary right posterior quadrant of a symptomatic patient with a possible crown or root fracture in the premolar/first molar area. Two scans were acquired—the first (**a**) was inadvertently taken at 180° rotational arc with the FOV centered too far posteriorly. The second scan (**b**) was taken at 360° rotational arc with the FOV centered on the region of interest (premolars/first molar). Notice the image clarity in identifying the palatal crown/root fracture on the second premolar in (**b**) compared with the noisier and poorer contrast image in (**a**)

1.4 Image Visualization

Image display is software-assisted and performed as an interactive process—the value of the voxels, such as image brightness and contrast, must be adjusted (data correction), the volumetric dataset reoriented, and the display adjusted and enhanced using task-specific protocols. Finally, the clinician interprets the findings demonstrated by the images, dynamically navigating through the imaging volume by scrolling through image stacks, adjusting thickness, and applying appropriate enhancements.

Endodontists are advised to adopt an efficient and consistent methodology to optimize image visualization prior to image interpretation. The following approach serves as a guide to improve the visibility of anatomic structures specifically for endodontics [48].

1.4.1 Re-Orient the Dataset

In endodontics, the ROI is most often a specific tooth or group of teeth within the dental arch. The first step is therefore to align each orthogonal multiplanar reformat (MPR) projection to the specific tooth under examination.

1.4.1.1 Recommendations for Endodontists

- **Adjust the sagittal plane.** In this projection, the vertical y-z axis should be adjusted to align with the long axis of the tooth such that the parasagittal plane transects both the middle of the occlusal surface/incisal edge and apical terminus of the root of the tooth labio-lingually.
- **Adjust the coronal plane.** In this projection, the vertical y-x axis should also be adjusted to align with the long axis of the tooth such that the paracoronal plane transects the middle of the occlusal surface/incisal edge and apical terminus of the root of the tooth mesio-distally.
- **Adjust the axial plane.** In this projection, the horizontal y-z axis should be adjusted to align with tooth such that the axial plane transects the cemento-enamel junction (CEJ) of the root of the tooth peri-circumferentially.

1.4.2 Correct the Data

The default display of orthogonal images may not be optimized for the visualization of dental anatomic structures and should be corrected using a sequential image enhancement protocol.

- **Adjust Contrast and Brightness.** Contrast and brightness are the principal methods for improving overall image detail. Contrast, also referred to as the window width (W), is adjusted to displaying only part of the available full gray value range. Brightness, also referred to as the window level (L), determines the central gray value within the window width. Dental imaging software often provides sliding bars with brightness and contrast options or allows direct alteration on the image using the mouse cursor where brightness and contrast adjustments are the vertical and horizontal motions on the display.
- **Sharpen Edges.** To improve the differentiation of, and detail related to, bony structures, it is necessary to sharpen the definition of edges. This can be achieved by applying edge detection enhancement filters. Combining histogram enhancement and sharpening filters in succession is the most efficient method of improving image quality for most clinical scenarios.
- **Reduce Noise.** The effect of noise on the image can be reduced by applying a smoothing enhancement algorithm. However, this will compete with edge enhancement algorithms. Increasing image section thickness from the sub-millimeter to millimeter range minimizes the effect of noise on the resulting image and maintains image sharpness.

1.4.2.1 Recommendations for Endodontics

The selection of an appropriate data correction enhancement for endodontics is CBCT system (model) specific and is determined by image thickness.

- **Adjust contrast and brightness for 1 mm sections, preferably using a histogram.** Image enhancements are highly slice thickness dependent. Adjustment of brightness and contrast can be performed empirically based on the visual appearance on the image and image thickness. However, a more reliable and consistent approach is to adjust the linear LUT to correspond to the available histogram (Fig. 1.9).
- **Review endodontic images at 1 mm section thickness initially and then reduce if necessary.** A 1 mm image slice provides optimal balance between resolution and noise and minimizes artifacts (Fig. 1.10). Decreasing slice thickness, even on high-resolution data, produces noisy images and worsens artifacts.
- **Use enhancement filters selectively.** Filters do not always improve the detection of root fractures [49–51] but can assist in distinguishing fractures from accessory root canals [52].
- **If enhancement filters are used, always compare the adjusted image with the original image.** Enhancements often introduce undesirable effects and artifacts. Overshoot or "Uberschwinger" artifacts are often prominent adjacent to high-density materials. Comparison of adjusted with original images is recommended (Fig. 1.11).

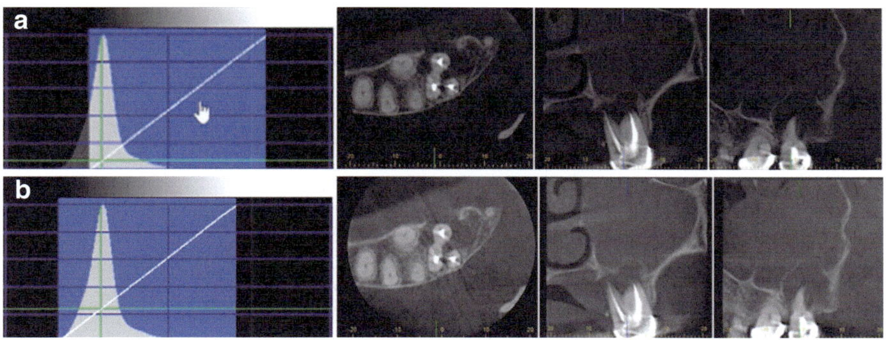

Fig. 1.9 Histogram of available CBCT volume pixel intensity values (i.e., shades) (gray area under the plot) and corresponding axial, cross-sectional, and parasagittal 1 mm sections (left to right) of the left posterior maxillary quadrant showing original default displayed images in the blue region, (**a**) which do not show all available pixel values at the lower end of the scale (gray area). Lookup table (LUT) adjusted images (**b**) move the blue region to the left and include all available pixel values. The adjusted images (**b**) clearly show perforation of the large expansile apical lesion through the floor of the maxillary sinus and soft tissue density material consistent with sinusitis of odontogenic origin

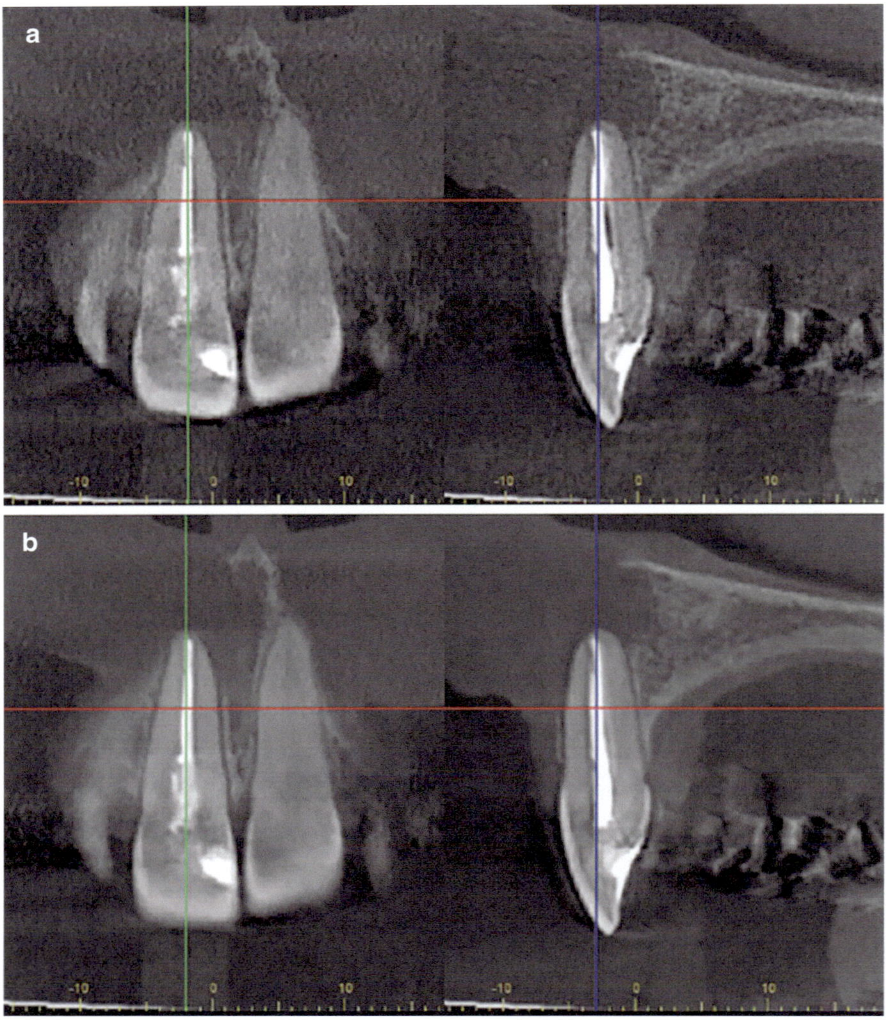

Fig. 1.10 Coronal and cross-sectional (left to right) images of the right maxillary central incisor at acquired 0.08 mm (**a**) and 1.0 mm (**b**) thickness. Increasing display thickness reduces noise and artifacts

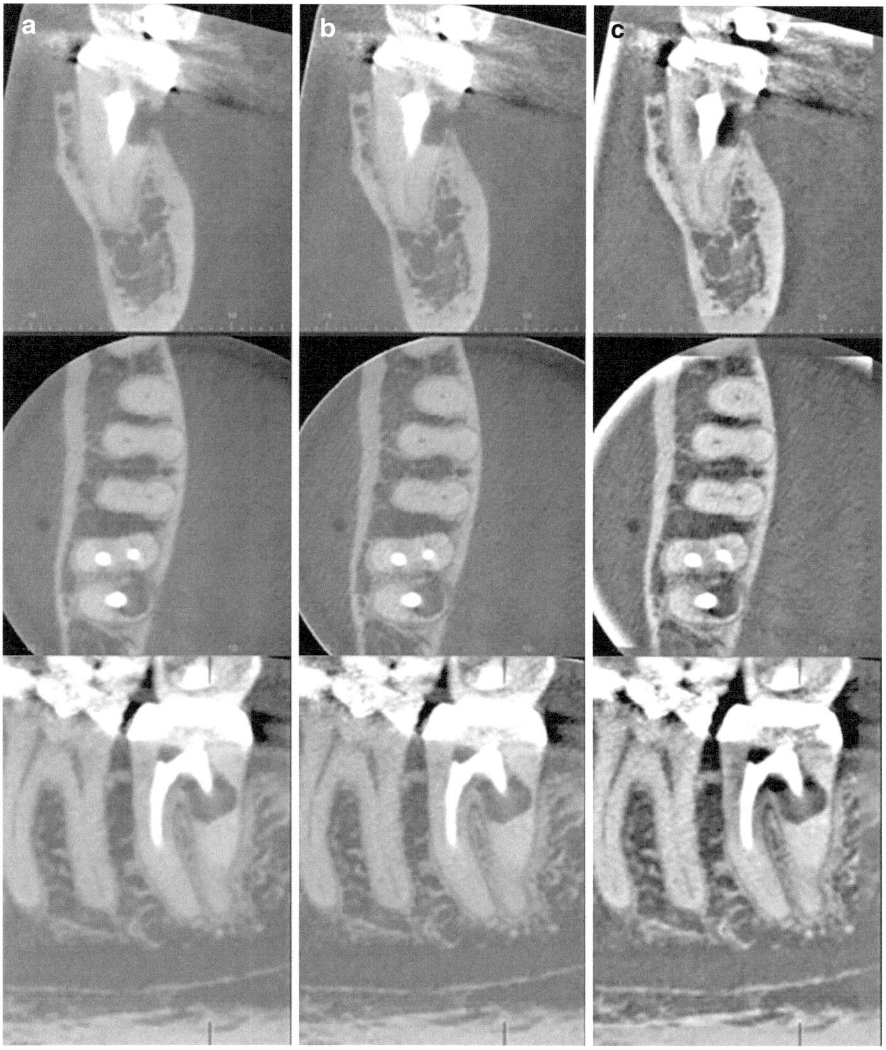

Fig. 1.11 Cross-sectional, axial, and para-sagittal (top to bottom) images of the mandibular left posterior quadrant with variable edge filter enhancement ranging from none (**a**), mild (**b**), and severe (**c**). Uniform peripheral dark banding adjacent to the root canal filling material (Uberschwinger artifact) increases with greater enhancement

1.4.3 Reformat the Data

Various options are available in the "radiographic toolbox" to reformat CBCT data and optimize CBCT image display specific to endodontics. These include multiplanar reformatting (MPR), aligning a curved or linear imaging plane with a specific anatomic structure and serial cross-sectional images perpendicular to the MPR, and various indirect (e.g., shaded surface display) and direct (e.g., ray sum and maximum intensity projection) volumetric techniques. Specific applications are described in Chaps. 2–10.

1.4.4 Explore the Data

CBCT software provides a graphic user interface for navigation and display of image data. Each window may be subdivided into two or a series of separate compartments referred to as frames, panels, or panes (consistent with the window analogy). The default window may allow selection or customization of the layout of the panes of that window. The most common default mode comprises four separate panels allowing viewing axial, coronal, and sagittal sections and either a custom MPR section or a 3D volumetric rendering which can be viewed simultaneously or individually.

Navigation refers to the process of reviewing each orthogonal series dynamically by scrolling through the consecutive image "stack" in a "cine" or "paging" mode. This can be performed either with mouse controls or by using a separate slider bar.

1.4.4.1 Recommendations for Endodontics

- **Explore volumetric data using orthogonal projections**. Viewing orthogonal projections is the principal technique for a systematic approach to interpretation of endodontic images.
- **Apply scrolling.** Scrolling should be performed cranio-caudally (i.e., in the axial plane from "head-to-toe") and then in reverse, slowing down in areas of greater complexity (e.g., apical terminus, area of external root resorption). Scrolling should be performed in at least two planes (e.g., coronal and axial).

1.5 Image Artifacts

Discrepancies between the reconstructed CBCT data and the physical state of the actual object that degrade the quality of CBCT images are termed artifacts. Additionally, structures that do not exist in the subject may appear within images [7]. These artifacts are due to x-ray-object interactions or are scanner, reconstruction, or patient based [53]. Based on appearance, artifacts (both white and dark) can present as follows:

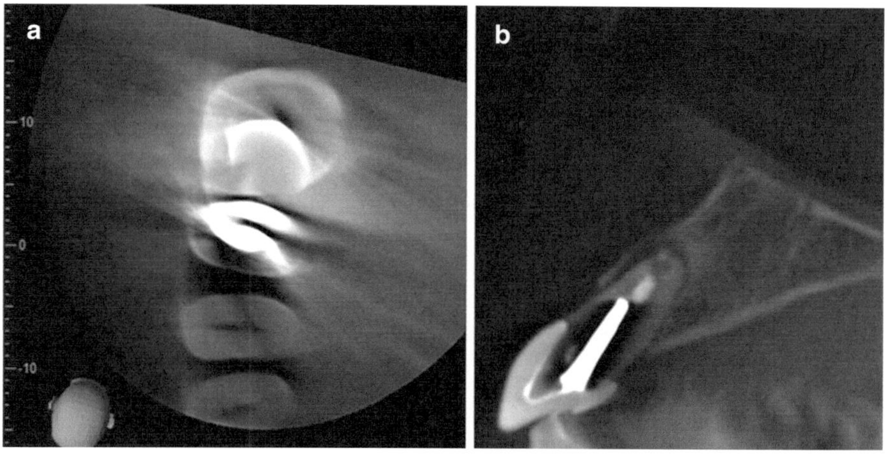

Fig. 1.12 (**a**) Axial slice demonstrating metallic restorations in the second premolar and first molar teeth. Note the radiating linear pattern of dark bands and streaks extending onto the root of the adjacent first premolar. (**b**) Sagittal CBCT section through the maxillary central incisor showing a dark zone adjacent to the metallic post, obscuring the root

- **Distortions and blur.** Due to patient movement or cupping artifacts.
- **Shading or graininess.** Due to noise within the system or effects of exomass.
- **Streaks.** Due to inadequate number of projections producing aliasing effects, partial volume averaging, and mechanical failure. Beam hardening artifacts are noted around dense bony structures, high-density restorative materials, and endodontic filling materials (Fig. 1.12).
- **Rings or bands.** Due to dexel defects or calibration error.

1.5.1 Recommendations for Endodontists

- **Exclusion of the crowns of the teeth from the FOV in heavily restored dentitions may improve image quality**. As beam hardening and scatter artifacts occur in the line of the divergent x-ray beam, adjusting the FOV to exclude restored crowns of the teeth may minimize the extension of these effects from both sides of the dentition onto the roots, improving image quality.
- **Become familiar with the appearance of artifacts as they may mimic fracture lines**. Metallic restorations produce dark bands and streaks which may be misinterpreted on restorations and adjacent teeth as dental caries. (Figs. 1.2, 1.3, and 1.4) or root fractures. Likewise, the region around metallic posts and gutta-percha yields dark bands, which may compromise the ability to detect fractures or resorption of the adjacent root structure.

1.6 Radiation Dose Considerations

The potential effects of x-ray photons on biologic molecules are mediated directly by ionizations of DNA or indirectly by the production of radicals via hydrolysis and may potentially produce biological damage which may manifest as radiation-induced effects.

1.6.1 Radiation-Induced Effects

There are two types of radiation-induced effects:

Tissue reactions, also referred to as deterministic effects, occur with high doses and only present when the radiation absorption in a tissue or organ exceeds a threshold level. Radiation doses from CBCT imaging are orders of magnitude lower than the threshold levels for deterministic effects in the various tissues exposed and can be considered essentially zero.

Stochastic effects involves irreversible alteration of the cell, usually from damage to cellular DNA resulting in cancer, leukemia, and genetic (i.e., heritable) effects, and is the only effect of possible significance in endodontic CBCT imaging as they theoretically have no minimum threshold dose and can therefore result from very low-dose levels. These effects are currently based on the linear non-threshold (LNT) hypothesis extrapolated from effects known to occur above 100,000 microsievert (μSv)—however, these effects have not been proven to occur in the dose range of small FOV CBCT (< 550 μSv).

1.6.2 Radiation Dose and Risk

Overall detriment associated with radiation doses for a specific diagnostic radiographic procedure is reported as effective dose, measured in sieverts (Sv). Effective dose is considered an estimate and does not consider the influences of age, gender, and other patient-specific risk factors and cannot be used to accurately specify risks to an individual patient.

Patient radiation dose for CBCT examinations is wide ranging and markedly influenced by the type and model of CBCT device, patient size (child vs. adult), region of interest (mandible vs. maxilla), exposure settings (kV, mA), and scan parameters (e.g., size of FOV, number of basis images, rotational arc, voxel size and resolution) [19, 54]. The range of effective dose for small FOV imaging used in endodontics averages 84 μSv (range, 7–521 μSv), equivalent to approximately 10 days of background radiation equivalent time. To make risk understandable to patients, the effective dose of CBCT can be described relative to median values of other dental radiographic procedures, including panoramic (20 μSv/2.5 days), cephalometric (4.5 μSv/0.5 days), bitewing (6 μSv/0.75 days), and full mouth series (177 μSv/22 days) radiography.

1.6.2.1 Methods to Minimize Patient Radiation Exposure

While the stochastic risks of radiation-induced cancer for a single CBCT procedure are small, patient exposure should be minimized to the greatest extent possible or "ALARA"—"as low as reasonably achievable." Methods to achieve dose reduction during CBCT imaging include:

- **Selection Criteria.** An important approach to prevent unnecessary patient radiation exposure is to select the most suitable procedure for the diagnostic task. The decision to prescribe CBCT examination should be based on the patient's history and clinical findings, with a high likelihood that the CBCT findings will influence the diagnostic and treatment planning process. Expert panels representing professional organizations have published remarkably similar consensus position statements on the use of CBCT in endodontics—clinical suggestions as to the when, where, why, what, how, and on whom (Table 1.1) [55, 56].
- **Optimization of Imaging Protocols.** In endodontics, small FOV scans should always be used as generally they provide adequate anatomic coverage. However, this requires careful technique so that the tooth segment under investigation is centered within the FOV and is perhaps the most effective method to achieve

Table 1.1 Indications for CBCT in Endodontics

		Organization	
Indication	Example	AAE/ AAOMR	ESE
Diagnosis of radiographic signs of periapical pathosis when there are contradictory or nonspecific signs and/ or symptoms	Symptomatic teeth with no signs of pathology, anatomic superimposition	✓	✓
Confirmation of non-odontogenic causes of pathosis	Sinusitis of maxillary origin	✓	✓
Assessment and/or management of complex dentoalveolar trauma	Severe luxation injuries, suspected alveolar fracture, horizontal root fractures	✓	✓
Appreciation of extremely complex root canal systems prior to endodontic management	Class III and IV dens invaginatus, accessory canals, root curvature, root canal system anomalies	✓	✓
Retreatment—Nonsurgical	Missed MB2, complex root canal anatomy		✓
Assessment of endodontic treatment complications	Post and root canal perforations, calcified canals, separated endodontic instruments	✓	✓
Assessment and/or management of root resorption,	Internal or external resorption	✓	✓
Presurgical assessment prior to complex periradicular surgery	Location of pathologic lesion, determine optimal surgical access	✓	✓
Presurgical dental implant planning	Immediate implant placement	✓	

AAE/AAOMR, The American Association of Endodontists and the American Academy of Oral and Maxillofacial Radiology [55]; ESE, European Society of Endodontology [56]

dose reduction by reducing the most common error for retakes [45, 57]. Recommended scan protocol exposure and acquisition settings have previously been described to provide a diagnostically optimal image.
- **Protective Aprons and Thyroid Collars.** The use of lead aprons in CBCT imaging is to reduce scatter radiation to radiosensitive tissues outside the head and neck region dose such as the thyroid, breast, and gonads. Recent authors have provided conflicting results on the effectiveness of lead aprons in CBCT procedures [58, 59]. Dentists should follow regional radiation safety regulations. A thyroid collar reduces the dose to the thyroid gland from the primary beam by almost 50% [60] and is recommended, especially in children, where the thyroid gland is highly radiosensitive. Care should be taken so that the thyroid collar is not in the path of the primary beam—this would lead to significant artifacts that may compromise the diagnostic quality of the image.

Acknowledgment The author is grateful to Dr. Sanjay M. Mallya (Los Angeles, California, USA), the author of this Chapter in the 2016 edition, for use of specific content and Fig. 1.12 for inclusion in this current chapter.

References

1. Azevedo B. Thanks but no thanks. Communique, American Association of Endodontists April 1, 2022. Accessed August 29, 2022. Available at https://www.aae.org/specialty/communique/thanks-but-no-thanks/.
2. Santaella GM, Rosalen PL, Queiroz PM, Haiter-Neto F, Wenzel A, Spin-Neto R. Quantitative assessment of variation in CBCT image technical parameters related to CBCT detector lateral-offset position. Dentomaxillofac Radiol. 2020;49(2):20190077.
3. Seibert JA. Flat-panel detectors: how much better are they? Pediatr Radiol. 2006;36(Suppl 14):173–81.
4. Hassan BA, Payam J, Juyanda B, van der Stelt P, Wesselink PR. Influence of scan setting selections on root canal visibility with cone beam CT. Dentomaxillofac Radiol. 2012;41(8):645–8.
5. Pauwels R, Silkosessak O, Jacobs R, Bogaerts R, Bosmans H, Panmekiate S. A pragmatic approach to determine the optimal kVp in cone beam CT: balancing contrast-to-noise ratio and radiation dose. Dentomaxillofac Radiol. 2014;43(5):20140059.
6. Goulston R, Davies J, Horner K, Murphy F. Dose optimization by altering the operating potential and tube current exposure time product in dental cone beam CT: a systematic review. Dentomaxillofac Radiol. 2016;45(3):20150254.
7. Bechara B, McMahan CA, Moore WS, Noujeim M, Geha H, Teixeira FB. Contrast-to-noise ratio difference in small field of view cone beam computed tomography machines. J Oral Sci. 2012;54(3):227–32.
8. Palomo JM, Rao PS, Hans MG. Influence of CBCT exposure conditions on radiation dose. Oral Surg Oral Med Oral Pathol Oral Radiol Endod. 2008;105(6):773–82.
9. Al-Okshi A, Lindh C, Salé H, Gunnarsson M, Rohlin M. Effective dose of cone beam CT (CBCT) of the facial skeleton: a systematic review. Br J Radiol. 2015;88(1045):20140658.
10. Pauwels R, Zhang G, Theodorakou C, Walker A, Bosmans H, Jacobs R, Bogaerts R, Horner K, SEDENTEXCT Project Consortium. Effective radiation dose and eye lens dose in dental cone beam CT: effect of field of view and angle of rotation. Br J Radiol. 2014;87(1042):20130654.

11. Panmekiate S, Rungwittayathon P, Suptaweeponboon W, Tangtraitham N, Pauwels R. Optimization of exposure parameters in dental cone beam computed tomography using a 3-step approach. Oral Surg Oral Med Oral Pathol Oral Radiol. 2018;126(6):545–52.
12. Chindasombatjaroen J, Kakimoto N, Shimamoto H, Murakami S, Furukawa S. Correlation between pixel values in a cone-beam computed tomographic scanner and the computed tomographic values in a multidetector row computed tomographic scanner. J Comput Assist Tomogr. 2011;35(5):662–5.
13. Vasconcelos KF, Nicolielo LF, Nascimento MC, Haiter-Neto F, Bóscolo FN, Van Dessel J, EzEldeen M, Lambrichts I, Jacobs R. Artefact expression associated with several cone-beam computed tomographic machines when imaging root filled teeth. Int Endod J. 2015;48(10):994–1000.
14. Helvacioglu-Yigit D, Demirturk Kocasarac H, Bechara B, Noujeim M. Evaluation and reduction of artifacts generated by 4 different root-end filling materials by using multiple cone-beam computed tomography imaging settings. J Endod. 2016;42(2):307–14.
15. Helvacioglu-Yigit D, Seki U, Kursun-Cakmak S, Demirturk Kocasarac H, Singh M. Comparative evaluation of artifacts originated by four different post materials using different CBCT settings. Tomography. 2022;8(6):2919–28.
16. Wang N, Zhang M, Zhu J, Zhu Y, Wu J. Multiple idiopathic cervical root resorption: a systematic review. Oral Dis. 2022;
17. Costa EDD, Queiroz PM, Santaella GM, Capelozza ALA, Ambrosano GMB, Freitas DQ. Influence of scan mode (partial/full rotations) and FOV size in the formation of artefacts in cone beam CT. Dentomaxillofac Radiol. 2019;48(4):20180340.
18. Kuo YF, Chen MH, Huang KH, Chang HH, Yeh CL, Lin CP. Comparing image qualities of dental cone-beam computed tomography with different scanning parameters for detecting root canals. J Formos Med Assoc. 2021;120(3):991–6.
19. Yeung AWK, Jacobs R, Bornstein MM. Novel low-dose protocols using cone beam computed tomography in dental medicine: a review focusing on indications, limitations, and future possibilities. Clin Oral Investig. 2019;23(6):2573–81.
20. Lennon S, Patel S, Foschi F, Wilson R, Davies J, Mannocci F. Diagnostic accuracy of limited-volume cone-beam computed tomography in the detection of periapical bone loss: 360° scans versus 180° scans. Int Endod J. 2011;44:1118–27.
21. Bechara B, McMahan CA, Nasseh I, Geha H, Hayek E, Khawam G, Raad M, Noujeim M. Number of basis images effect on detection of root fractures in endodontically treated teeth using a cone beam computed tomography machine: an in vitro study. Oral Surg Oral Med Oral Pathol Oral Radiol. 2013;115(5):676–81.
22. Jones D, Mannocci F, Andiappan M, Brown J, Patel S. The effect of alteration of the exposure parameters of a cone-beam computed tomographic scan on the diagnosis of simulated horizontal root fractures. J Endod. 2015;41:520–5.
23. Durack C, Patel S, Davies J, Wilson R, Mannocci F. Diagnostic accuracy of small volume cone beam computed tomography and intraoral periapical radiography for the detection of simulated external inflammatory root resorption. Int Endod J. 2011;44:136–47.
24. Hashem D, Brown JE, Patel S, Mannocci F, Donaldson AN, Watson TF, Banerjee A. An in vitro comparison of the accuracy of measurements obtained from high-and low-resolution cone-beam computed tomography scans. J Endod. 2013;39:394–7.
25. Costa ED, Brasil DM, Queiroz PM, Verner FS, Junqueira RB, Freitas DQ. Use of the metal artefact reduction tool in the identification of fractured endodontic instruments in cone-beam computed tomography. Int Endod J. 2020;53(4):506–12.
26. Bauman R, Scarfe W, Clark S, Morelli J, Scheetz J, Farman A. Ex vivo detection of mesiobuccal canals in maxillary molars using CBCT at four different isotropic voxel dimensions. Int Endod J. 2011;44(8):752–8.
27. Vizzotto MB, Silveira PF, Arús NA, Montagner F, Gomes BP, da Silveira HE. CBCT for the assessment of second mesiobuccal (MB2) canals in maxillary molar teeth: effect of voxel size and presence of root filling. Int Endod J. 2013;46(9):870–6.

28. Martins JNR, Marques D, Silva EJNL, Caramês J, Mata A, Versiani MA. Second mesiobuccal root canal in maxillary molars-A systematic review and meta-analysis of prevalence studies using cone beam computed tomography. Arch Oral Biol. 2020;113:104589.
29. Mouzinho-Machado S, Rosado LPL, Coelho-Silva F, Neves FS, Haiter-Neto F, de-Azevedo-Vaz SL. Influence of voxel size and filter application in detecting second Mesiobuccal canals in cone-beam computed tomographic images. J Endod. 2021;47(9):1391–7.
30. Aktan AM, Yildirim C, Karataşlıoğlu E, Çiftçi ME, Aksoy F. Effects of voxel size and resolution on the accuracy of endodontic length measurement using cone beam computed tomography. Ann Anat. 2016;208:96–102.
31. Van Pham K. Endodontic length measurements using cone beam computed tomography with dedicated or conventional software at different voxel sizes. Sci Rep. 2021;11(1):9432.
32. De Martin E, Silva D, Campos CN, Pires Carvalho AC, Devito KL. Diagnosis of mesiodistal vertical root fractures in teeth with metal posts: influence of applying filters in cone-beam computed tomography images at different resolutions. J Endod. 2018;44(3):470–4.
33. Guo XL, Li G, Zheng JQ, Ma RH, Liu FC, Yuan FS, Lyu PJ, Guo YJ, Yin S. Accuracy of detecting vertical root fractures in non-root filled teeth using cone beam computed tomography: effect of voxel size and fracture width. Int Endod J. 2019;52(6):887–98.
34. Kolsuz ME, Eren H, Çelikten B, Dalgali Evli P, Demirtürk Kocasaraç H, Orhan K. Influence of cone-beam computed tomography voxel sizes in the detection of chemically induced external root resorptions. Med Sci Monit. 2022;28:e936160.
35. Liedke GS, da Silveira HE, da Silveira HL, Dutra V, de Figueiredo JA. Influence of voxel size in the diagnostic ability of cone beam tomography to evaluate simulated external root resorption. J Endod. 2009;35(2):233–5.
36. Neves F, Vasconcelos T, Vaz S, Freitas D, Haiter-Neto F. Evaluation of reconstructed images with different voxel sizes of acquisition in the diagnosis of simulated external root resorption using cone beam computed tomography. Int Endod J. 2012;45:234–9.
37. Rosado LPL, Fagundes FB, Freitas DQ, Oliveira ML, Neves FS. Influence of the intracanal material and metal artifact reduction tool in the detection of the second Mesiobuccal Canal in cone-beam computed tomographic examinations. J Endod. 2020;46(8):1067–73.
38. Kamburoğlu K, Yılmaz F, Yeta EN, Özen D. Assessment of furcal perforations in the vicinity of different root canal sealers using a cone beam computed tomography system with and without the application of artifact reduction mode: an ex vivo investigation on extracted human teeth. Oral Surg Oral Med Oral Pathol Oral Radiol. 2016;121(6):657–65.
39. Nikbin A, Dalili Kajan Z, Taramsari M, Khosravifard N. Effect of object position in the field of view and application of a metal artifact reduction algorithm on the detection of vertical root fractures on cone-beam computed tomography scans: an in vitro study. Imaging Sci Dent. 2018;48(4):245–54.
40. Saati S, Eskandarloo A, Falahi A, Tapak L, Hekmat B. Evaluation of the efficacy of the metal artifact reduction algorithm in the detection of a vertical root fracture in endodontically treated teeth in cone-beam computed tomography images: an in vitro study. Dent Med Probl. 2019;56(4):357–63.
41. Dalili Kajan Z, Taramsari M, Khosravi Fard N, Khaksari F, Moghasem HF. The efficacy of metal artifact reduction mode in cone-beam computed tomography images on diagnostic accuracy of root fractures in teeth with intracanal posts. Iran Endod J. 2018;13(1):47–53.
42. Farias-Gomes A, Fontenele RC, Rosado LPL, Neves FS, Freitas DQ. The metal post material influences the performance of artefact reduction algorithms in CBCT images. Braz Dent J. 2022;33(1):31–40.
43. Santaella GM, Wenzel A, Haiter-Neto F, Rosalen PL, Spin-Neto R. Impact of movement and motion-artefact correction on image quality and interpretability in CBCT units with aligned and lateral-offset detectors. Dentomaxillofac Radiol. 2020;49(1):20190240.
44. Moratin J, Berger M, Rückschloss T, Metzger K, Berger H, Gottsauner M, Engel M, Hoffmann J, Freudlsperger C, Ristow O. Head motion during cone-beam computed tomography: analysis of frequency and influence on image quality. Imaging Sci Dent. 2020;50(3):227–36.

45. Spin-Neto R, Matzen LH, Schropp L, Gotfredsen E, Wenzel A. Factors affecting patient movement and re-exposure in cone beam computed tomography examination. Oral Surg Oral Med Oral Pathol Oral Radiol. 2015;119(5):572–8.
46. Valizadeh S, Vasegh Z, Rezapanah S, Safi Y, Khaeazifard MJ. Effect of object position in cone beam computed tomography field of view for detection of root fractures in teeth with intracanal posts. Iran J Radiol. 2015;12(4):e25272.
47. Iikubo M, Nishioka T, Okura S, Kobayashi K, Sano T, Katsumata A, Ariji E, Kojima I, Sakamoto M, Sasano T. Influence of voxel size and scan field of view on fracture-like artifacts from gutta-percha obturated endodontically treated teeth on cone-beam computed tomography images. Oral Surg Oral Med Oral Pathol Oral Radiol. 2016;122(5):631–7.
48. Scarfe WC, Angelopoulos C. Chapter 5: CBCT in daily use. Chapter. In: Scarfe WC, Angelopoulos C, editors. Maxillofacial cone beam computed tomography: principles, techniques and clinical applications. Springer International Publishing AG; 2018. p. 115–90.
49. Ferreira LM, Visconti MA, Nascimento HA, Dallemolle RR, Ambrosano GM, Freitas DQ. Influence of CBCT enhancement filters on diagnosis of vertical root fractures: a simulation study in endodontically treated teeth with and without intracanal posts. Dentomaxillofac Radiol. 2015;44(5):20140352.
50. González AR, Tosoni GM, Freitas DQ, Oliveira ML. Influence of sharpening filters on the detection of root fractures using low-dose cone-beam computed tomography. Clin Oral Investig. 2022;26(7):4797–803.
51. Nascimento MC, Nejaim Y, de Almeida SM, Bóscolo FN, Haiter-Neto F, Sobrinho LC, Silva EJ. Influence of cone beam CT enhancement filters on diagnosis ability of longitudinal root fractures. Dentomaxillofac Radiol. 2014;43(3):20130374.
52. Bueno MR, Azevedo BC, Estrela CRA, Sousa-Neto MD, Estrela C. Method to identify accessory root canals using a new CBCT software. Braz Dent J. 2021;32(6):28–35.
53. Schulze R, Heil U, Groβ D, Bruellmann DD, Dranischnikow E, Schwanecke U, Schoemer E. Artefacts in CBCT: a review. Dentomaxillofac Radiol. 2011;40(5):265–73.
54. Ludlow JB, Timothy R, Walker C, Hunter R, Benavides E, Samuelson DB, Scheske MJ. Effective dose of dental CBCT-a meta analysis of published data and additional data for nine CBCT units. Dentomaxillofac Radiol. 2015;44(1):20140197.
55. AAE and AAOMR Joint Position Statement: Use of Cone Beam Computed Tomography in Endodontics 2015 Update. (2015). http://www.aae.org/uploadedfiles/clinical_resources/guidelines_and_position_statements/cbctstatement_2015update.pdf. Accessed 30 Dec 2022.
56. Patel S, Brown J, Semper M, Abella F, Mannocci F. European Society of Endodontology position statement: use of cone beam computed tomography in endodontics: European Society of Endodontology (ESE) developed by. Int Endod J. 2019;52(12):1675–8.
57. Hung K, Hui L, Yeung AWK, Scarfe WC, Bornstein MM. Image retake rates of cone beam computed tomography in a dental institution. Clin Oral Investig. 2020;24(12):4501–10.
58. Rottke D, Andersson J, Ejima KI, Sawada K, Schulze D. Influence of lead apron shielding on absorbed doses from cone-beam computed tomography. Radiat Prot Dosim. 2017;175(1):110–7.
59. Schulze RKW, Sazgar M, Karle H, de Las Heras Gala H. Influence of a commercial lead apron on patient skin dose delivered during oral and maxillofacial examinations under cone beam computed tomography (CBCT). Health Phys. 2017;113(2):129–34.
60. Pauwels R, Horner K, Vassileva J, Rehani MM. Thyroid shielding in cone beam computed tomography: recommendations towards appropriate use. Dentomaxillofac Radiol. 2019;48(7):20190014.

New Software for Endodontic Diagnosis and Treatment: The e-Vol DXS

2

Mike Bueno and Carlos Estrela

Abstract

The applications of a new CBCT software to help resolve routine clinical cases in endodontics are presented in this chapter. The need for high-quality images to visualize complex anatomical structures has led to the development of the e-Vol DXS software. The unique feature of this CBCT software is the ability to import and use DICOM files and enhance the imaging adjustments capabilities to analyze CBCT volumes from different CBCT scanners. This novel CBCT software is designed with unique features to improve image quality such as task-specific brightness and contrast adjustment, custom image thickness control, a custom image sharpening filter, a proprietary noise reduction filter, and the ability to automatically recognize and apply imaging filters to scanner-specific data, saving time in data correction, and data imaging navigation. These tools and specially designed 3D rendering filters reduce artifacts that can interfere with making accurate diagnoses.

2.1 Introduction

Diagnosing oral cavity diseases has become increasingly important as it plays a crucial role in successful endodontic treatment. Misdiagnosis can be fatal for the preservation of the tooth and is also responsible for several errors in invasive

M. Bueno (✉)
Department of Radiology, School of Dentistry São Leopoldo Mandic, Campinas, SP, Brazil

CROIF, Diagnostic Imaging Center, Cuiabá, Brazil
e-mail: mike@croif.com.br

C. Estrela
Department of Stomatologic Sciences, Federal University of Goiás, Goiânia, Brazil

M. I. Fayad, B. R. Johnson (eds.), *3D Imaging in Endodontics*,
https://doi.org/10.1007/978-3-031-32755-1_2

therapeutic procedures. Consequently, incorrect treatment can lead to an unfavorable prognosis and result in sequelae that have led to severe legal issues.

The scientific advances of the last decades have opened several perspectives to increase the success rates of endodontic diagnosis and treatment [1–43]. The introduction of cone-beam computed tomography (CBCT) into the clinical practice of endodontics has dramatically improved planning and diagnosis, facilitated clinical decision-making, increased confidence in professionals, and improved the predictability of prognosis for different clinical conditions [1, 14, 42].

This chapter describes directly and concisely the applications of a new CBCT software to help resolve routine clinical cases in endodontics and further increase success rates. Various CBCT scanners have been introduced in the dental market to meet the needs of professionals. They all have their native software for the necessary adjustments of the acquired images. Recently, a sophisticated post-processing software, e-Vol DXS (CDT Software, São José dos Campos, SP, Brazil), with multiple task-specific-rendering features, has been introduced to enhance the data of CBCT scans [4, 5, 7, 10].

The need for high-quality images to visualize complex anatomical structures, precise identification of lesions, and reduced artifacts has led to the development of the e-Vol DXS software [4]. The unique feature of this CBCT software is the ability to import and use DICOM files and enhance the imaging adjustment capabilities to analyze CBCT volumes from different CBCT scanners. The original CBCT data may not be well-suited for diagnosis of fine detail, depending on the native CBCT software. They may be blurred, may not be sharp enough, and may contain numerous artifacts. These images require a series of adjustments to improve image quality. This novel CBCT software is designed with unique features to improve image quality such as: task-specific brightness and contrast adjustment, custom image thickness control, a custom image sharpening filter, a proprietary noise reduction filter, and the ability to automatically recognize and apply imaging filters to scanner-specific data, saving time in data correction and data imaging navigation. These tools and specially designed 3D rendering filters reduce artifacts that can interfere with making accurate diagnoses [4].

2.2 Quality in the CBCT Scan Acquisition for Endodontics

Across the healthcare field, dentistry is most concerned with the high quality of the minute details of CBCT images. Endodontics, in particular, requires CBCT scans of exceptionally high quality, as the doubts are usually for features with a size much smaller than 1 mm [1–42].

Obtaining a CBCT scan with a clear image is essential for endodontic procedures. This requires a set of factors, such as a very well-designed CBCT scanner that produces CBCT scans with small voxels (high voxel resolution, equal to or less than 0.1 mm), a small field of view (FOV), high contrast resolution, and low noise [4, 5].

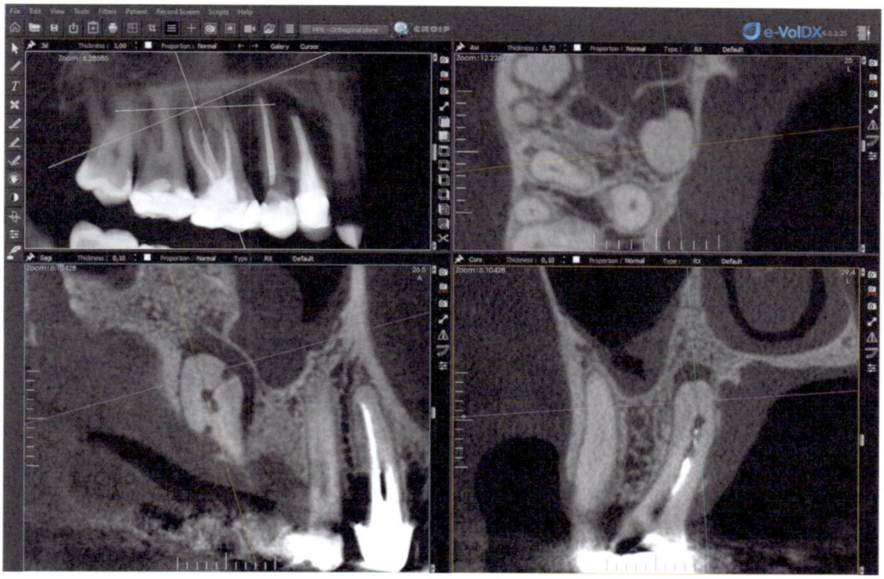

Fig. 2.1 CBCT scan—high spatial resolution is essential for evaluating details in endodontics. In this high spatial resolution, CBCT scan of a routine clinical patient, even tiny accessory root canals of the apical delta are visible. In addition, several other findings, such as root resorption and apical osteolysis, can be seen (technical specifications: CBCT FOV 5 × 5 cm; voxel 100 μ) (Coloca o KV o mA e o tempo de acquisicao)

In CBCT examinations, the milliamperage (mA) and the number of basis images, usually associated with exposure time, must be adjusted to meet the interpretation needs. These settings are generally higher for endodontic images to reduce noise and thus avoid false-positive findings in the images, such as false-positive root fractures [11].

Features such as voxel size, FOV, contrast resolution, number of basis images, noise, and patient stabilization are interdependent, and the final product is named "spatial resolution." High spatial resolution means a sharp image, which is fundamental in endodontics. A high dynamic range of images is also required to reduce the risk of artifacts [4].

The features of the e-Vol DXS software are better suited when high image quality is available. CBCT scans with high spatial resolution and high dynamic range are indicated. The images used in this chapter follow this principle [4] (Fig. 2.1).

2.3 Management of Large DICOM Files

Some of the current CBCT scanners can acquire medium FOV images for specific endodontic applications. Medium FOV sizes, such as 8 × 8 cm or 10 × 10 cm, can be reconstructed with small voxel sizes as small as 75 μ voxel. The final file sizes on

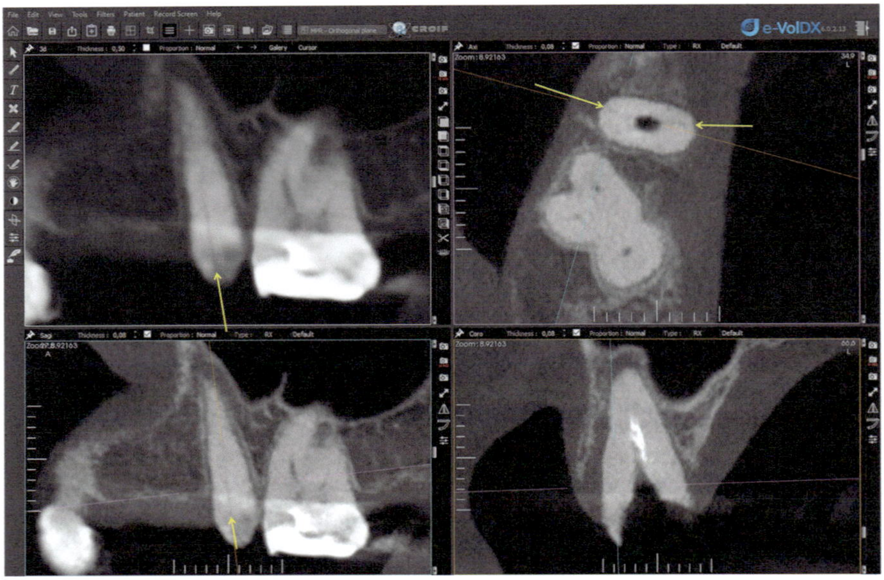

Fig. 2.2 Management of a large DICOM file. Medium volume CBCT with 10 × 10 cm FOV and 75 μ voxel. A discrete fracture line (yellow arrow) is visible in the image. CBCT with a compressed DICOM file eight times smaller than the original file without losing important details like this discreet fracture line

those volumes are exponentially larger than the smaller FOV ones and cause computer crashes or slow down networks. The e-Vol DXS software has a tool that converts multi-file DICOM files into a single DICOM file with three-dimensional architecture that is 2 to 8 times smaller than the original DICOM file, with no detectable loss of image quality. The e-Vol DXS software preserves all the dynamic ranges of the DICOM files [4] (Fig. 2.2).

2.4 Adjustment of CBCT Images

When opening a CBCT scan on the computer, the professional has to adjust the original image to improve sharpness and gray level for diagnosis. This correction may be laborious and challenging to reproduce in every volume.

The e-Vol DXS software has an interesting feature; it allows presetting an adjustment procedure for the CBCT DICOM images. The professional makes careful adjustments to the image, such as brightness, contrast, sharpness, and thickness, and clicks the save button at the end. When another image is acquired with the same CBCT scanner model and parameters, the e-Vol DXS software automatically recognizes the characteristics of the CBCT scan (the DICOM). It applies the pre-recorded adjustments. This makes the process much easier and standardizes the visualization of CBCT scans to the preferred adjustments. The preset settings can be shared with other users so that all users in a larger practice can have the same DICOM adjustment pattern. In the e-Vol DXS software, the sharpness tool has been built in a sophisticated way with control of the intensity and thickness of the edge, generally not found in other software [4].

2.5 Noise Control

Noise is digital pollution, usually appearing as grains or small lines in CBCT images. When noise is high, it interferes with the interpretation of the CBCT image. In some situations, noise can lead to false positives for small canals or cracks [4, 11] (Fig. 2.3).

In the vast majority of cases, the best way to attenuate noise is to use the native software of the CBCT scanner to increase slice thickness. Increasing the thickness results in overlapping voxel layers, which attenuates noise but with the side effect of masking small structures, such as accessory root canals [12] (Fig. 2.4).

In addition to total thickness control, the e-Vol DXS software has a sophisticated noise control tool that does not increase thickness. The "multi-CDT" tool reduces noise (Fig. 2.5) by controlling sensitivity. We can navigate the image with noise attenuation and reduced thickness, which is an ideal strategy for image navigation in endodontics [3, 4, 8, 13, 25].

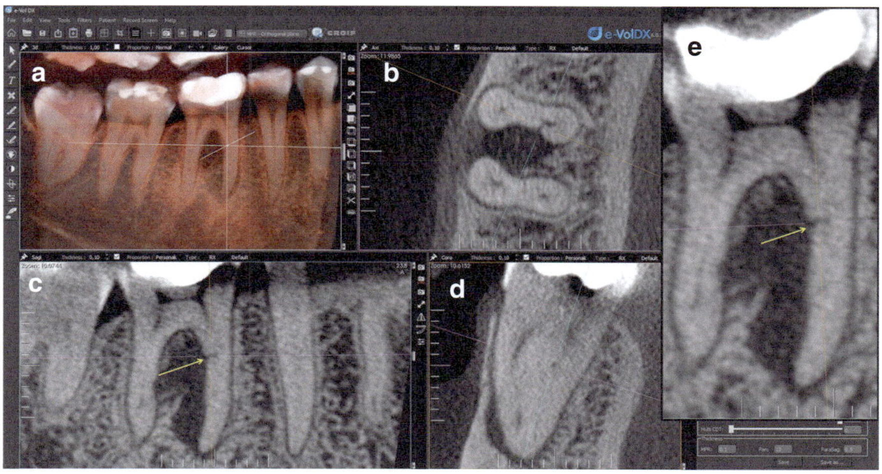

Fig. 2.3 Navigation lines with parallax adjustment indicating two lines and a point on the MPR slices (**b**, **c**, **d**). However, there are many other small dots and lines due to noise in the CBCT image. It is important to compare the region indicated by the yellow arrow of the cross-section (**c**) and the enlarged cross-section (**e**) with the other images in Figs. 2.4 and 2.5. 3D image with slice position indexing (**a**). Technical specifications: CBCT FOV 5x5 cm; voxel 100 μ

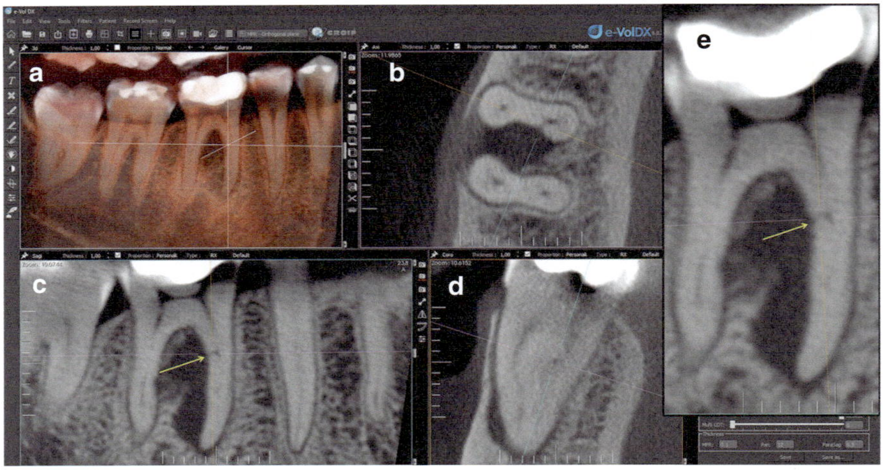

Fig. 2.4 The same CBCT image shown in Fig. 2.3 with an increase in slice thickness from 0.1 mm (Fig. 2.3) to 1 mm (Fig. 2.4). In Fig. 2.4, noise attenuation was performed, improving the image's appearance, but the lines indicated at the tooth's root (yellow arrow) are also attenuated, which could lead to diagnostic doubts. Greater thickness can lead to false negatives for thin root canals. It is important to compare the region indicated by the yellow arrow of the cross-section (**c**) and the enlarged cross-section (**e**) with the other images in Figs. 2.3 and 2.5. MPR slices (**b**, **c**, **d**). Magnification section (**e**). 3D image with slice position indexing (**a**). Technical specifications: CBCT FOV 5 × 5 cm; voxel 100 μ

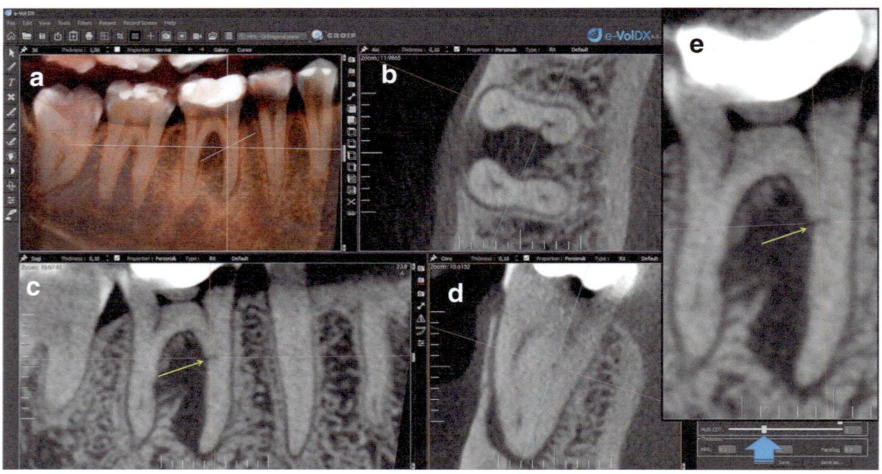

Fig. 2.5 The same CBCT scans are shown in Figs. 2.3 and 2.4. The native thickness is 0.1 mm, and the multi-CDT noise reduction filter (broad blue arrow below) was applied, leading to noise attenuation and improving the image appearance while keeping the lines indicated at the root (yellow arrows) evident, with a better result than in Fig. 2.4. It is essential to compare the region indicated by the yellow arrow of the cross-section (**c**) and enlarged cross-section (**e**) with the other images in Figs. 2.3 and 2.4. Multiplanar reconstruction (MPR) slices (**b**, **c**, **d**). Magnification section (**e**). 3D image with slice position indexing (**a**). Technical specifications: CBCT FOV 5 × 5 cm; voxel 100 μ

2.6 Image Navigation Dynamics

The navigation dynamics follow the sequence of capturing and adjusting the CBCT image, followed by the parallax correction that must be performed so that the area to be analyzed, such as a root canal, has lines perpendicular and parallel to the area of interest. If the parallax is not adequately corrected, the root canal will have an incorrect shape (Fig. 2.6), and if it is correctly adjusted, the root canal will be positioned perfectly (Fig. 2.7) and will be more evident. The thickness of 1 mm exacerbates the parallax error. Parallax adjustment needs to be refined, allowing the control of the thickness of the navigation lines, the slope of the lines or the volume of the CBCT image, the distance between the lines, the presence or absence of the central point (Fig. 2.8), and many other vital customizations that improve navigation in endodontics [3, 4, 8, 12, 13, 25, 26].

Unlimited zooming can be performed independently for each multiplanar reconstruction (MPR) slice window. The cursor lines can be tilted like in a static volume, and another option is to tilt the entire volume. In the e-Vol DXS software, there is an important tool that indexes the 2D images of the MPR with the 3D images, allowing the browsing of 2D MPR images by visualizing the spatial position of the cursor in the 3D image. The quality, easiness, and speed of navigation of the CBCT scan are essential for solving endodontic problems [4, 5, 10].

The vast majority of native CBCT software uses a screen capturing resolution of 96 dpi for images to be used in emails, presentations, or referral letters. The capture imaging tool of the e-Vol DXS software can capture much higher-resolution images varying between 192 dpi and 384 dpi [4].

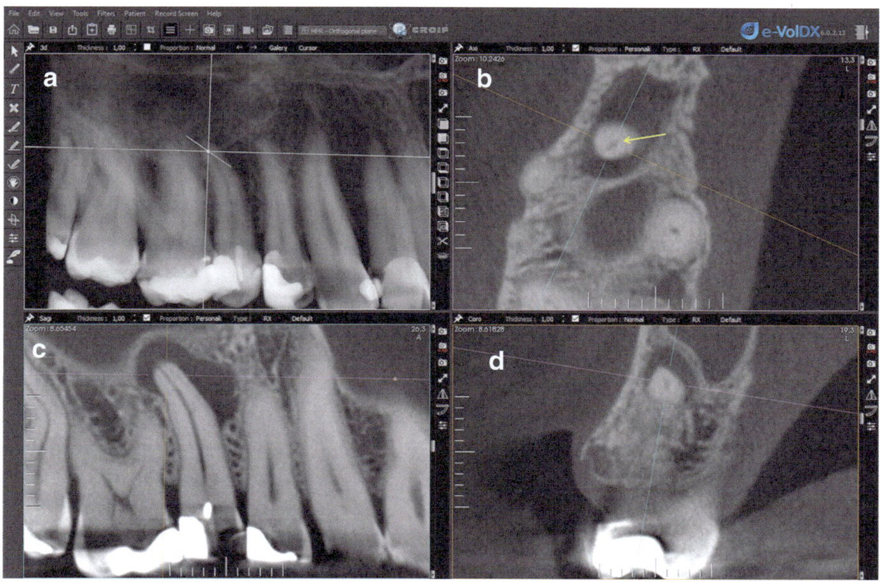

Fig. 2.6 In the axial slice (**b**), the root canal (yellow arrow) is not clearly visible and presents an elongated shape in the middle-distal direction (slice thickness of 1 mm). MPR slices (**b**, **c**, **d**). 3D image with slice position indexing (**a**)

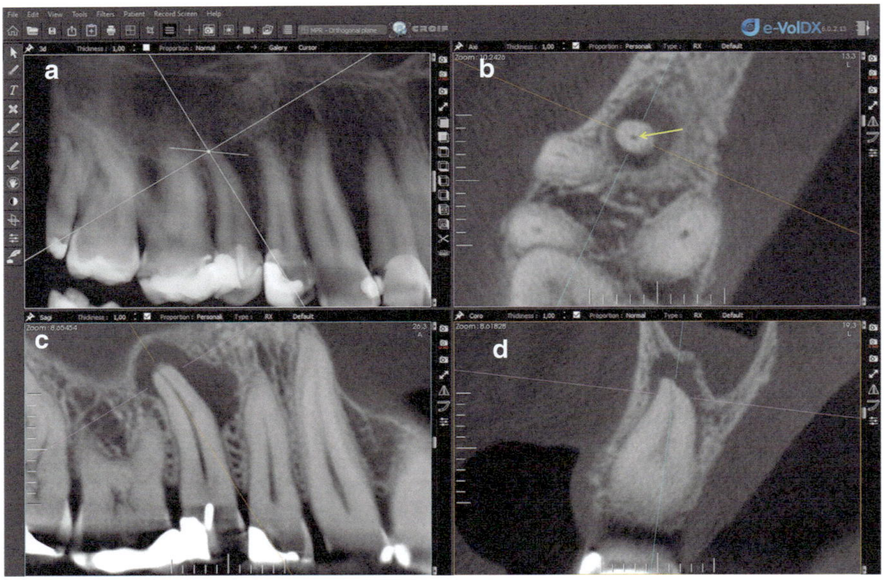

Fig. 2.7 This is the same CBCT scan as in the previous figure. Here, the parallax adjustment was performed with a slice perpendicular to the root canal. The root canal was more visible in the axial section (**b**) (yellow arrow), showing a circular shape, slightly elongated in the buccal-palatal direction. The result was a significant improvement in the root canal visibility and the fidelity of root canal shape by comparing Fig. 2.7 with Fig. 2.6. MPR slices (**b**, **c**, **d**), 3D image (**a**)

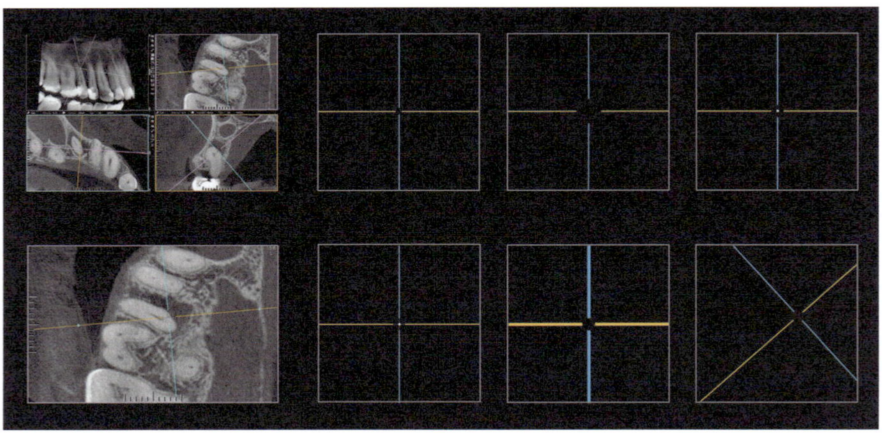

Fig. 2.8 Parallax correction is essential in endodontics. On the left, line sharpness adjustments in the e-Vol DXS software were important for locating the accessory root canal on the side of the root. On the right, some of the navigation line configuration options for endodontics are shown. Hotkeys can be used for quick configuration switching. Versatility, easiness, and high speed are important in these diagnostic maneuvers

2.7 White Contrast Artifacts

In professional photography and video production, the dynamic range of an image is one of the most studied and coveted properties due to its importance for image quality. A high dynamic range image has a wide recording range of dark and light tones. The more extensive the dynamic range, the greater the possibility of capturing details in the light and dark extremes. An image can have a high specific dynamic range only in light tones or only in dark tones [4].

Surprisingly, the dynamic range of a CBCT scan is a subject that is rarely discussed. Many scanners capture images with a high dynamic range for light colors and are not adequately explored by the scanner's native software or the user. This can result in a type of artifact named "blooming artifact," a white artifact larger than its true size caused by high-density bodies such as intracanal posts, root canal filling material, or other high-density materials. Considering the characteristics of the dynamic range of CBCT images and the properties of a blooming artifact, a filter named blooming artifact reduction (BAR) was developed for the e-Vol DXS software [4].

The BAR filter of the e-Vol DXS software acts on the image contrast and uses an algorithm with amplification of the reading signal of the entire bright range of the image recorded in the dynamic range and helps with the correct visualization in the margins with white contrast artifacts (Figs. 2.9, 2.10, 2.11, 2.12, 2.13 and 2.14). The BAR filter in the e-Vol DXS software takes the information potential of a CBCT image in dentistry to a new level [4, 27, 40].

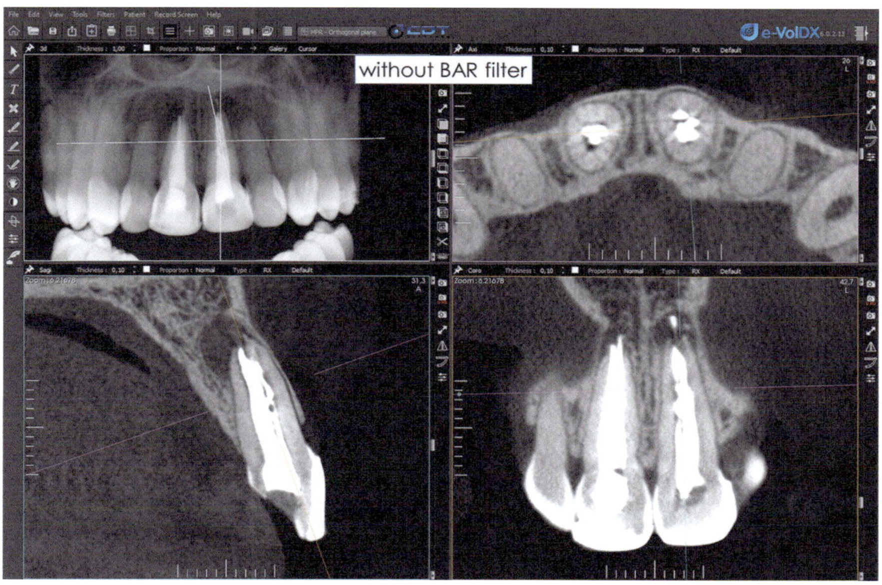

Fig. 2.9 CBCT image without the BAR (blooming artifact reduction) filter. A CBCT image with medium contrast such as this is generally used for good visualization of dental and bone details. In dense structures, like dental materials, blooming artifacts are seen

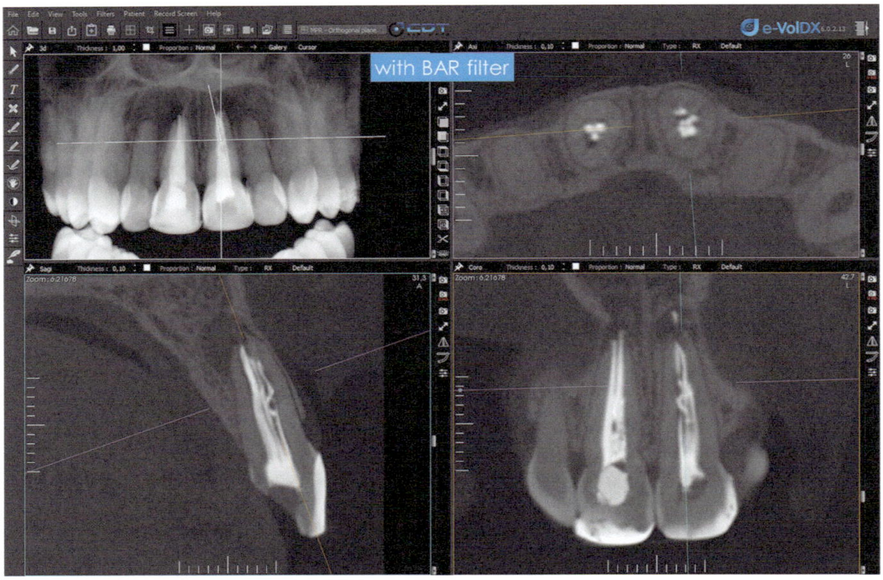

Fig. 2.10 CBCT image with the BAR (blooming artifact reduction) filter. The application of the BAR filter in the e-Vol software reduced white contrast artifacts, enabling the visualization of details in the margins of the materials. The individualization of gutta-percha cones in the root canal filling and the spaces between them are important details in endodontics

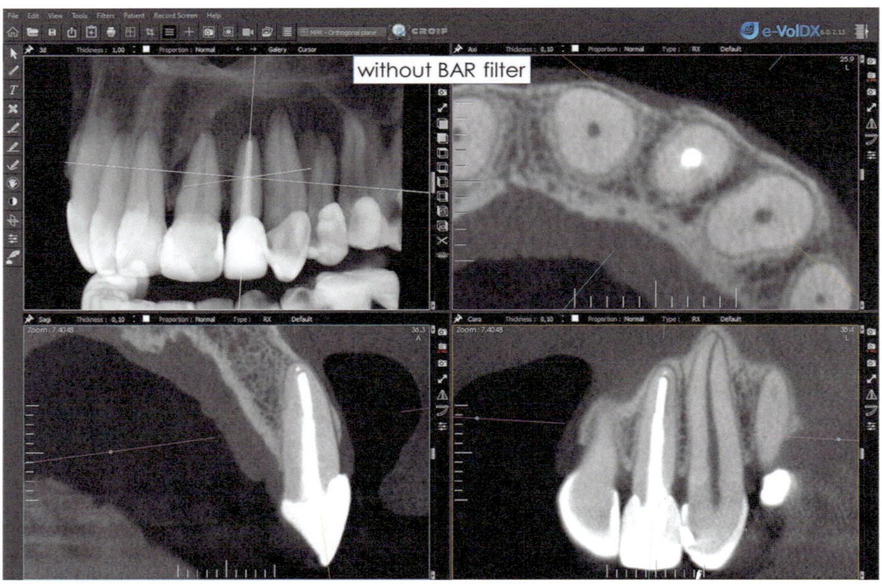

Fig. 2.11 CBCT image without the BAR (blooming artifact reduction) filter. Dense bodies such as dental materials exhibit blooming artifacts

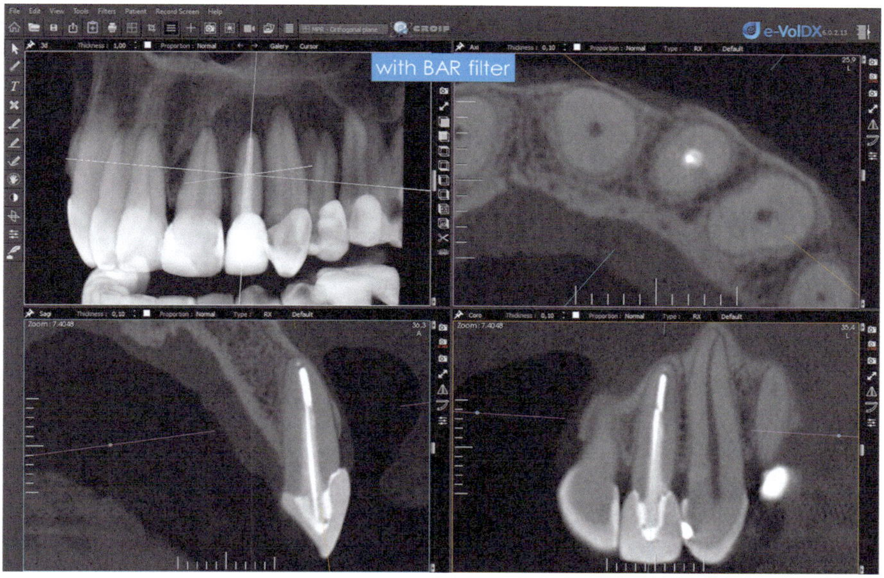

Fig. 2.12 CBCT image with the BAR (blooming artifact reduction) filter. The application of the BAR filter in the e-Vol software reduced white artifacts, enabling the visualization of details in the margins of the materials. The visualization of the intracanal fiber post and the margin seal of the prosthetic crown are important details in endodontics

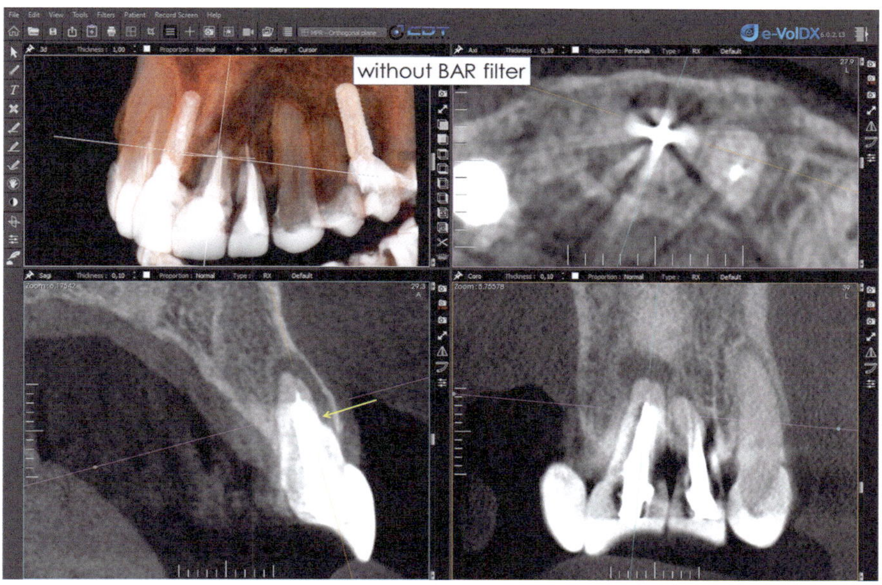

Fig. 2.13 CBCT image without the BAR (blooming artifact reduction) filter. It is not clear whether or not there is a perforation in the buccal root (yellow arrow) in the region of the intracanal post

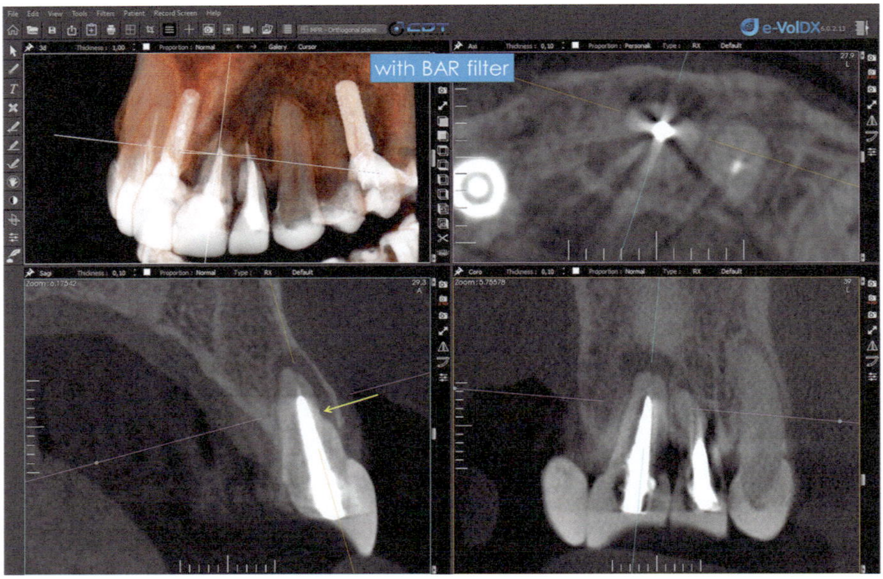

Fig. 2.14 CBCT image with the BAR (blooming artifact reduction) filter. The application of the BAR filter in the e-Vol software led to the reduction of white artifacts, enabling the visualization of details in the margins of the materials. With the reduction of the blooming of the intracanal post, it becomes clearly visible that there was no perforation in the buccal root (yellow arrow)

2.8 Density

By understanding the dynamic range of the CBCT scan and using the BAR filter in the e-Vol DXS software, the density analysis function of materials and tissues becomes much more subtle and sophisticated [4, 27, 40] (Figs. 2.15, 2.16, 2.17, 2.18, 2.19, 2.20 and 2.21).

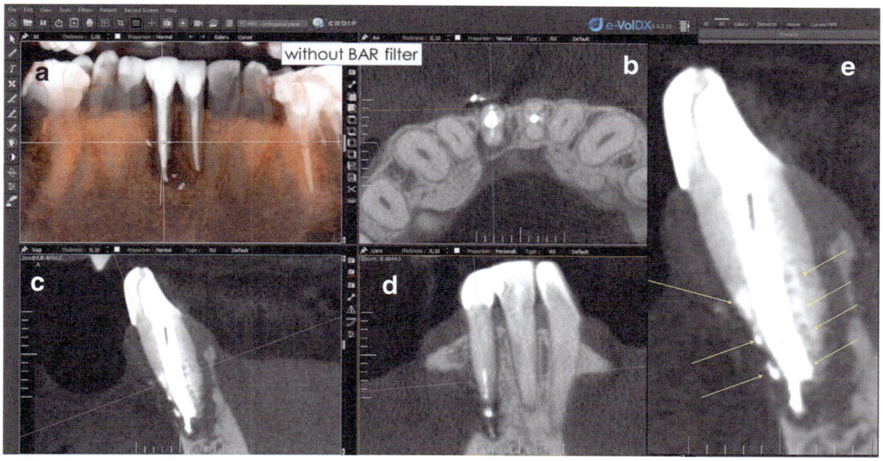

Fig. 2.15 CBCT image without the BAR (blooming artifact reduction) filter. White areas in the image (yellow arrows) similar to artifacts are shown. MPR slices (**b**, **c**, **d**). Magnification section (**e**). 3D image with slice position indexing (**a**)

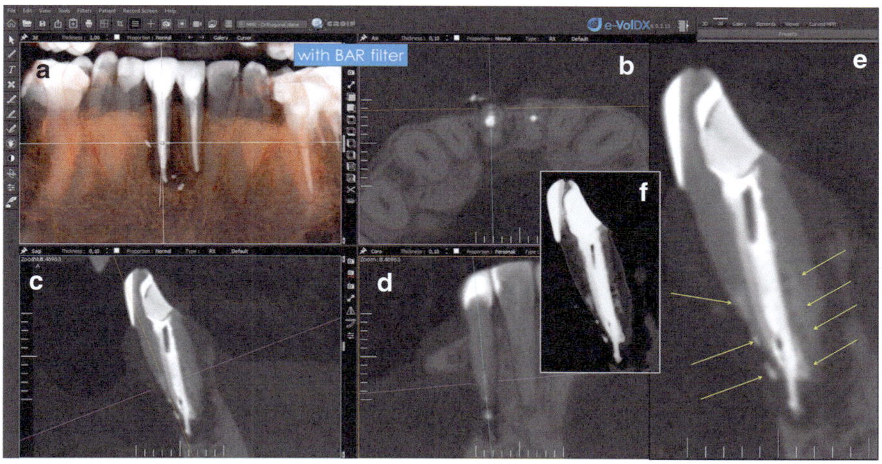

Fig. 2.16 CBCT image with the BAR (blooming artifact reduction) filter. The use of the BAR filter in the e-Vol DXS software led to the reduction of white artifacts, allowing the visualization of the reticulated aspect of the material, which is not characteristic of an artifact, but of a filling material failure in the root fracture line. MPR slices (**b**, **c**, **d**). Magnification section (**e**). 3D image with slice position indexing (**a**). 3D section of the specific e-Vol DXS for material evaluation (**f**)

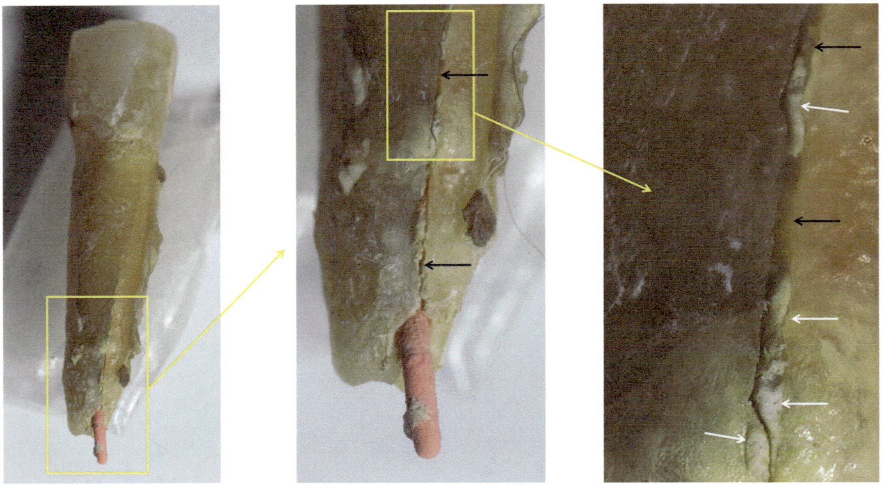

Fig. 2.17 This is the same region as that in Figs. 2.15 and 2.16, but after tooth extraction. A fracture line was confirmed (black arrow), which can be seen on the buccal and lingual aspects of the root. Reticulated material was confirmed (white arrow) with higher magnification of the microphotograph image

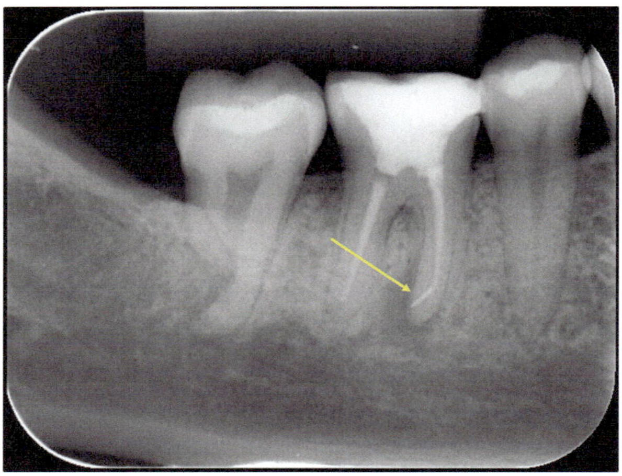

Fig. 2.18 Periapical radiograph of a mandibular first molar with a clinical history of a fractured endodontic instrument fragment (apical region of the mesial root; yellow arrow)

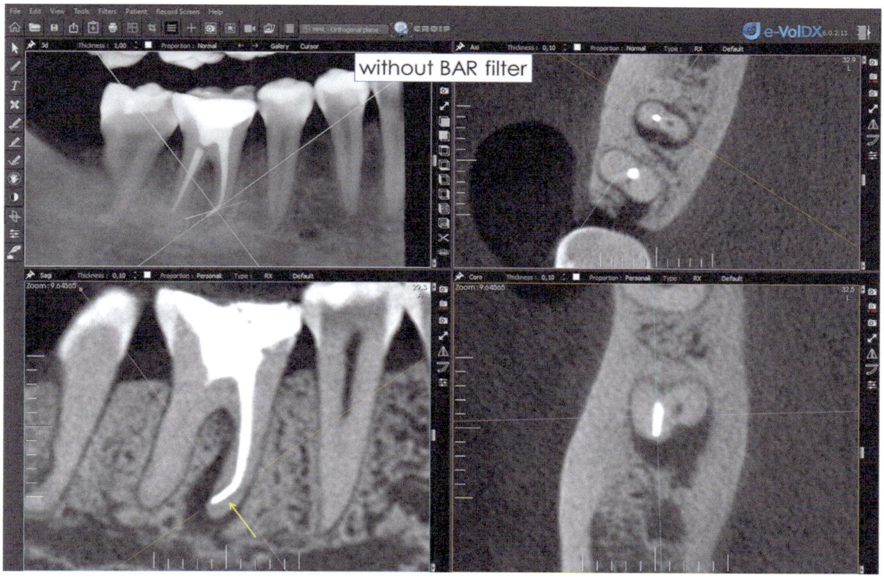

Fig. 2.19 The presence of white expansion artifacts (blooming artifact) makes it difficult to distinguish between the fractured endodontic instrument fragment (yellow arrow) and the root canal filling material

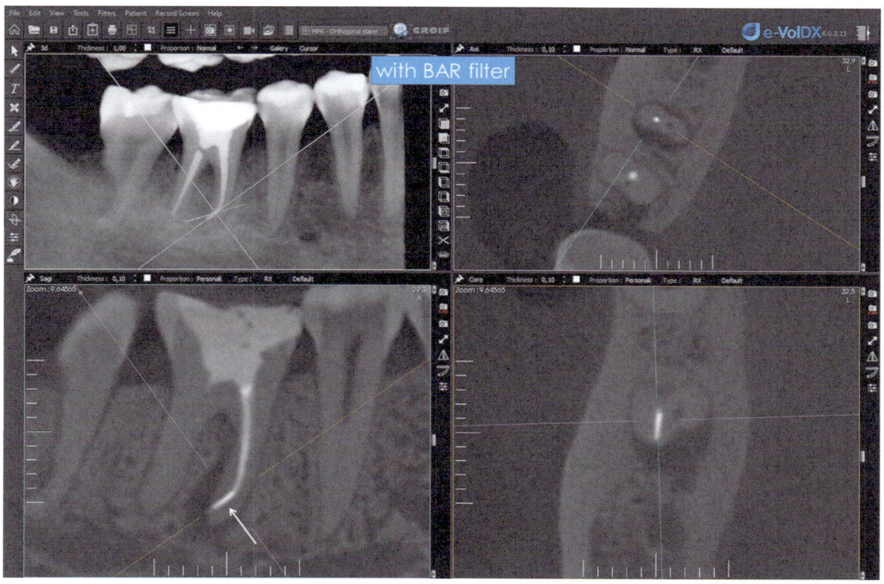

Fig. 2.20 The application of the BAR (blooming artifact reduction) filter in the e-Vol software led to the reduction of white artifacts, allowing the partial distinction of the fractured endodontic instrument fragment (white arrow), which has a lighter shade than the root canal filling material

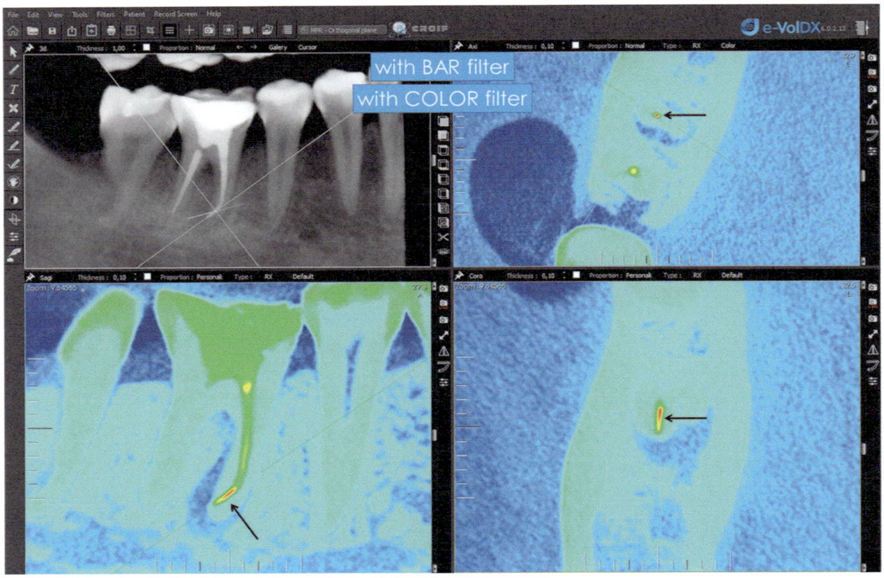

Fig. 2.21 The application of the BAR filter associated with the "Color Map" tool in the e-Vol DXS causes the white color to be replaced by the red color, increasing the sensitivity for detecting the fragment of the endodontic instrument (black arrow)

2.9 Dark Artifacts

The information from the dark parts of a DICOM file is not recorded in the image's dynamic range due to beam hardening from dark artifacts. Without data, lost artifacts cannot be recovered after the primary reconstruction of CBCT scans [4, 9].

Some specific algorithms perform the primary reconstruction through mathematical calculations from the RAW files (before the DICOM formation) of the CBCT scan, removing most of the dark areas of the tomography like the Carestream's metal artifact reduction (MAR) filter [4, 9].

In the e-Vol DXS software, opening two overlapping DICOM files and switching between them to compare the visualization with and without applying filters such as MAR is possible. It is essential to visualize the two volumes because filters such as MAR reduce the contrast, which can lead to diagnostic doubts. The two visualizations can be used to get the most out of each DICOM file (Figs. 2.22, 2.23 and 2.24). Because two DICOMs are loaded from the same CBCT, compression of the image in the e-Vol DXS, as mentioned earlier, becomes even more important.

Since the early days of CBCT, 3D rendering has mostly been used for overviews rather than as a complementary diagnostic. However, this has changed in recent years with advanced software producing high-quality 3D images, and in some cases, 3D has been fully used as a diagnostic tool. In the e-Vol DXS software, there are more than 100 3D filters, many of which are targeted at specific endodontic conditions, such as for evidencing root canals (Figs. 2.25 and 2.26), root fractures (Fig. 2.27), bone (Fig. 2.28), etc.

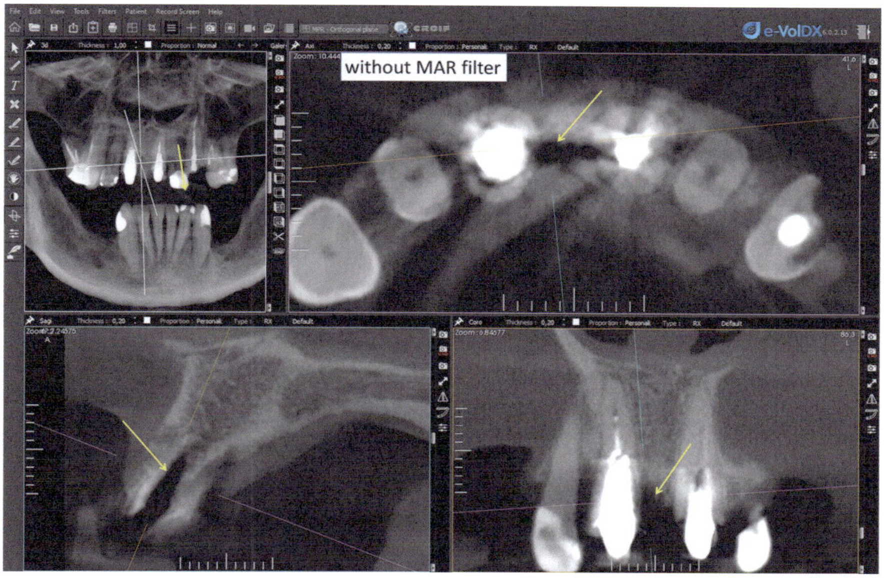

Fig. 2.22 Dark artifacts (yellow arrows) greatly impair the interpretation of CT images

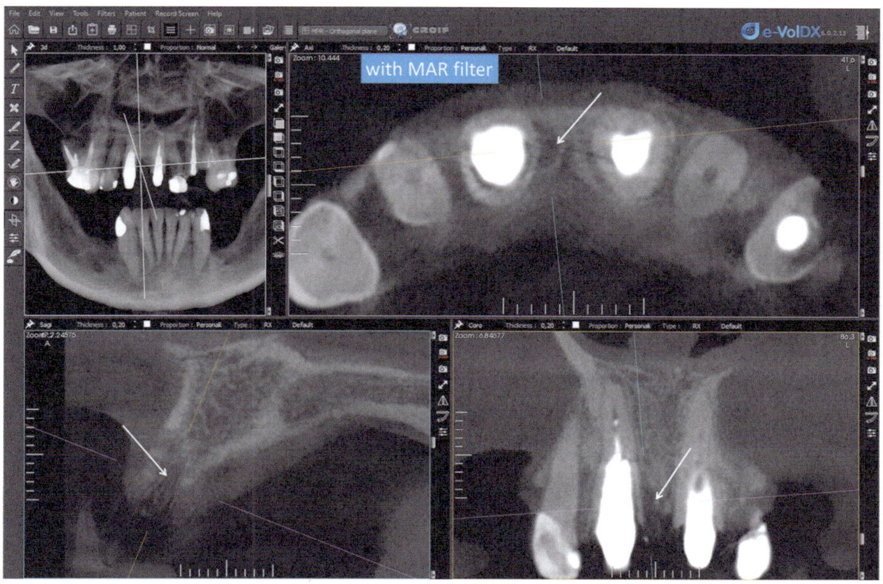

Fig. 2.23 Filters such as the Carestream's MAR (metal artifact reduction) filter can reduce dark artifacts helping endodontic diagnosis in some specific cases such as this one that revealed a vertical bone loss in the mesial aspect of a maxillary central incisor (white arrow) that was hidden by an artifact in the tomography without the MAR filter (Fig. 2.22). In e-Vol DXS, it is common to open two CBCT volumes on the same screen, one without the MAR filter and the other with the MAR filter. Using the "V" key on the keyboard, the user can switch between the volume with (Fig. 2.23) and without the MAR filter (Fig. 2.22) in any navigation position and inclination

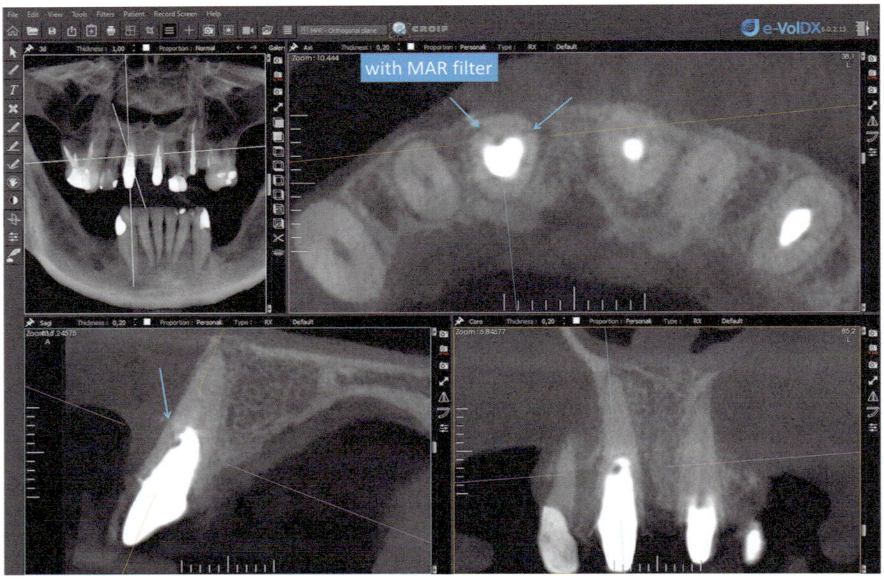

Fig. 2.24 In the same case as in the previous figure, with the reduction of dark artifacts by the MAR filter, dark images that were not artifacts, such as the root fracture line (blue arrow), were not removed

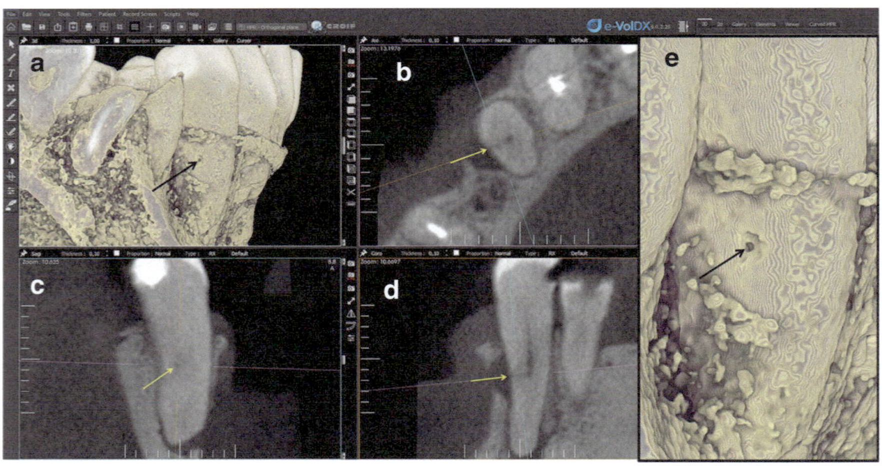

Fig. 2.25 A discrete lateral accessory root canal visible in MPR slices (**b**, **c**, **d**) (yellow arrows) is best seen from 3D reconstruction (**a**) and the magnified 3D view (**e**). This 3D reconstruction of the e-Vol software is specific for the evaluation of accessory canals and can be used with enormous magnification in high quality

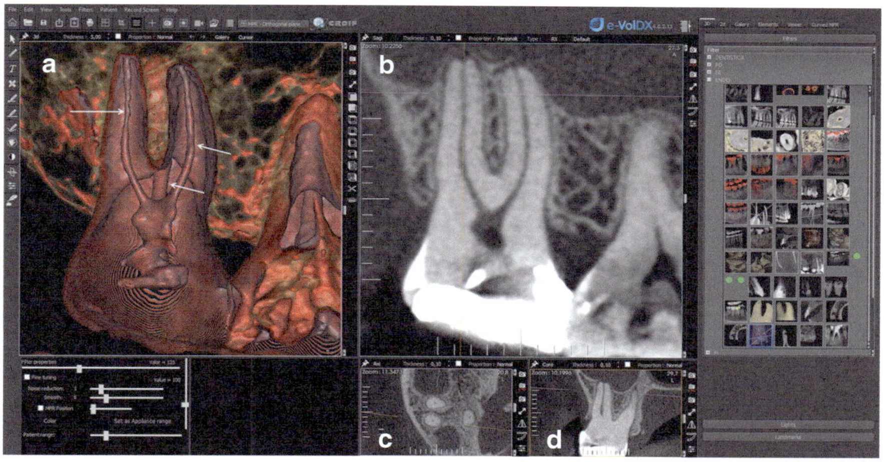

Fig. 2.26 The "Dental Pulp" filter from e-Vol DXS is a special 3D filter that leaves the dentin transparent in the CBCT image and leaves the pulp space (white arrow) in the 3D reconstruction (**a**). It is a very interesting filter for pulp microanatomy evaluation. MPR slices (**b**, **c**, **d**)

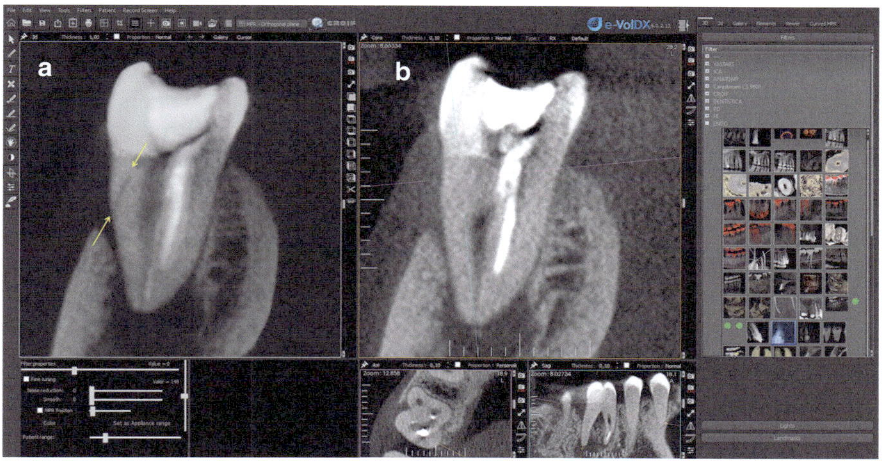

Fig. 2.27 The "FTF" filter of e-Vol DXS is a special filter that generates a slice in the 3D image (**a**) with transparency and greater dynamic range than the MPR slice, increasing the visibility of the fracture line (yellow arrow) compared to the traditional MPR slice (**b**)

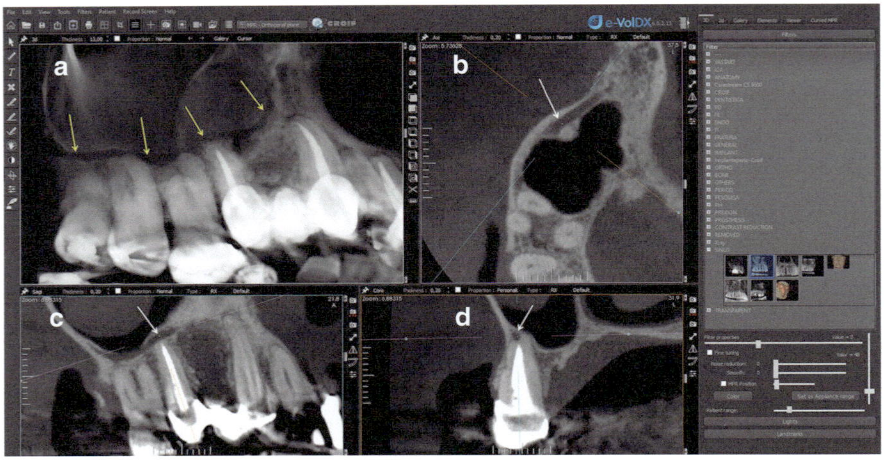

Fig. 2.28 Many filters from e-Vol DXS are dedicated to bone anatomical assessment, such as the "SMX" filter for assessing the microanatomy structures of maxillary sinus. The posterior superior alveolar neurovascular canal, which in this patient passes very close to the root apex of the maxillary second premolar in the MPR slices (**b**, **c**, **d**) (white arrow), is very clearly and continuously visible in the 3D image with the SMX filter (**a**) (yellow arrow)

2.10 3D

Since the early days of CBCT, 3D reconstruction has mostly been used for overviews rather than as a complementary diagnostic tool. However, this has changed in recent years with advanced software producing high-quality 3D images, and in some cases, 3D has been fully used as a diagnostic tool. In the e-Vol DXS software, there are more than 100 3D filters, many of which are targeted at specific endodontic conditions, such as for evidencing root canals (Figs. 2.25 and 2.26), root fractures (Fig. 2.27), bone (Fig. 2.28), etc.

2.11 Realistic 3D

The e-Vol DXS software has an advanced method of 3D reconstruction with the application of artificial intelligence algorithms that produce a realistic 3D image. This cinematographic rendering technique can generate photorealistic 3D images (Figs. 2.29, 2.30, 2.31, 2.32, 2.33, 2.34, 2.35, 2.36, 2.37 and 2.38) that have great potential for application in clinical practice, research, and teaching in endodontics [8, 10, 25, 26].

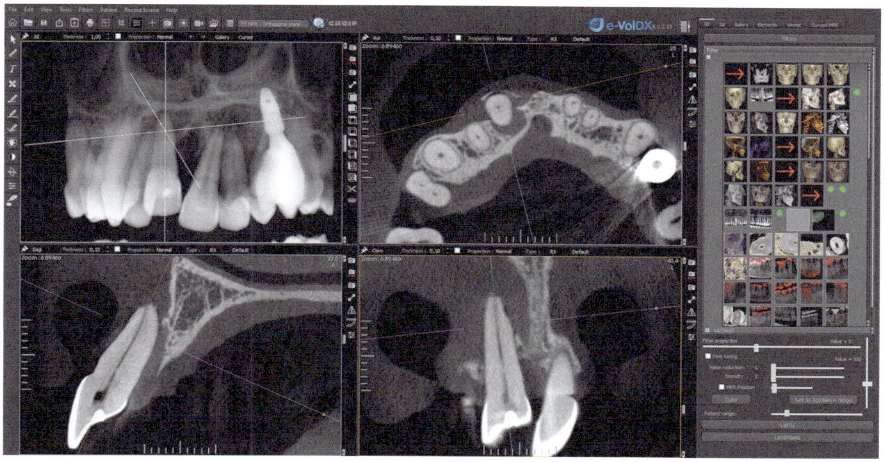

Fig. 2.29 CBCT image of a case with lateral dislocation and fracture of the alveolar ridge

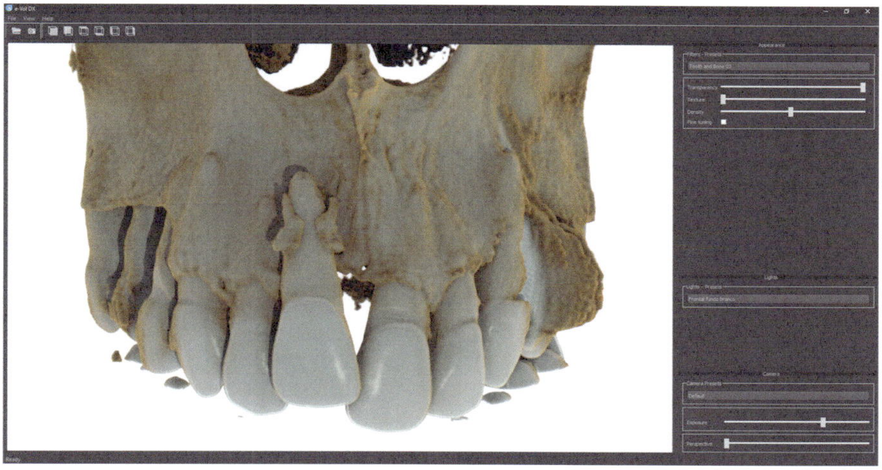

Fig. 2.30 Realistic 3D image from e-Vol DXS. Fracture and bone displacement are highlighted in the realistic 3D reconstruction (same as in Fig. 2.29) by the depth view, projection of shadows, and high image sharpness

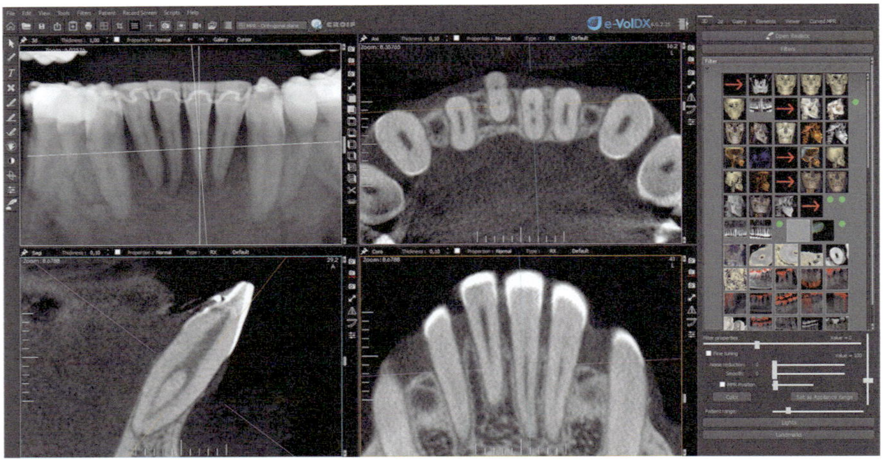

Fig. 2.31 CBCT image with mandibular central incisors with two root canals

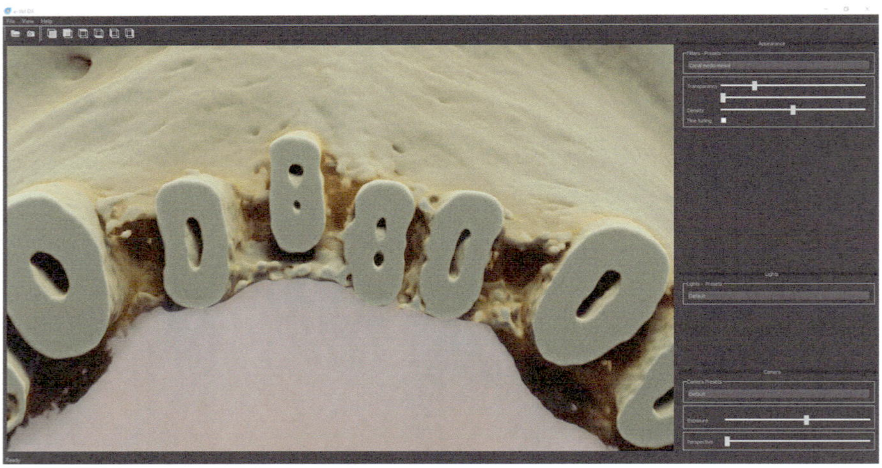

Fig. 2.32 Realistic 3D image of e-Vol DXS. Realistic 3D evaluation (same as in Fig. 2.31) can be performed in the form of cuts with high magnification and high image sharpness

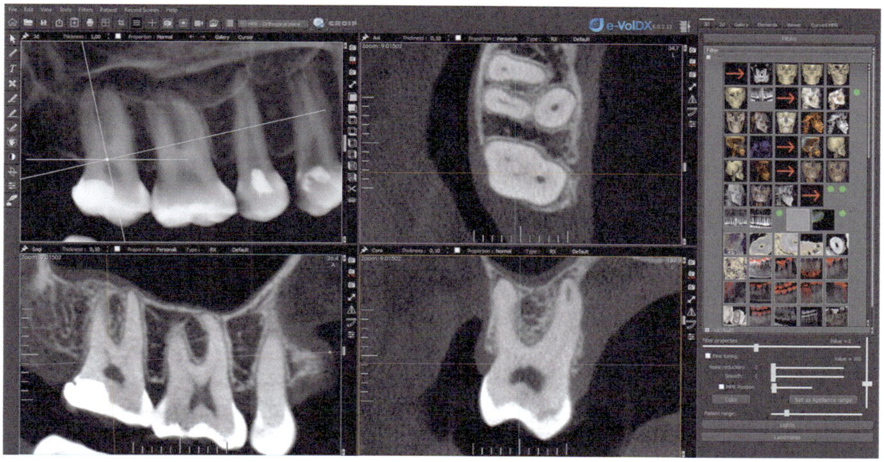

Fig. 2.33 Atretic vestibular canals in the maxillary second molar

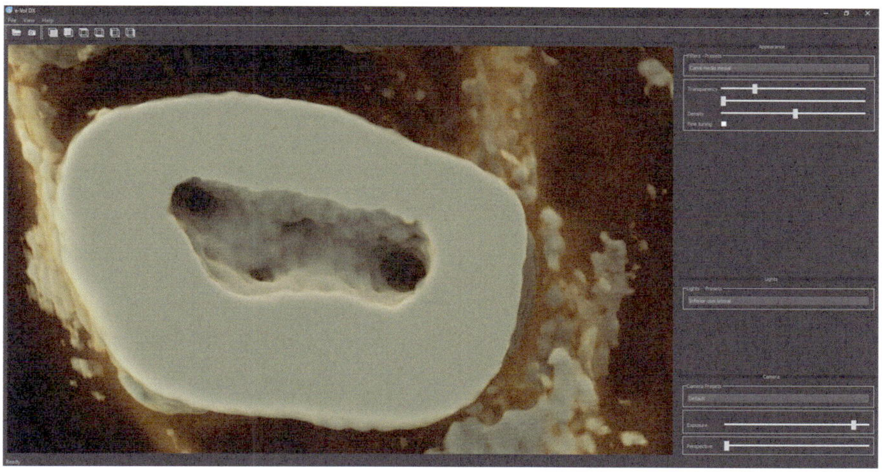

Fig. 2.34 Realistic 3D of e-Vol DXS. Realistic view of the floor of the maxillary second molar pulp chamber (same as in Fig. 2.33) with high magnification and high image sharpness

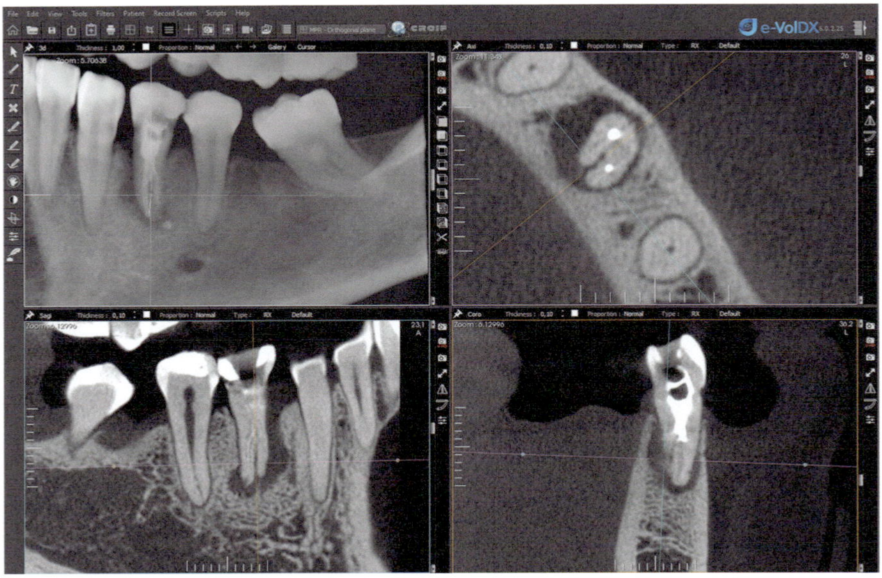

Fig. 2.35 CBCT image of a mandibular first premolar with a deep anatomical root groove. The sulcus line could be confused with a root fracture

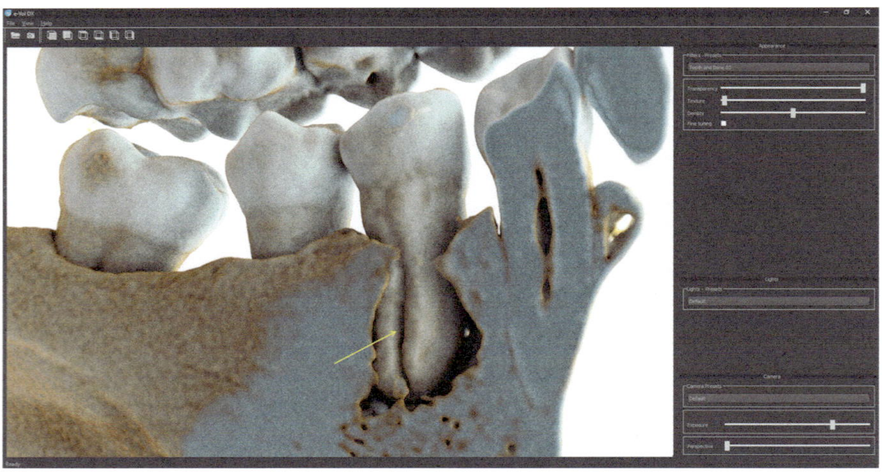

Fig. 2.36 Realistic 3D image from e-Vol DXS. The anatomical root groove observed in the previous tomographic sections of Fig. 2.35 is shown here with realistic 3D reconstruction, a very sharp image, revealing the rounded edges of the root, which is a characteristic that distinguishes from the edges of a root fracture that are not rounded

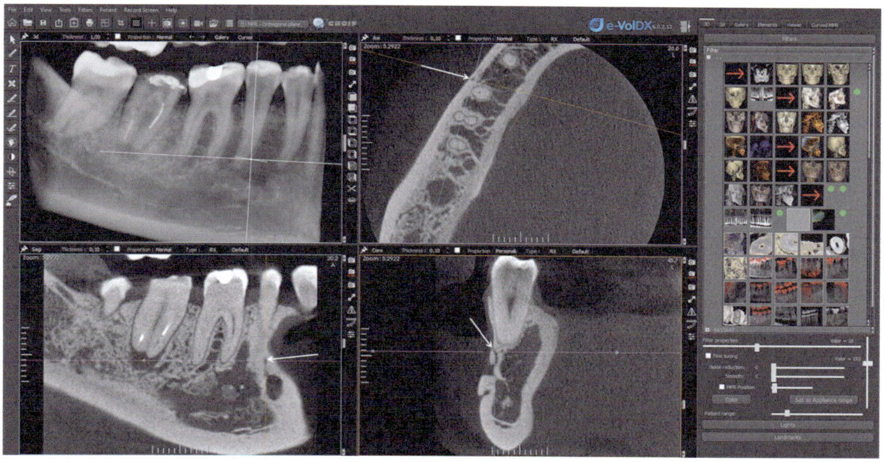

Fig. 2.37 Neurovascular ramifications are important structures to be identified especially when planning for apical endodontic microsurgery. Tiny neurovascular canals can be difficult to identify in MPR sections in routine tomographic analysis. In this case, there is a tiny accessory neurovascular canal (white arrow) above the mental foramen

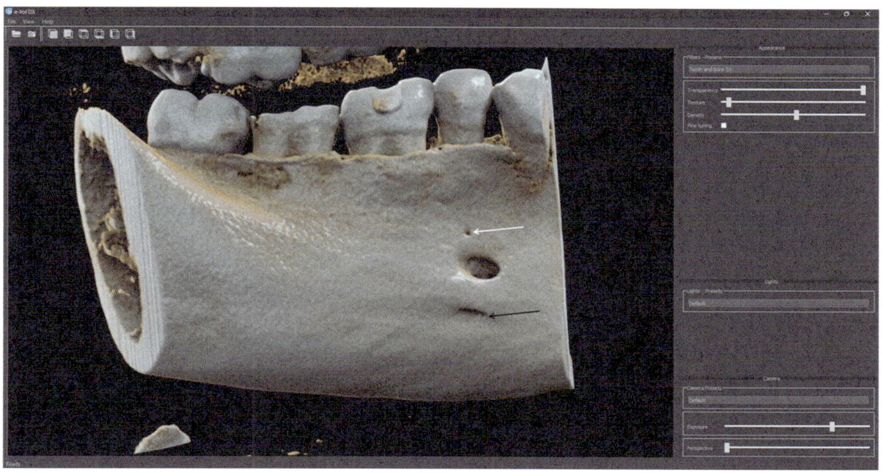

Fig. 2.38 Realistic 3D from e-Vol DXS. The tiny accessory neurovascular canal foramen above the mental foramen (white arrow) is easily located in the realistic 3D image (same as in Fig. 2.37). There is another major accessory foramen (black arrow) located below the mental foramen

2.12 e-Vol DXS Viewer

Navigating a CBCT scan is challenging, and returning exactly to a previous position can be difficult. The e-Vol DXS Viewer is a communication tool that records screen data such as XYZ coordinates, zoom level, brightness, contrast, and more information. With this tool, the user can click on the descriptions and access the exact image that was previously recorded. This facilitates complex diagnoses, allows communication between professionals and the patient, and takes CBCT navigation to a new level of sophistication.

Another feature is the possibility of creating a group of images, such as the image of a tooth and images of all findings of this tooth (Figs. 2.39, 2.40 and 2.41).

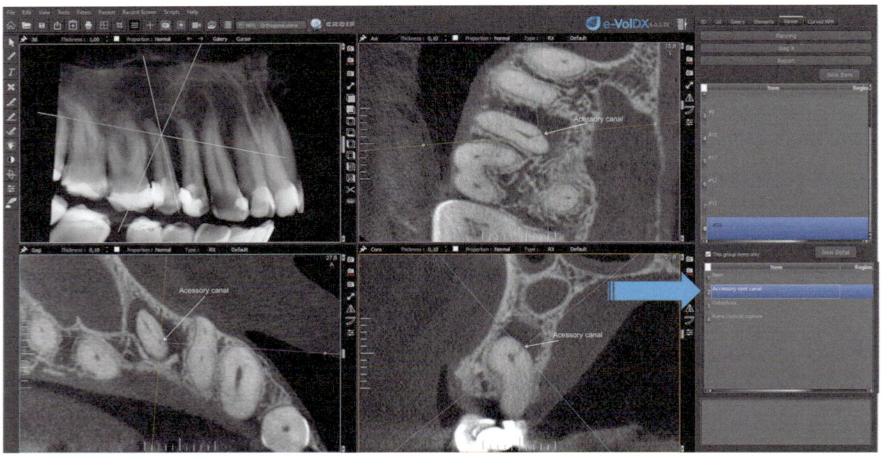

Fig. 2.39 Viewer tool—a lateral accessory canal in the maxillary second premolar is seen. The e-Vol DXS Viewer tool records coordinates, brightness, contrast, and zoom logs. With one click (big blue arrow), the screen returns to this exact image. There is the option to engrave an arrow and/or indication text

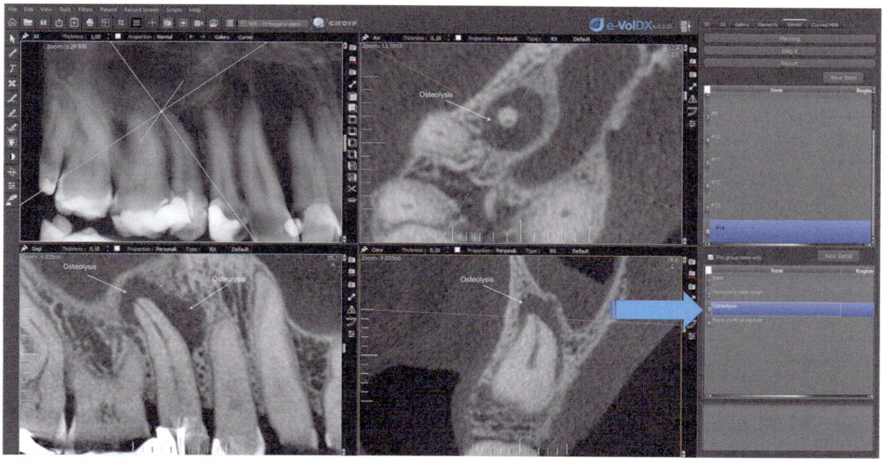

Fig. 2.40 Viewer tool—area of osteolysis in the apical and lateral region of the maxillary second premolar. The e-Vol DXS Viewer tool records coordinates, brightness, contrast, and zoom logs. With one click (big blue arrow), the screen returns to this exact image. There is the option to engrave an arrow and/or indication text

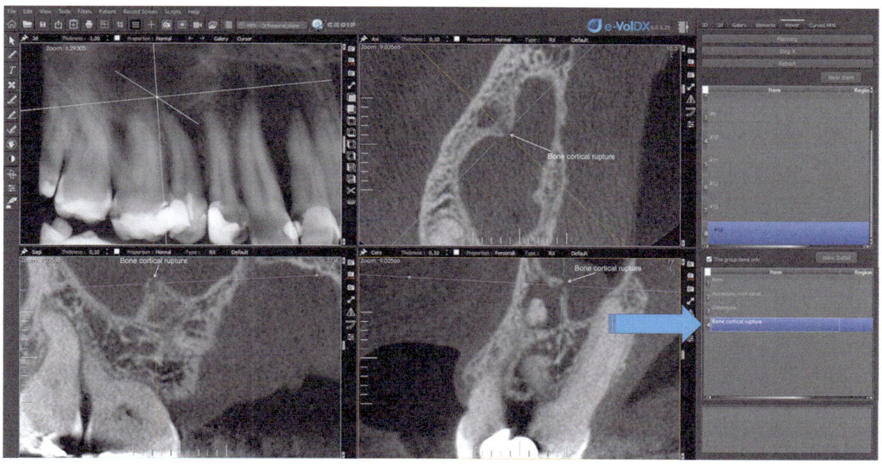

Fig. 2.41 Viewer tool—area of osteolysis in the apical region of the maxillary second premolar led to the rupture of the cortical floor of the maxillary sinus. The e-Vol viewer tool records coordinates, brightness, contrast, and zoom logs. With one click (big blue arrow), the screen returns to this exact image. There is the option to engrave an arrow and/or indication text

2.13 General Considerations

Modern technologies associated with information technology were responsible for revolutions in all areas of human knowledge. The health field's benefits influence individuals' quality of life by assisting in diagnosing, planning, and treating pathological changes. The industrial revolution changed the way many people lived. Today's world is experiencing significant change enabled by the speed and quality of information, and financial and time savings, benefiting the health fields in particular. Biotechnology has revolutionized the way of thinking and living of our time.

The application of CBCT in endodontics can make clinical management more reliable in structuring diagnosis, decision-making, and strategic planning, thereby improving the predictability of outcomes [1–43]. The incorporation and mastery of new skills to current technologies of health professionals, especially endodontists, is increasingly a requirement to overcome the challenges they face daily in complex root canal treatments.

Therefore, new strategic planning models have been incorporated into clinical practice to improve the quality of life of individuals requiring root canal treatment, provide the professionals with greater confidence in operative procedures, improve predictability, and achieve a higher success rate. Knowledge and mastery of new CBCT image post-processing software such as e-Vol DXS encourage the endodontist to increasingly address challenging clinical cases that otherwise seem impossible to solve.

References

1. Arai Y, Tammisalo E, Iwai K, et al. Development of a compact computed tomographic apparatus for dental use. Dentomaxillofac Radiol. 1999;28:245–8.
2. Bueno MR, Estrela C, Azevedo BC, et al. Cone beam computed tomography: revolution in dentistry. Rev Ass Paul Cir Dent. 2007;61:325–8.
3. Bueno MR, Estrela C, De Figueiredo JA, Azevedo BC. Map-reading strategy to diagnose root perforations near metallic intracanal posts by using cone beam computed tomography. J Endod. 2011;37:85–90.
4. Bueno MR, Estrela C, Azevedo BC, Diogenes A. Development of a new cone-beam computed tomography software for endodontic diagnosis. Braz Dent J. 2018;29:517–29.
5. Bueno MR, Estrela C. Incorporation of cone beam computed tomography in dental research. In: Estrela C, editor. Scientific methodology: science, teaching, research. 3rd ed. Porto Alegre, RS, Brazil: Artmed; 2018. p. 667–84.
6. Bueno MR, Estrela CRA, Granjeiro JM, Sousa-Neto MD, Estrela C. Method to determine the root canal anatomic dimension by using a new cone-beam computed tomography software. Braz Dent J. 2019;30:3–11.
7. Bueno MR, Estrela C. Impact of a new cone beam computed tomography software on clinical decision making in endodontics. Den Press Endod. 2019;9:20–8.
8. Bueno MR, Estrela C, Azevedo BC, Cintra JLJ. Root canal shape of human permanent teeth determined by new cone-beam computed tomographic software. J Endod. 2020;46:1662–74.
9. Bueno MR, Estrela C, Azevedo B, Diogenes A. Application of a new CBCT software with specific filters for blooming artifact reduction: case series. Dent Press Endod. 2020;10:27–35.
10. Bueno MR, Estrela C, Granjeiro JM, Estrela MRA, Azevedo BC, Diogenes A. Cone-beam computed tomography cinematic rendering: clinical, teaching and research applications. Braz Oral Res. 2021;35:e024.

11. Bueno MR, Azevedo BC, Estrela C. A critical review of the differential diagnosis of root fracture line in CBCT scans. Braz Dent J. 2021;32:114–28.
12. Bueno MR, Azevedo BC, Estrela CRA, Sousa-Neto MD, Estrela C. Method to identify accessory root canals using a new CBCT software. Braz Dent J. 2021;32:28–35.
13. Bueno MR, Estrela C. A computational modeling method for root canal endoscopy using a specific CBCT filter: a new era in the metaverse of endodontics begins. Braz Dent J. 2022;33:21–30.
14. Cotton TP, Geisler TM, Holden DT, et al. Endodontic applications of cone beam volumetric tomography. J Endod. 2007;33:1121–32.
15. Estrela C, Bueno MR, Leles CR, Azevedo B, Azevedo JR. Accuracy of cone beam computed tomography and panoramic and periapical radiography for detection of apical periodontitis. J Endod. 2008;34:273–9.
16. Estrela C, Bueno MR, Azevedo BC, Azevedo JR, Pécora JD. A new periapical index based on cone beam computed tomography. J Endod. 2008;34:1325–31.
17. Estrela C, Bueno MR, Sousa-Neto MD, Pécora JD. Method for determination of root curvature radius using cone-beam computed tomography images. Braz Dent J. 2008;19:114–8.
18. Estrela C, Bueno MR, De Alencar AH, Mattar R, Valladares Neto J, Azevedo BC, De Araújo Estrela CR. Method to evaluate inflammatory root resorption by using cone beam computed tomography. J Endod. 2009;35:1491–7.
19. Estrela C, Bueno MR, Porto OC, Rodrigues CD, Pécora JD. Influence of intracanal post on apical periodontitis identified by cone-beam computed tomography. Braz Dent J. 2009;20:370–5.
20. Estrela C, Valladares Neto J, Bueno MR, Guedes OA, Porto OCL, Pecora JD. Linear measurements of human permanent dental development stages using cone-beam computed tomography: a preliminary study. Dent Press J Orthod. 2010;15:44–78.
21. Estrela C, Rabelo LE, de Souza JB, Alencar AH, Estrela CR, Sousa Neto MD, Pécora JD. Frequency of root canal isthmi in human permanent teeth determined by cone-beam computed tomography. J Endod. 2015;41:1535–9.
22. Estrela C, Bueno MR, Couto GS, Rabelo LE, Alencar AH, Silva RG, Pécora JD, Sousa-Neto MD. Study of root canal anatomy in human permanent teeth in a subpopulation of Brazil's center region using Cone-Beam Computed Tomography—part 1. Braz Dent J. 2015;26:530–6.
23. Estrela C, Porto OC, Costa NL, Garrote Mda S, Decurcio DA, Bueno MR, Silva BS. Large reactional osteogenesis in maxillary sinus associated with secondary root canal infection detected using Cone-beam Computed Tomography. J Endod. 2015;41:2068–78.
24. Estrela C, Nunes CA, Guedes OA, Alencar AH, Estrela CR, Silva RG, Pécora JD, Sousa-Neto MD. Study of anatomical relationship between posterior teeth and maxillary sinus floor in a subpopulation of the Brazilian central region using Cone-Beam Computed Tomography—part 2. Braz Dent J. 2016;27:9–15.
25. Estrela C, Couto GS, Bueno MR, Bueno KG, Estrela LRA, Porto OCL, Diogenes A. Apical foramen position in relation to proximal root surfaces of human permanent teeth determined by using a new Cone-beam Computed Tomographic Software. J Endod. 2018;44:1741–8.
26. Estrela CRA, Bueno MR, Estrela MRA, Estrela LRA, Guedes OA, Azevedo BC, Cintra LTA, Estrela C. Frequency and risk factors of maxillary sinusitis of endodontic origin evaluated by a dynamic navigation and a new filter of Cone-Beam Computed Tomography. J Endod. 2022;48:1263–72.
27. Estrela C, Costa MVC, Bueno MR, Rabelo LEG, Decurcio DA, Silva JA, Estrela CRA. Potential of a new Cone-Beam CT software for blooming artifact reduction. Braz Dent J. 2020;31:582–8.
28. Moura MS, Guedes OA, De Alencar AH, Azevedo BC, Estrela C. Influence of length of root canal obturation on apical periodontitis detected by periapical radiography and cone beam computed tomography. J Endod. 2009;35:805–9.
29. Faitaroni LA, Bueno MR, Carvalhosa AA, Mendonça EF, Estrela C. Differential diagnosis of apical periodontitis and nasopalatine duct cyst. J Endod. 2011;37:403–10.
30. Alencar AH, Dummer PM, Oliveira HC, Pécora JD, Estrela C. Procedural errors during root canal preparation using rotary NiTi instruments detected by periapical radiography and cone beam computed tomography. Braz Dent J. 2010;21:543–9.

31. Valladares-Neto J, Estrela C, Bueno MR, Guedes OA, Porto OCL, Pecora JD. Mandibular condyle dimensional changes in subjects from 3 to 20 years of age using Cone-Beam Computed Tomography: a preliminary study. Dent Press J Orthod. 2010;15:172–81.
32. Decurcio DA, Bueno MR, de Alencar AH, Porto OC, Azevedo BC, Estrela C. Effect of root canal filling materials on dimensions of cone-beam computed tomography images. J Appl Oral Sci. 2012;20:260–7.
33. Pécora JD, Estrela C, Bueno MR, Porto OC, Alencar AH, Sousa-Neto MD, Estrela CR. Detection of root canal isthmuses in molars by map-reading dynamic using CBCT images. Braz Dent J. 2013;24:569–74.
34. Nunes CA, Guedes OA, Alencar AH, Peters OA, Estrela CR, Estrela C. Evaluation of periapical lesions and their association with maxillary sinus abnormalities on Cone-beam Computed Tomographic images. J Endod. 2016;42:42–6.
35. Silva BSF, Bueno MR, Yamamoto-Silva FP, Gomez RS, Peters OA, Estrela C. Differential diagnosis and clinical management of periapical radiopaque/hyperdense jaw lesions. Braz Oral Res. 2017;31:e52.
36. Benjamin G, Ather A, Bueno MR, Estrela C, Diogenes A. Preserving the neurovascular bundle in targeted endodontic microsurgery: a case series. J Endod. 2021;47:509–19.
37. Porto OCL, Silva BSF, Silva JA, Estrela CRA, Alencar AHG, Bueno MR, Estrela C. CBCT assessment of bone thickness in maxillary and mandibular teeth: an anatomic study. J Appl Oral Sci. 2020;28:e20190148.
38. Soares PBF, Vilela ABF, Moura CCG, Estrela C, Bueno MR, Soares CJ. Lateral luxation of incisor—a case report of using a new Cone-Beam Computed Tomography software and reposition guideline. Braz Dent J. 2020;31:337–43.
39. Decurcio DA, Bueno MR, Silva JA, Loureiro MAZ, Damião Sousa-Neto M, Estrela C. Digital planning on guided endodontics technology. Braz Dent J. 2021;32:23–33.
40. Gregoris Rabelo LE, Bueno MDR, Costa MVCD, de Musis CR, Estrela CRA, Guedes OA, Gavini G, Estrela C. Blooming artifact reduction using different cone-beam computed tomography software to analyze endodontically treated teeth with intracanal posts. Comput Biol Med. 2021;136:104679.
41. Pacheco-Yanes J, Gazzaneo I, Campello AF, Marceliano-Alves MF, Estrela C, Bueno MR, Lopes RT, Rôças IN, Alves FRF, Siqueira JF Jr. Planned apical preparation using Cone-Beam Computed Tomographic measures: a micro-computed tomographic proof of concept in human cadavers. J Endod. 2022;48:280–6.
42. Scarfe WC, Farman AG, Sukovic P. Clinical applications of cone-beam computed tomography in dental practice. J Can Dent Assoc. 2007;72:75–80.
43. Sousa VC, Alencar AHG, Bueno MR, Decurcio DA, Estrela CRA, Estrela C. Evaluation in the danger zone of mandibular molars after root canal preparation using novel CBCT software. Braz Oral Res. 2022;36:e038.

3 Utilization of Cone Beam Computed Tomography in Endodontic Diagnosis

Mohamed I. Fayad and Bradford R. Johnson

Abstract

Endodontic diagnosis is dependent upon evaluation of the patient's chief complaint, medical and dental history, and clinical and radiographic examination. A clinical examination must be performed before considering any radiographic examination. Imaging is an essential part of endodontic practice, from diagnosis and treatment planning to outcome assessment. Intraoral radiographs have inherent limitations due to the compression of three-dimensional (3D) structures in a two-dimensional (2D) image. Superimposition of anatomic structures and image noise results in distortion of the area of interest. The use of cone beam computed tomography (CBCT) could overcome these issues by visualizing the dentition and the relationship of anatomic structures in three dimensions. CBCT units reconstruct the projection data to provide inter-relational images in three orthogonal planes (axial, sagittal, and coronal). For most endodontic applications, limited or focused field of view (FOV) CBCT is preferred over large volume CBCT. This chapter will review the utilization of CBCT in endodontic diagnosis and management of periapical pathosis, diagnosis of pain, cracked teeth and vertical root fractures, internal and external resorptive defects, and traumatic injuries. A new CBCT software package (e-Vol DX, CDT-Brazil) that has been developed to overcome CBCT software limitations and support diagnosis, treatment planning, and management of endodontic cases will be presented.

M. I. Fayad (✉) · B. R. Johnson
Department of Endodontics, University of Illinois Chicago, Chicago, IL, USA
e-mail: mfayad1@uic.edu; bjohnson@uic.edu

M. I. Fayad, B. R. Johnson (eds.), *3D Imaging in Endodontics*,
https://doi.org/10.1007/978-3-031-32755-1_3

3.1 Introduction

Radiographic interpretation is a critical component in diagnosis, treatment, and evaluation of healing. Interpreting a film-based radiograph or digital image continues to be a somewhat subjective process. Goldman et al. [1] showed that agreement between 6 examiners was only 47% when evaluating healing of periapical lesions using 2D periapical radiographs. In a follow-up study, Goldman et al. [2] also reported that when examiners evaluated the same images at two different times, they only had 19–80% agreement with their previous interpretations. In a more recent study, inter-observer and intra-observer reliability in detecting periradicular radiolucencies by using a digital radiograph system was evaluated. Agreement among all six observers for all radiographs was less than 25%, and agreement for 5 of 6 observers was approximately 50% [3].

3.2 Detection of Periapical Lesions

CBCT imaging has the ability to detect small areas of periapical pathosis prior to being apparent on 2D radiographs [4], as well as differentiating larger, indistinct periapical radiolucent areas from normal variations in bone density (Figs. 3.1

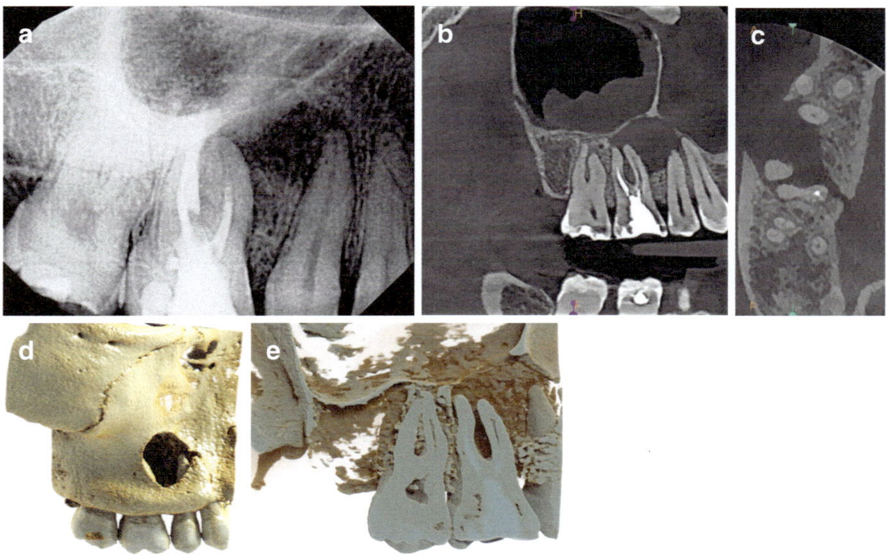

Fig. 3.1 A 31-year-old female was referred to consultation for tooth #3. Tooth #3 had a previous root canal therapy and symptomatic apical periodontitis. (**a**) Periapical radiograph of teeth #2, 3, 4, and 5. Tooth #3 presented with an under-filled mesiobuccal canal. (**b**) Sagittal CBCT view of the upper left quadrant showing a low-density area related to tooth #3 and extending to teeth #4 and 5. Perforation of the sinus floor and maxillary sinus mucositis were noted. Both teeth (4 and 5) tested positive for vitality testing. (**c**) Axial view demonstrating the extent of the unilocular, expansile, and perforating low-density area. (**d**) 3D realistic rendering of the defect in the e-VOLDX software. (**e**) e-VOLDX realistic rendering utilizing the canal anatomy filter demonstrating the etiology of the lateral nature of the defect to be due to the lateral canal in the apical one-third of the MB root

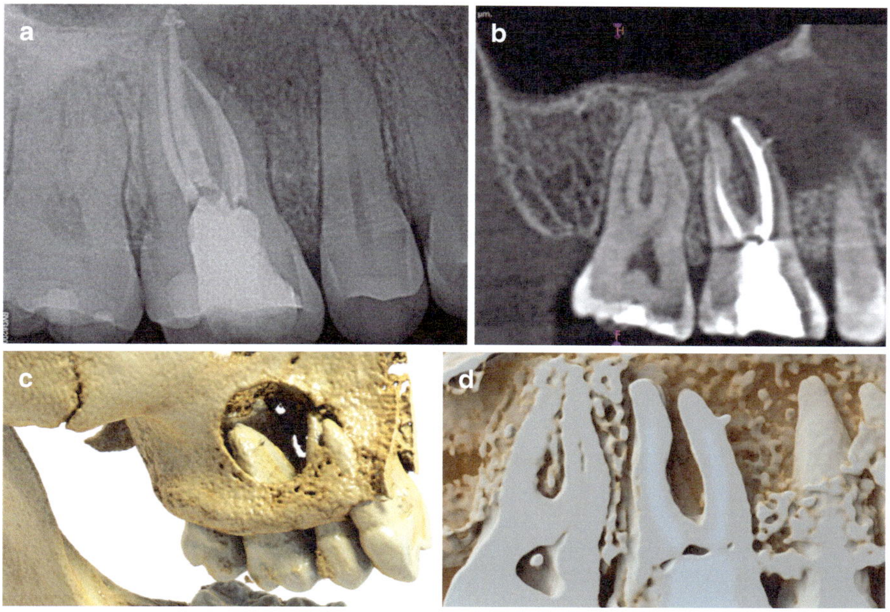

Fig. 3.2 Continuation of case 2.1. (**a**) Postoperative radiograph of the final obturation of tooth #3. (**b**) Sagittal CBCT view of the final obturation demonstrating the obturation of the lateral canal and the sealer extrusion. (**c**) e-VOLDX realistic rendering demonstrating the sealer extrusion from the lateral canal. (**d**) e-VOLDX cropped realistic rendering demonstrating the obturation in the buccal canals and sealer extrusion from the lateral canal

and 3.2). This finding was validated in clinical studies in which periapical periodontitis detected in intraoral radiographs and CBCT was 20% and 48%, respectively [5]. In a 1-year posttreatment study by the same authors, absence of a periapical radiolucency was found in 93% of the cases when evaluated by 2D radiographs but only 74% when using CBCT [6]. Ex vivo studies in which simulated periapical lesions were created showed similar findings [7, 8].

However, some caution is warranted in the interpretation of CBCT periapical findings since the CBCT-PAI score is commonly greater than the 2D Periapical Index (PAI) score and some teeth with healthy pulps may demonstrate a widened apical periodontal ligament (PDL) space on CBCT [9].

3.3 Differential Diagnosis of Pain when Etiology Is Unclear and Identification of Unusual Anatomical Relationships

Diagnosis of orofacial pain can be a challenging process for the clinician prior to and after endodontic treatment. In challenging diagnostic pain cases, the clinical and radiographic findings are often inconclusive. Inability to determine the true source of pain can be attributed in part to limitations in both pulp sensibility testing and 2D intraoral radiographic imaging (Figs. 3.3, 3.4, 3.5, 3.6, 3.7, 3.8 and 3.9).

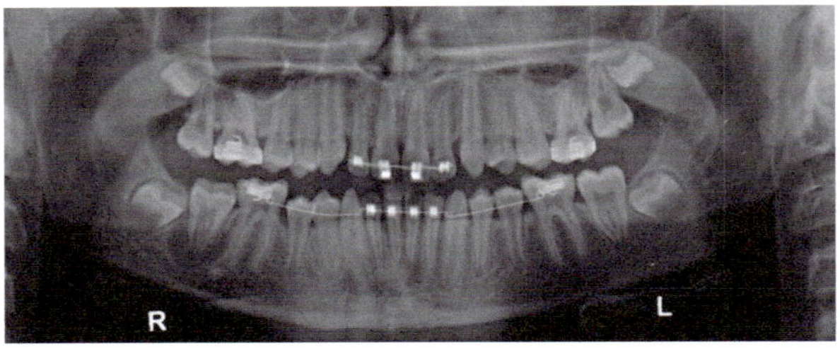

Fig. 3.3 A 14-year-old female was referred to consultation for tooth #31. The panoramic radiograph revealed a radiolucency related to tooth #31. The tooth responded positively to pulp sensibility tests and periodontal probing was WNL except for an 8-mm pocket on the mid-buccal surface. The patient was previously seen by two other dental specialists and extraction of #31 had been recommended by both

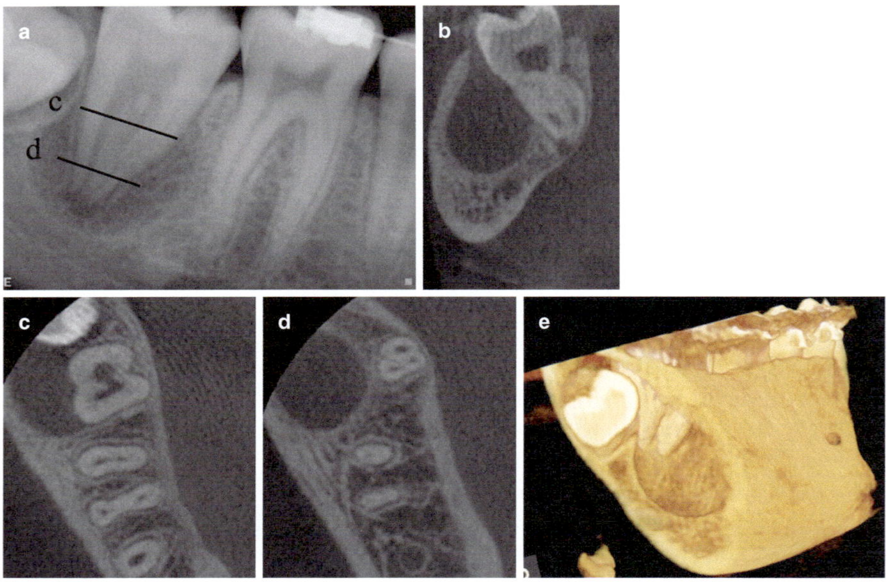

Fig. 3.4 Continuation of case from Fig. 3.3. (**a**) Periapical radiograph of tooth #31. (**b**) Coronal view showing the buccal location of the periapical radiolucency in relation to tooth #31. Notice the apical one-third of the root is surrounded by bone which explains the positive response to cold and EPT. The lines on the periapical radiograph correspond to the axial section views **c** and **d**. Axial sections **c** and demonstrate the origin of the lesion as tooth #32. 3D reconstruction (**e**) demonstrates the buccal location of the lesion and explains the isolated deep periodontal probing on the buccal aspect of tooth #31

Persistent pain following root canal therapy or other therapeutic dental intervention can present a diagnostic challenge. Atypical odontalgia (AO), atypical facial pain (AFP), and persistent dentoalveolar pain (PDAP) are often used interchangeably to describe orofacial pain of uncertain etiology, although PDAP seems to be emerging as the preferred term [10, 11]. The diagnostic yield of intraoral

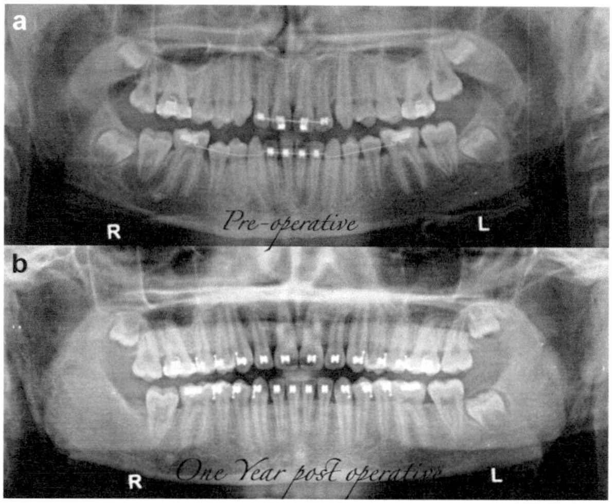

Fig. 3.5 Continuation of case from Fig. 3.3. Tooth #32 was extracted, and the lesion was submitted for biopsy. The biopsy result was a dentigerous cyst. Panoramic images (**a**) and (**b**) are pre-operative and 1-year recall, respectively. Good bony healing around #31 is evident

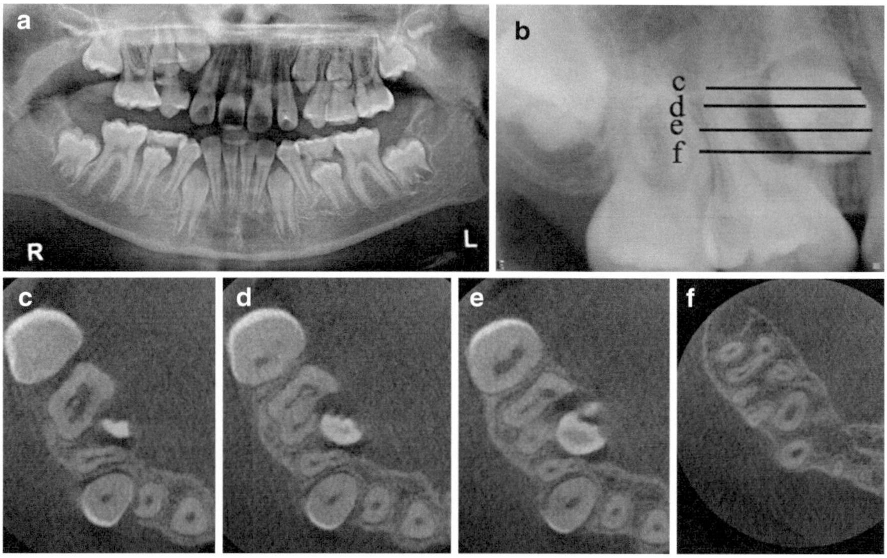

Fig. 3.6 (**a**) Panoramic radiograph of a 9-year-old patient who was referred to evaluate the path of eruption of tooth #4 as part of orthodontic treatment planning. (**b**) Periapical radiograph of tooth #4. The lines on the periapical radiograph correspond to the axial section views **c**, **d**, **e**, and **f**. (**c**), (**d**), and (**e**) are the different coronal-apical cross-section levels demonstrating the ectopic resorption of the mesio-palatal aspect of tooth #3 by the cusp tip of tooth #4. The resorptive pattern seen on the CBCT axial images cannot be detected on either the panoramic or periapical radiographs. (**f**) The most apical cross-section shows no resorption at that level

radiographs and CBCT was evaluated in the differentiation between patients presenting with apical periodontitis and suspected PDAP without the evidence of periapical bone destruction. CBCT imaging detected 17% more teeth with apical bone loss (apical periodontitis) than intraoral radiographs [12].

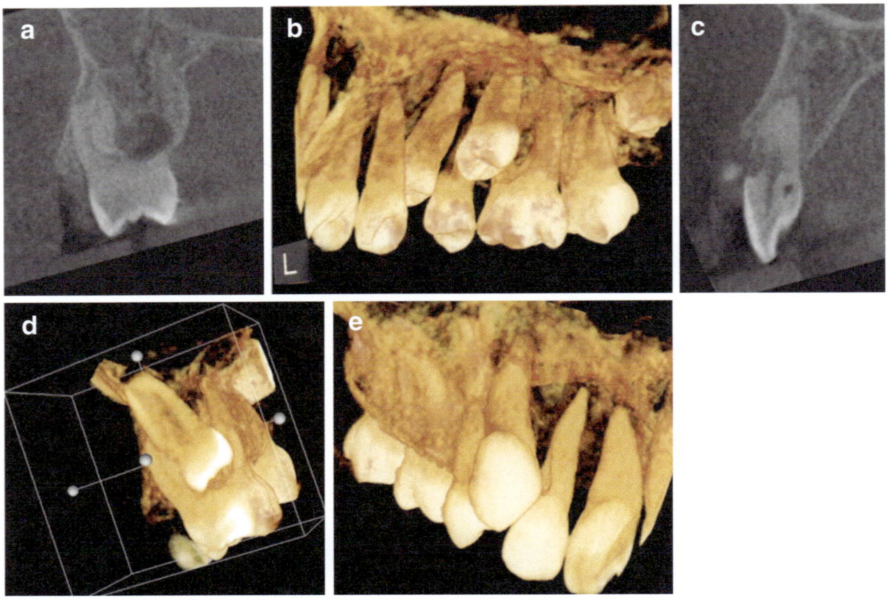

Fig. 3.7 Continuation of case from Fig. 3.6. (**a**) Coronal view of the mesial furcation of tooth #3 demonstrating the resorptive defect in the furcation and mesio-palatal aspect. (**b**) and (**d**) are 3D reconstructions demonstrating the same pattern from the palatal and mesial views, respectively. (**c**) Sagittal view of tooth #7 demonstrating resorption caused by the ectopic eruption of tooth #6. (**e**) 3D reconstruction demonstrating the relationship between teeth #6 and 7. The information obtained from this CBCT scan will have a significant impact on orthodontic treatment planning

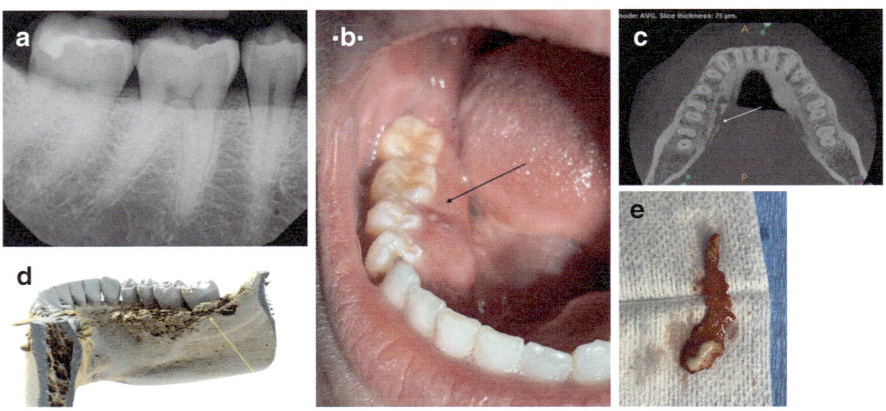

Fig. 3.8 A 33-year-old female presented with pain related to the lower left quadrant. (**a**) Periapical radiograph of teeth #29, 30, and 31. All teeth tested positive to vitality testing and were tender to percussion. (**b**) A lingual swelling adjacent to teeth # 28, 29, and 30. (**c**) Axial view of the lower arch demonstrating lingual bone sequestration (white arrow). (**d**) e-VOLDX realistic rendering demonstrating the lingual bone sequestration. (**e**) The sequestrated lingual bone after surgical removal. Patient lingual soft tissue healed to normal color, texture, and architecture and presented for follow-up appointments asymptomatic

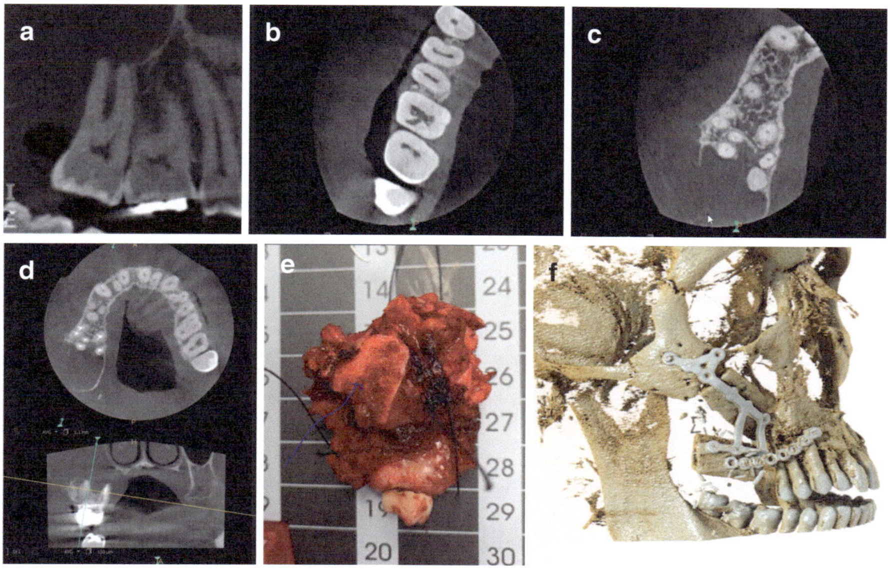

Fig. 3.9 A 44-year-old male presented for evaluation of pain related to the upper right quadrant. Teeth #2 and 3 had a previous root canal treatment and symptomatic apical periodontitis. (**a**, **b**, and **c**) Sagittal CBCT view was requested from the previous endodontist. A distal resorptive defect with pulpal exposure was noted and was the reason tooth #3 received root canal therapy. The patient continued to be symptomatic and tooth #2 was tender to percussion. A week later, tooth #2 received root canal therapy. Pain subsided but returned 6 months later and the patient was referred for a second opinion. (**d**) Axial and Sagittal CBCT view demonstrating a multilocular, expansile, and perforating lesion that was noted in the preoperative CBCT axial view (**c**). Diagnosis was ameloblastoma of the maxilla (**e** and **f**). Resected portion of the maxilla and maxilla reconstruction

3.4 Detection of Cracked Teeth and Root Fractures

Cracked teeth can present a diagnostic challenge, a restorative dilemma, and often a source of frustration for both clinicians and patients because of the vague symptoms, low sensitivity of available imaging modalities, and unpredictable prognosis. Problems related to cracked teeth are the third leading cause of tooth loss after caries and periodontal disease [13].

Cracks and root fractures generally develop slowly over time. By the time a crack is visible, it has progressed through three stages: initiation, propagation, and manifestation. Once a crack has initiated, it can remain asymptomatic for several years. An asymptomatic phase can change drastically over time as the crack is subjected to repetitive parafunctional habits, occlusal stress, thermal cycling, and colonization with bacterial biofilms [14–16].

Cracked teeth may present with crack lines present in the vertical plane. Several terminologies and classifications have been proposed to describe the characteristics of cracked teeth. The American Association of Endodontists (AAE) categorizes cracks into five types: craze lines, fractured cusp, cracked tooth, split tooth, and vertical root fracture (VRF). The term longitudinal fracture is used because it typically represents vertical extension of fractures over distance and time. These five categories of longitudinal fractures have been devised to provide global definitions that researchers and clinicians can use to make the various conditions more widely understandable [17].

Cracked teeth are diagnosed based on clinical manifestations and clinical exam testing, such as transillumination, periodontal probing depths, biting stress test, magnification, and staining with methylene blue. Although these tests are useful, there is no standard examination that can predict the long-term outcome of cracked tooth treatment. The AAE Colleagues for Excellence classified treatable versus untreatable cracked teeth based on longitudinal marginal ridge crack (MRC) extension apically into the root in relation to the cementoenamel junction (CEJ). The ability to assess the apical extent of a MRC would be a great diagnostic aid for clinicians to support case selection and clinical decision-making.

Assessment of the extent of a MRC is critical for predicting the most likely treatment outcome. For years, endodontists were accustomed to evaluating the internal extent of the MRC using methylene blue staining and operating microscopes. On the other hand, the external extension of the MRC on the root surface was proposed to be a more accurate predictor of the prognosis of a MRC tooth and would allow clinicians to make a better pretreatment decision regarding treatment outcome [18]. Alternative radiographic imaging systems have recently become available for use in dentistry. Among these new imaging technologies is cone beam computed tomography (CBCT). CBCT technology allows the precise visualization and evaluation of teeth and the surrounding structures. The use of CBCT has great potential as a diagnostic tool to assist in the detection of the external extent of MRC and VRF by detecting early patterns of bony changes adjacent to the MRC and VRF.

A joint position statement by the American Association of Endodontists and the American Academy of Oral and Maxillofacial Radiology (AAE/AAOMR) recommends CBCT as the imaging modality of choice for such cases [19].

CBCT imaging has the diagnostic capability to detect early patterns of bony changes adjacent to marginal ridge cracks and vertical root fractures. Based on these early patterns of bony changes, the clinician can determine the extension of the MRC on the external surface of the root and its location prior to initiating treatment. If left untreated, the MRC will propagate on the external surface of the root and will result in breakdown of periodontal attachment and periodontal defect formation.

Despite technological advancements in CBCT hardware, the interpretation of the acquired images is still compromised by viewing software packages that often have limited navigational tools and lack adequate filters to overcome some challenges of CBCT technology such as artifacts. A new CBCT software package (e-Vol DX, CDT-Brazil) has been developed to overcome these software limitations and support diagnosis, treatment planning, and management of endodontic cases [20]. This imaging method provides high-resolution images due to submillimeter voxel sizes, dynamic multiplane imaging navigation, the ability to change the volume

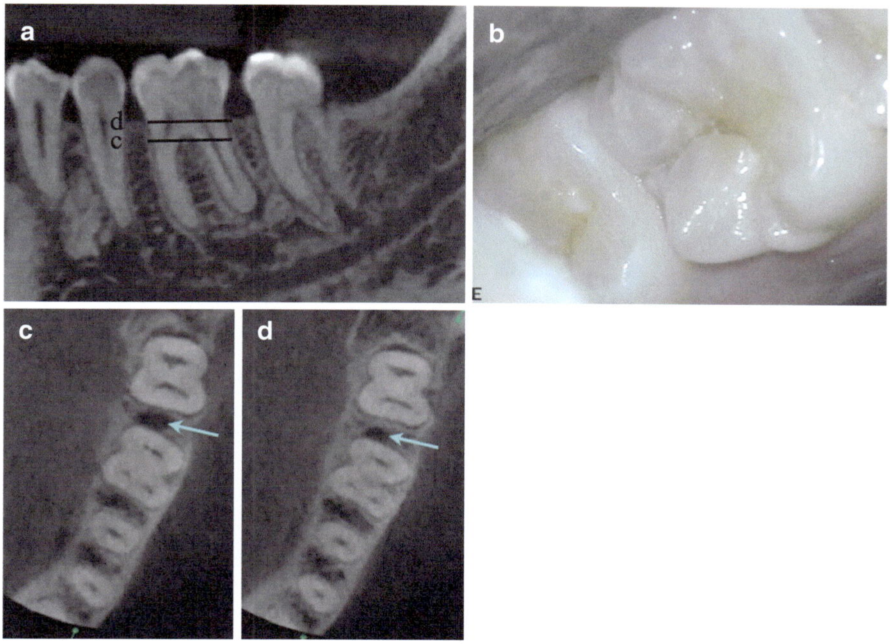

Fig. 3.10 Patient presented for evaluation and treatment of tooth #19. The chief complaint was pain on biting and sensitivity to hot drinks. Clinical findings: no response to cold and positive response to bite stress testing. A diagnosis of a necrotic pulp and symptomatic apical periodontitis was established. The presumed etiology was an extension of a distal marginal ridge crack. (**a**) Sagittal view of tooth #19 showing a distal root periapical radiolucency. The lines on the sagittal view correspond to the axial section views (**c**) and (**d**). (**b**) Clinical image (occlusal view) demonstrating the distal marginal ridge crack. Axial views (**c**) and (**d**) demonstrate the distal bone loss associated with the fracture (blue arrows) and unfavorable prognosis

parameters such as slice thickness and slice intervals, and data correction applying imaging filters and manipulation of brightness and contrast. With CBCT DICOM images and the combination of CBCT DICOM images imported into e-Vol DX, clinicians can visualize marginal ridge crack extension in relation to the CEJ for the first time.

The combination of early patterns of bony changes and the actual visualization of the MRC extension as well as VRF has been a breakthrough in CBCT imaging, providing the clinician with more accurate 3D information. Based on this enhanced information, the clinician can make an accurate diagnosis, leading to a more predictable outcome (Figs. 3.10, 3.11, 3.12, 3.13 and 3.14).

When teeth present with MRCs that are considered treatable, it is generally accepted that early restorative intervention is recommended to prevent irreversible damage, such as pulpal inflammation/necrosis and/or structural failure. Historically, various forms of dental intervention from occlusal adjustment to indirect and direct restorations to orthodontic bands have been advocated. Although many options have been proposed for the treatment of posterior MRC, most of the treatment

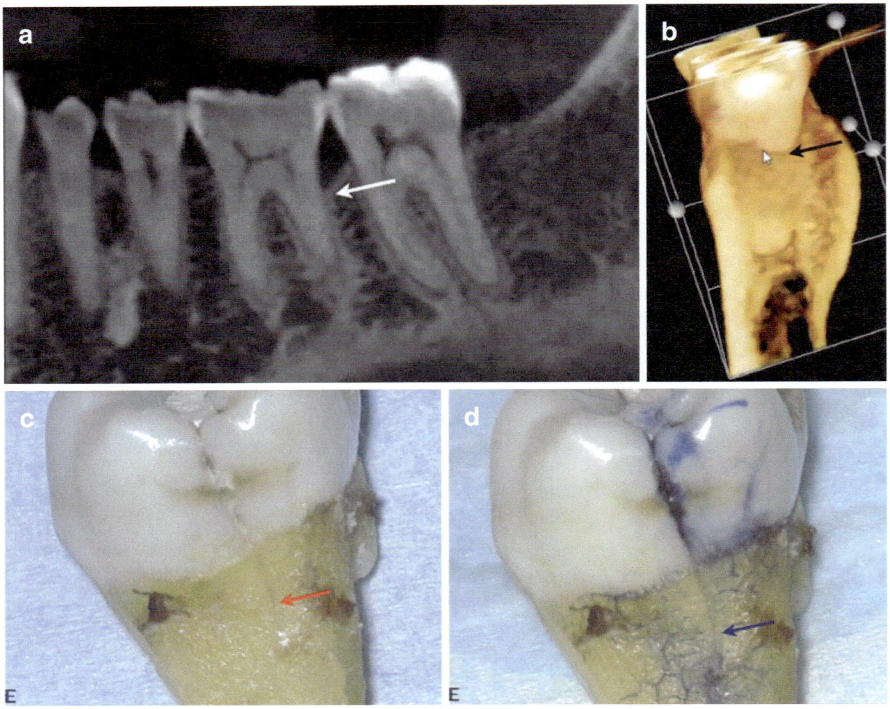

Fig. 3.11 Continuation of case from Fig. 3.10; (**a**) Sagittal view demonstrating an angled distal bony defect. (**b**) 3D reconstruction view demonstrating the angled distal bony defect seen in (**a**). (**c**) and (**d**) show the extracted tooth before and after staining the longitudinal distal root fracture (red and blue arrows)

recommendations are not evidence based. In a study that evaluated the differences in treatment approach of dental practitioners toward different cracked teeth scenarios, a large difference in the approach and treatment planning between dental practitioners and specialists was observed [21]. Although there are no universally accepted restorative protocols, the aim of restorative therapy is to immobilize the segments of the tooth that flex on loading [22].

Improved understanding of the microanatomy of tooth structure has led to a revolution in dentistry that is known by several names, including micro dentistry, minimally invasive dentistry, biomimetic dentistry, and bio-emulation dentistry. These treatment concepts have developed due to a coalescence of principles of tooth microanatomy, materials science, adhesive dentistry, and reinforcing techniques that, when applied together, will allow dentists to predictably repair and restore teeth. Evidence now supports the concept that the enamel on a tooth acts like a compression dome protecting the underlying dentin from damaging tensile forces (compression dome concept). Disruption of the compression system, such as MRC, leads to significant shifts in occlusal loads, resulting in crack propagation, flexural pain, and fracture loss of tooth structure [23].

Teeth with MRC can present as asymptomatic or symptomatic. To date, studies have evaluated the prognosis of symptomatic cracked teeth and cracked teeth that

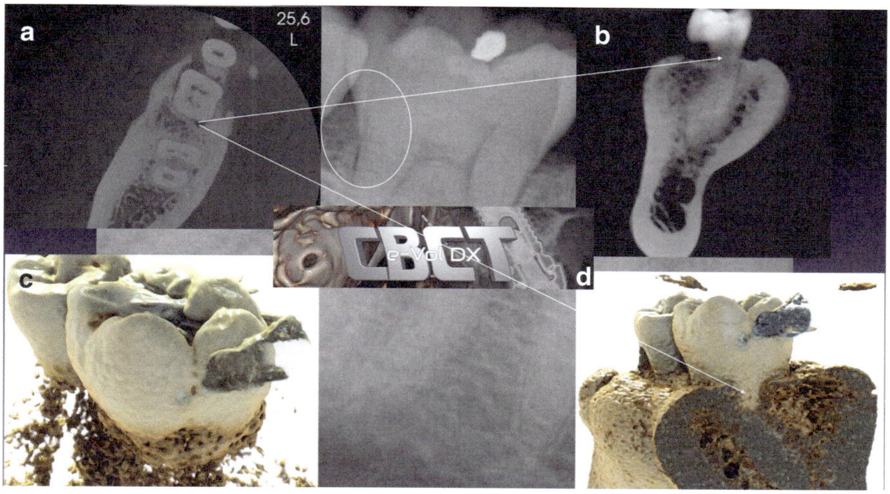

Fig. 3.12 Tooth #30 presents with a distal marginal ridge crack. The periapical radiograph demonstrated normal distal root bone pattern and periodontal probings were within normal limits (WNL). (**a**) Axial CBCT view demonstrating the distal bony changes adjacent to the distal marginal ridge crack. (**b**) CBCT DICOM images imported into e-VolDX software and utilizing the fracture filter. The distal marginal ridge crack extending below the CEJ can be visualized. (**c** and **d**) Applying the realistic rendering function and visualizing the distal marginal ridge crack extension as well as the early distal bony changes adjacent to the distal marginal ridge crack. All views confirm that the distal marginal ridge crack has extended below the CEJ

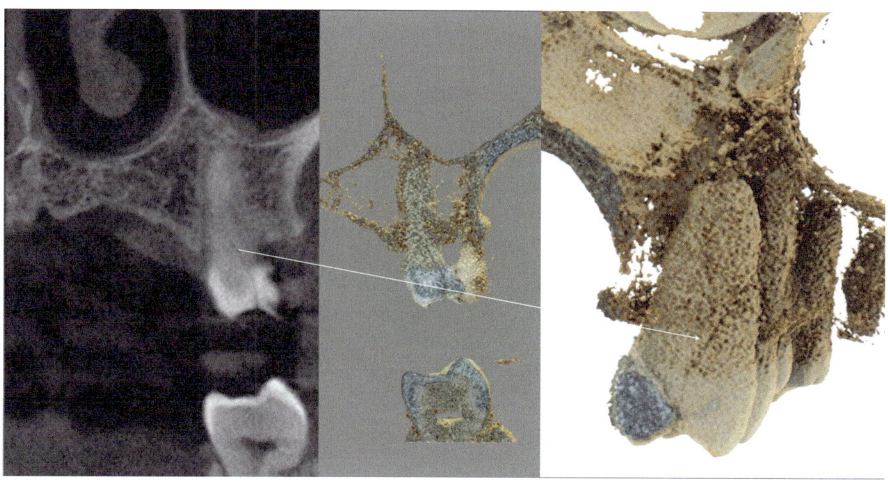

Fig. 3.13 An example of tooth #13 presenting with a distal marginal ridge crack extending below the CEJ and halfway into the root. CBCT Dicom images imported into e-VOLDX software and utilizing both the fracture filter and realistic rendering enabling the visualization of the extent of the distal marginal ridge crack (white arrow)

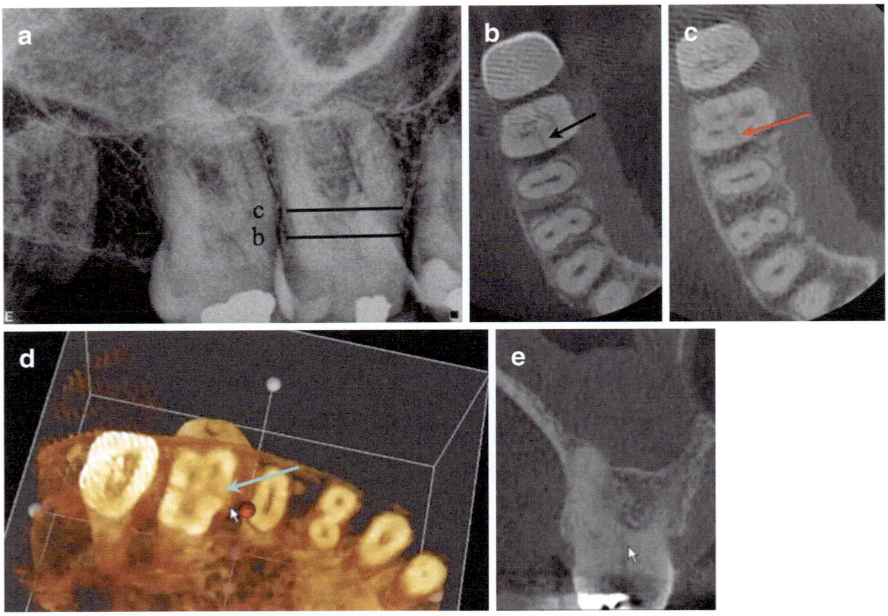

Fig. 3.14 (**a**) Periapical radiograph of tooth #3. The patient presented complaining of pain to cold and biting. Periodontal probing depths were WNL. Lines correspond to the axial sections in (**b**) and (**c**). (**b**) and (**c**) are axial views showing the extent of the fracture (black and red arrows in (**b**) and (**c**), respectively). (**d**) 3D reconstruction, axial view of (**c**) showing the mesial-distal crack (blue arrow). (**e**) A coronal view demonstrating extension of the fracture into the furcation

were retained by endodontic treatment. Clinical outcomes of cracked teeth diagnosed with reversible pulpitis were evaluated [24]. It was concluded that if marginal ridge cracks were identified early enough in teeth diagnosed with reversible pulpitis and a crown was placed, root canal treatment was necessary in only about 20% of the cases within a 6-month period. A similar study evaluated pulpal complications after diagnosis of vital cracked teeth [25]. Fifty-eight out of 199 (29.1%) teeth had pulpal complications. Thirty-eight of 58 (65.5%) were diagnosed with irreversible pulpitis after 1.2 years, and 20 of 58 (34.5%) were diagnosed with necrotic pulp after 2 years. It was concluded that the absence of a full-coverage crown increased the risk of pulpal complications. These studies confirm that it is essential to brace the cracked tooth to minimize cusp flexion and to provide full coverage that will protect the structural integrity and protect the pulp from the oral environment and bacterial contamination of the pulp.

The outcome and survival of endodontically treated cracked posterior teeth was evaluated in several recent studies [26–28]. One study concluded that survival for cracked teeth at 2 years was 100% and declined to 96.6% at 4 years. Success at 4 years was 90.6% [27]. Studies evaluating the success and survival rates of endodontically cracked teeth without a preoperative CBCT is a major limitation in most studies. The results of the previous studies can be skewed dramatically based on the unknown external extension of the MRC.

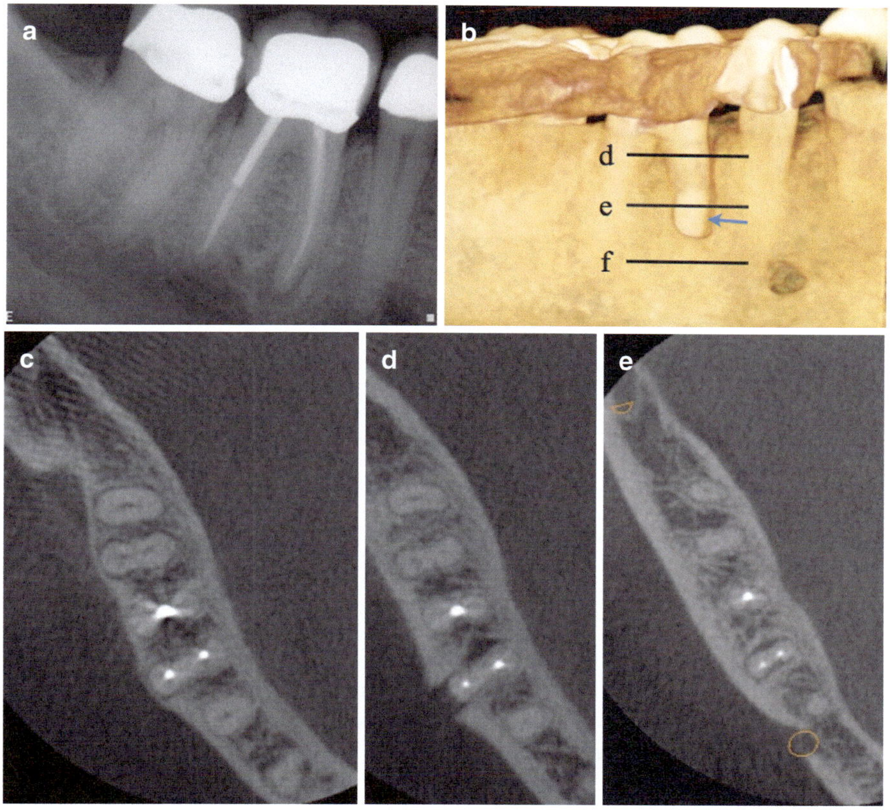

Fig. 3.15 (**a**) Periapical radiograph of tooth #30. (**b**) 3D reconstruction demonstrating the mid-root buccal defect (arrow). Lines correspond to the axial section views (**c**), (**d**), and (**e**). Note axial view demonstrating the mid-root buccal bone loss in (**d**)

Clinically, a thorough dental history and classic clinical and radiographic signs and symptoms, such as pain, swelling, presence of a sinus tract, and/or presence of an isolated deep periodontal pocket, can be helpful hints to suggest the presence of a VRF. Radiographically, a combination of periapical and lateral root radiolucency "halo" appearance is valuable information indicating the possible presence of VRF. Several of the previously mentioned clinical and radiographic elements have to align to establish a presumptive diagnosis of VRF; however, direct visual examination, usually requiring surgical exposure, is still the reference standard for diagnosis of VRF.

In a case series, the following five findings on CBCT exam were consistent with confirmed VRF [29]:

1. Loss of bone in the mid-root area with intact bone coronal and apical to the defect (Figs. 3.15 and 3.16).

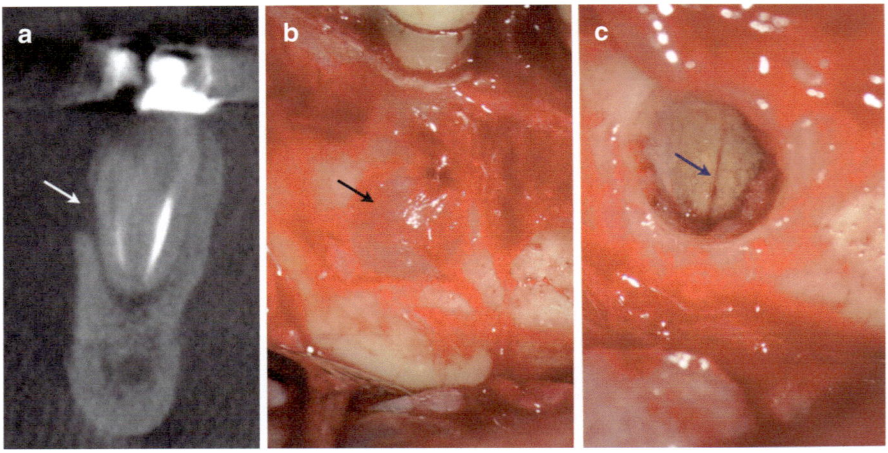

Fig. 3.16 Continuation of case in Fig. 3.15. (**a**) Coronal view demonstrating the mid-root buccal bone loss (arrow). Surgical exploration was performed to confirm the presence of a vertical root fracture. (**b**) Note the granulation tissue at mid-root level(arrow). (**c**) Surgical degranulation of the defect demonstrates the vertical root fracture in the mesial root (arrow)

2. Absence of the entire buccal plate of bone in axial, coronal, and/or 3D reconstruction.
3. Radiolucency around a root where a post terminates (Fig. 3.17).
4. Space between the buccal and lingual plate of bone and fractured root surface (Figs. 3.18, 3.19 and 3.20).
5. Visualization of the VRF on the CBCT spatial projection views.

The combination of CBCT DICOM images and e-Vol DX software is a great imaging tool when evaluating cases presenting with cuspal fractures. Based on this enhanced information, the clinician can make an accurate diagnosis on the extent of the apical extent of the cuspal fracture in relation to the crestal bone, leading to a more predictable outcome (Figs. 3.21, 3.22 and 3.23).

In summary, the prognosis for teeth with MRCs is determined by three principal factors: the extent and location of the crack, the point in time when restorative intervention is initiated, and the type of restoration. For teeth presenting with MRCs, early restoration with full cuspal coverage can improve the outcome. MRCs above the CEJ may be predictably treated, whereas radicular cracks extending below the CEJ have a lower prognosis with an increased probability of extraction. Teeth presenting with MRCs are more often lost due to periodontal breakdown than structural failure. For cracked teeth presenting with irreversible pulpitis, research has shown that endodontic treatment is an option and has a favorable prognosis when the MRC has not extended below the CEJ. CBCT imaging and a new software such as e-Vol DX aid in diagnosis and treatment planning for teeth with MRCs and VRFs.

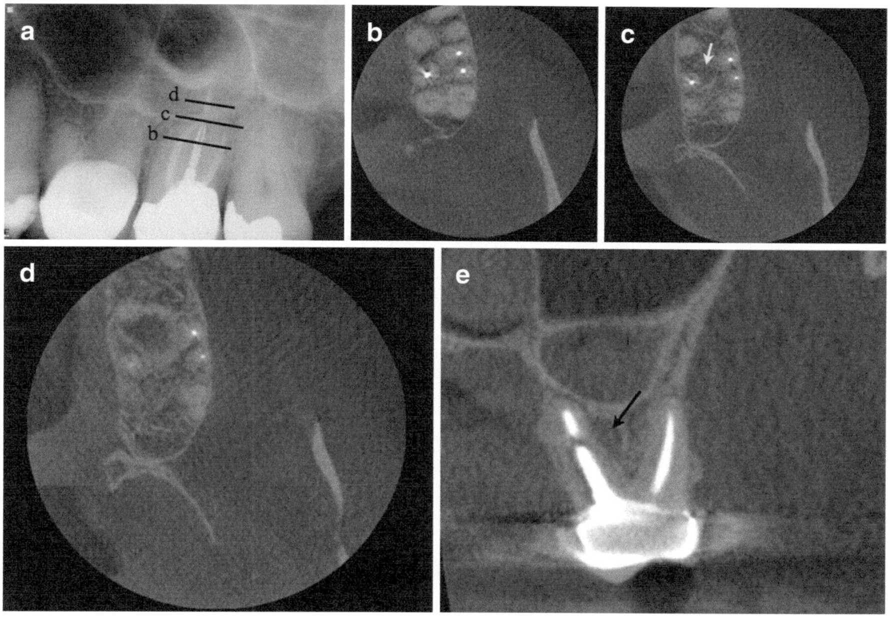

Fig. 3.17 (**a**) Periapical radiograph of tooth #14. The three lines correspond to the axial section views in (**b**), (**c**), and (**d**). Note mid-root radiolucency (**c**) in relation to the palatal root at the apical level of the post (blue arrow). Intact palatal bone was observed coronal and apical to the mid root level (**b** and **d**). (**e**) Coronal view showing the distal-buccal and palatal roots of #14. The arrow demonstrates the lateral radiolucency in relation to the palatal root. Vertical root fracture of the palatal root was determined, and patient was referred for extraction

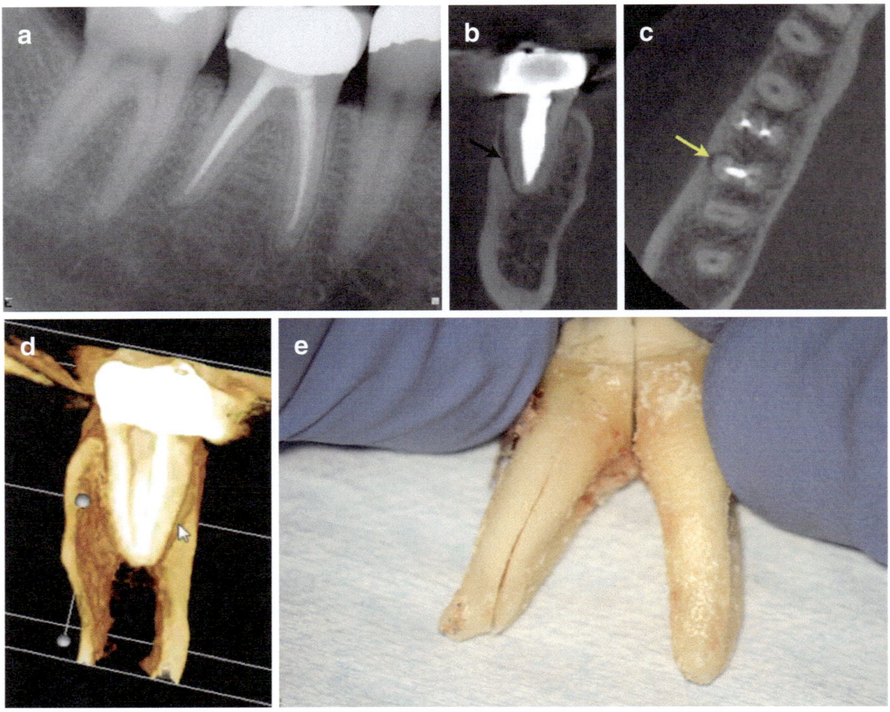

Fig. 3.18 (**a**) Periapical radiograph of tooth #30. (**b**) Coronal view of the distal root demonstrating the space between the distal root and the buccal cortical plate (black arrow). (**c**) Axial view of the distal root demonstrating the space between the distal root and the buccal cortical plate (yellow arrow). (**d**) 3D reconstruction of the distal root demonstrating the space between the distal root and the buccal cortical plate. (**e**) Clinical image after surgical sectioning and extraction and confirmation of distal root vertical fracture

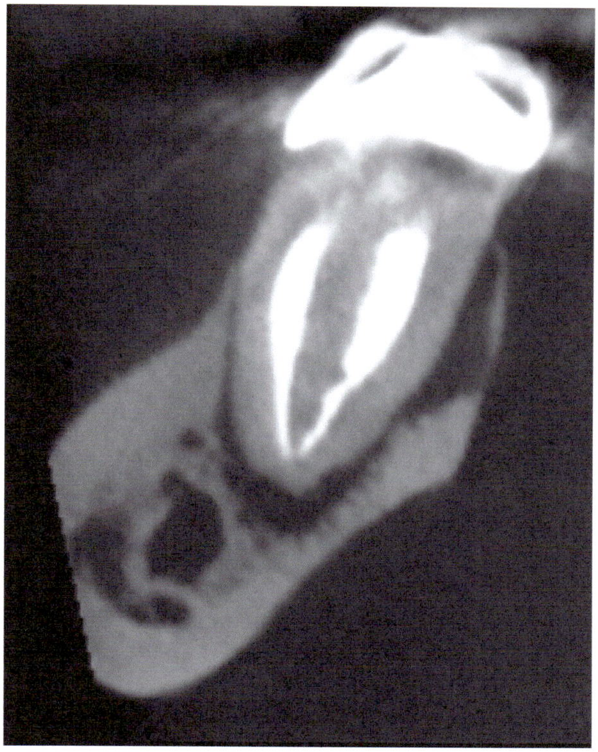

Fig. 3.19 Tooth #30 was referred for nonsurgical / surgical retreatment. The coronal view demonstrated a low-density area associated with the root apex as well as early bone changes adjacent to the lingual aspect of mesial root. At the time of the clinical examination, the lingual aspect of the mesial root presented with no abnormal periodontal probing due to the intact lingual collar of bone

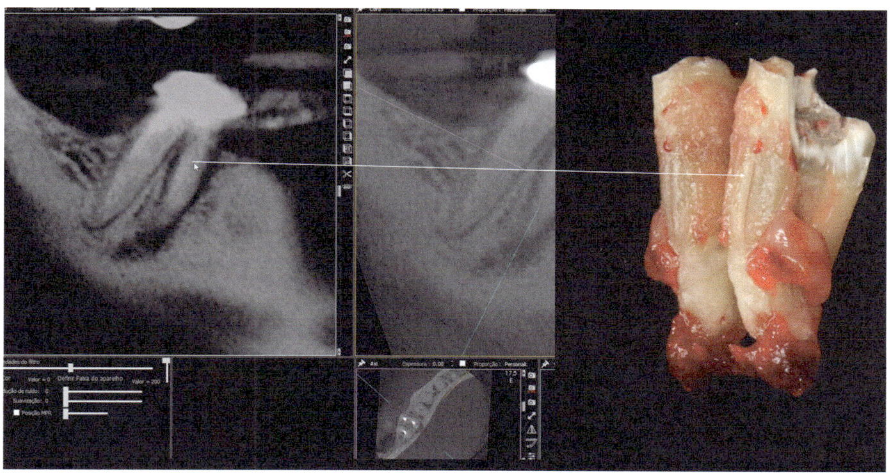

Fig. 3.20 Continuation of case in Fig. 3.19. DICOM CBCT images were imported into e-VolDX software and utilized the fractured filter. The lingual VRF of the mesial root can be visualized and coincides with the VRF present on the lingual root after tooth #30 was extracted. Note the fine size of VRF on the extracted mesial root and the sensitivity of the e-VolDX filter demonstrating the VRF

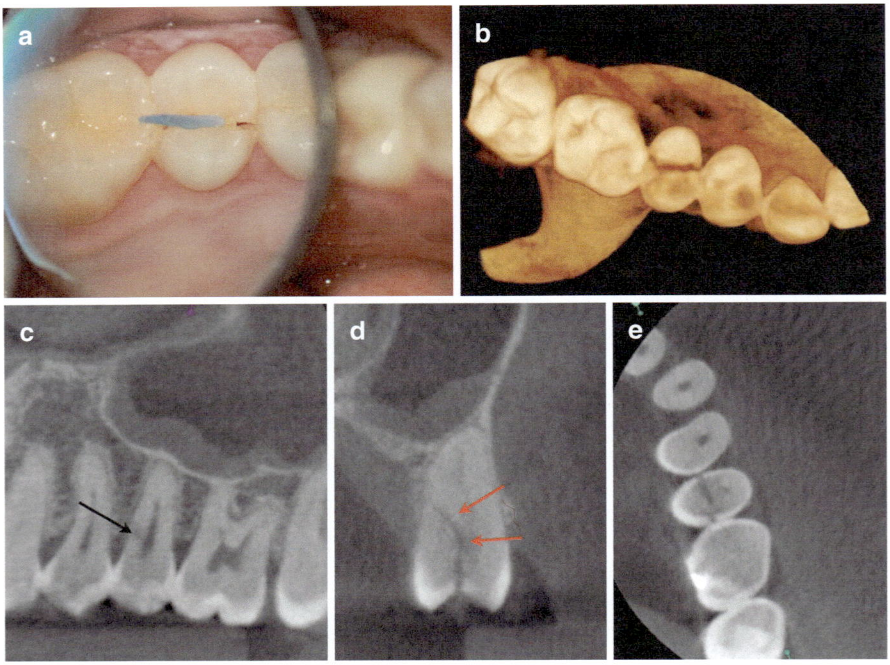

Fig. 3.21 Patient presented for evaluation of a mesial-distal fracture, tooth #13. In order to determine restorability and the extent of the palatal cusp fracture, a CBCT was recommended. (**a**) Clinical picture with a wedge slightly separating the buccal and palatal cusps. (**b**) 3D reconstruction of the split tooth after placing the wedge. (**c**) Sagittal view of tooth #13 demonstrates the subosseous extent of the fracture (black arrow). (**d**) Coronal view demonstrating the palatal extent of the fracture (red arrow). (**e**) Axial view demonstrating the split nature of both cusps. Tooth #13 was determined to be non-restorable, and extraction was recommended

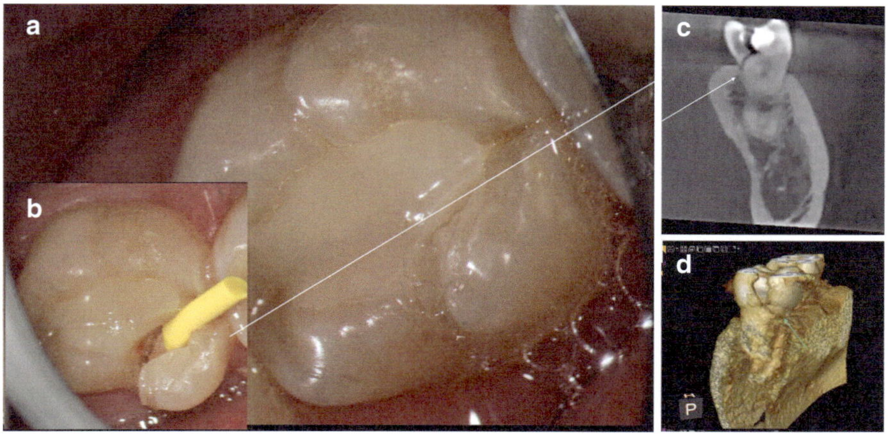

Fig. 3.22 Patient presented for evaluation of a disto-lingual cuspal fracture, tooth #18. In order to determine restorability and the extent of the disto-lingual cuspal fracture, a CBCT was recommended. (**a**) Clinical picture of the disto-lingual cuspal fracture. (**b**) Clinical picture with a wedge slightly separating the disto-lingual cuspal fracture. (**c**) Coronal view demonstrating the palatal extent of the fracture (red arrow). (**d**) 3D reconstruction of the wedged disto-lingual cusp fracture demonstrating the sub-gingival and supra-osseous extent of the cuspal fracture. Tooth #18 was determined to be restorable and root canal therapy was recommended

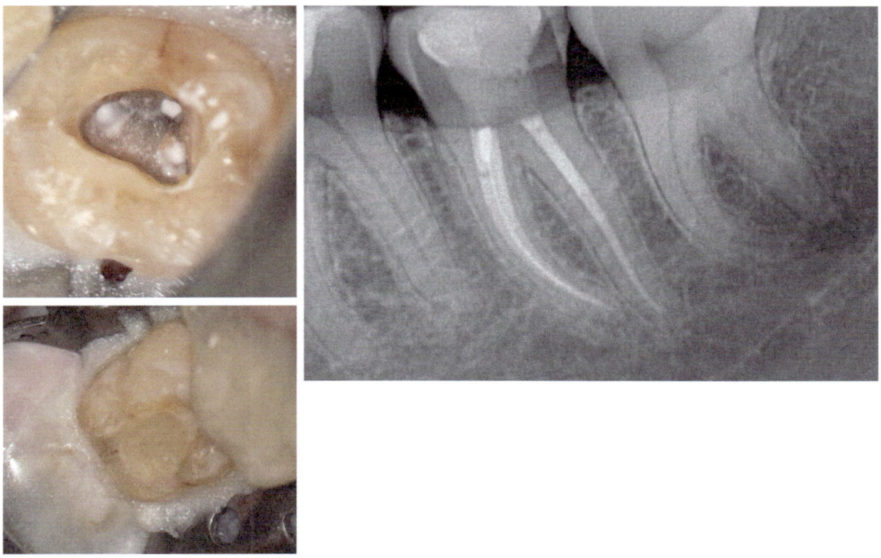

Fig. 3.23 Continuation of Fig. 3.22. The tooth was clamped to hold the fractured cusps together and root canal therapy was initiated. A 2-visit root canal therapy was performed and on the second visit tooth #18 presented with the disto-lingual cusp bonded to the rest of tooth. Access cavity was restored with composite resin restoration, occlusion was adjusted, and referred to the general dentist for the final restoration

3.5 Detection and Diagnosis of Inflammatory Resorptive Defects

Diagnosis of root resorption is often challenging due to the typically quiescent onset and varying clinical presentation (Figs. 3.24, 3.25 and 3.26). Definitive diagnosis and treatment planning are ultimately dependent on the radiographic representation of the disease. Two-dimensional imaging offers limited diagnostic potential when compared to 3D imaging [30, 31, 32]. Chap. 12 will explore diagnosis and treatment of resorptive defects in greater detail.

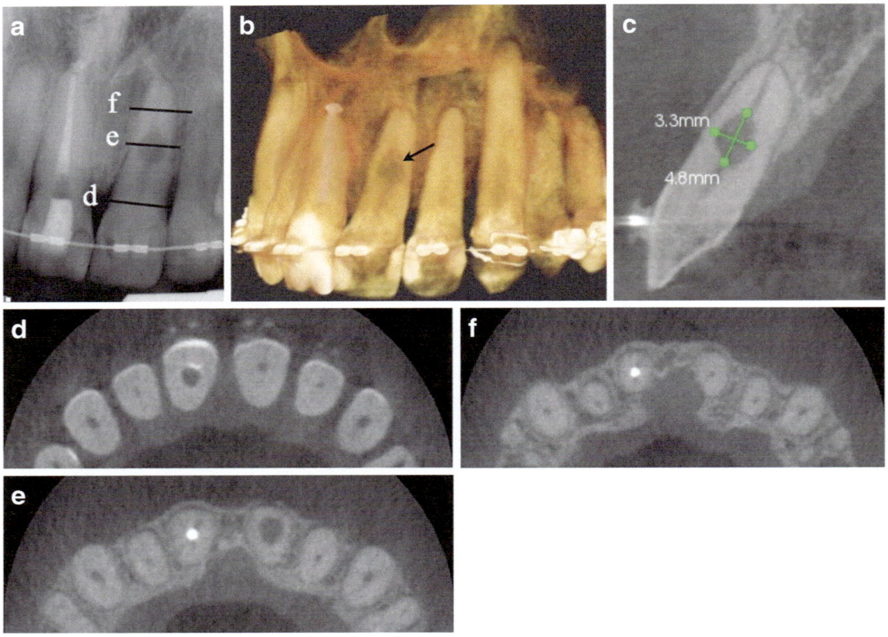

Fig. 3.24 Patient was referred for evaluation and treatment of an internal resorptive defect on tooth #9. (**a**) Periapical radiograph of tooth #9. The three lines correspond to the axial section views in (**d**), (**e**), and (**f**). (**b**) 3D reconstruction of maxillary anterior teeth demonstrating the internal resorptive defect (black arrow). (**c**) Sagittal view of tooth #9 with the 3.3 × 4.8 mm measurement of the defect. (**d**), (**e**), and (**f**) are axial views of tooth #9. Note the normal canal anatomy coronal and apical to the defect (**d**, **f**). The maximum width of the defect is demonstrated in axial view (**e**)

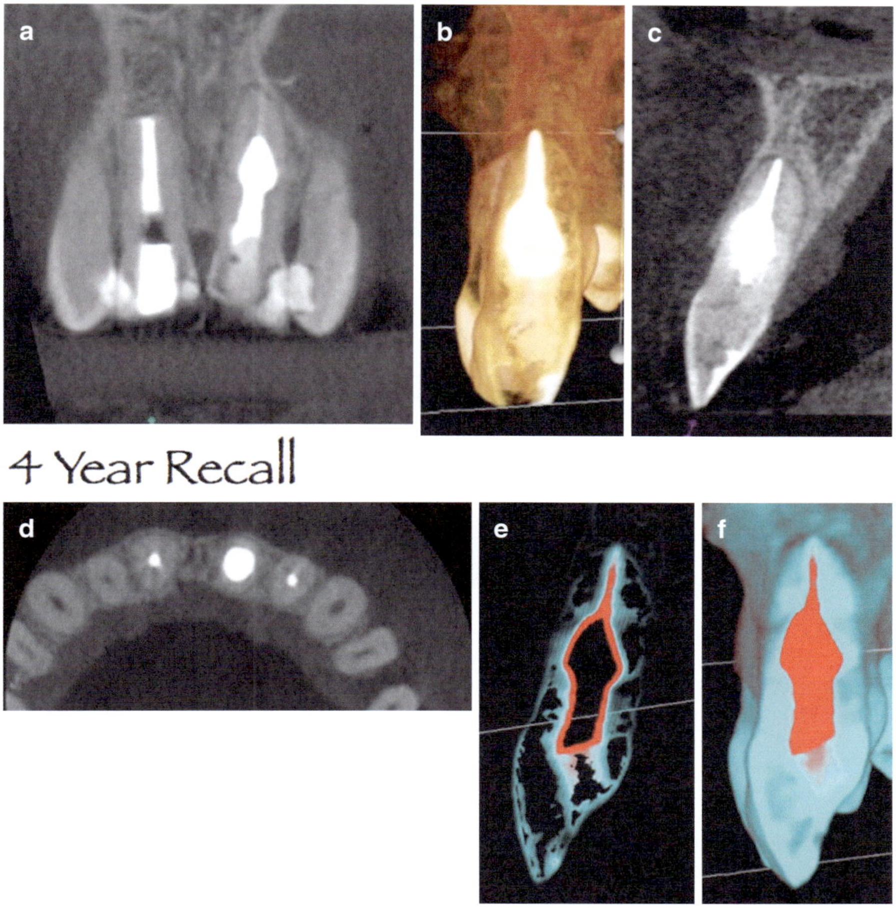

Fig. 3.25 Continuation of case in Fig. 3.24: (**a**) Coronal view, 4-year recall of tooth# 9 and healing of previous periapical surgery on tooth #8. (**b**, **e**, **f**) are 3D reconstructions of tooth #9. (**e**) and (**f**) are 3D templates constructed to determine the interface and adaptability of the root canal filling to the resorptive defect canal walls. (**c**) is a sagittal view and (**d**) is an axial view through the widest section of the resorptive defect

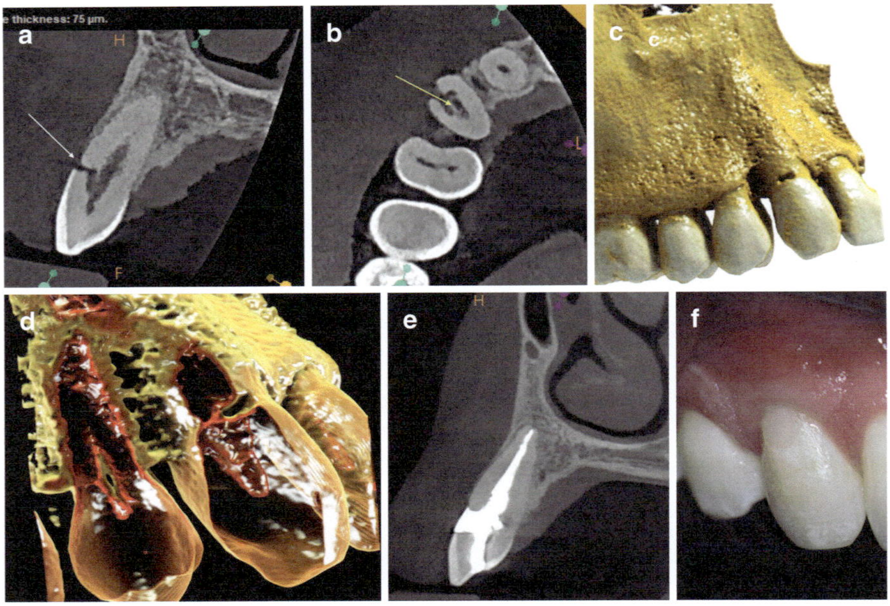

Fig. 3.26 A 44-old male presented for consultation and treatment of tooth #6. Tooth #6 presented with a class III Heather say Invasive cervical resorption (ICR). (**a**) Sagittal CBCT view demonstrating the extent of the ICR defect. (**b**) Axial view demonstrating the coronal extent of the ICR defect. The protective peri canalar resorption resistant sheet (PRRS) can be noted (white arrow). (**c**) A realistic rendering e-VOLDX image demonstrating the buccal defect location. (**d**) A realistic e-VOLDX rendering utilizing the pulp filter. The extent of the ICR defect in relation to the buccal marginal bone as well as relation to the dental pulp can be determined. The PRRS can be noted. (**e**, **f**) A sagittal CBCT view and clinical image of 1 year follow-up. The soft tissue healed to normal color, texture, and contour

3.6 Traumatic Dental Injuries (TDI)

Traumatic dental injuries present a clinical challenge with regard to diagnosis, treatment planning, and prognosis. Radiographic assessment is important to identify the location, type, and severity of TDI (Figs. 3.27 and 3.28). According to the 2012 International Association of Dental Traumatology guidelines [33], a series of periapical radiographs from different angulations and an occlusal film are recommended for evaluation of TDI. CBCT was recommended as well for the visualization of TDI, particularly root fractures and lateral luxations, and monitoring of healing and complications.

Unfortunately, 2D imaging has limitations in the diagnosis and detection of TDI due to projection geometry, magnification, superimposition of anatomic structures, distortion, and processing errors.

In the diagnosis of horizontal root fractures (HRF) utilizing 2D imaging, the fracture line will only be detected if the X-ray beam passes directly through it. The

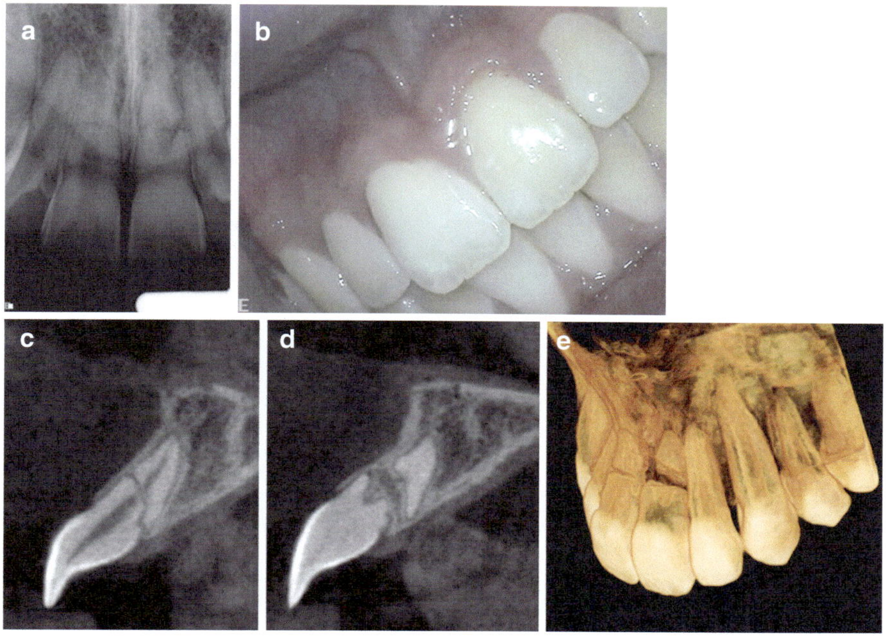

Fig. 3.27 A 15-year-old patient with a history of trauma to the anterior maxilla was referred for consultation for teeth #8 and 9. Tooth #8 had a grade I mobility and tooth #9 had a grade II + mobility. (**a**) Periapical radiograph for teeth #8 and 9. Horizontal root fractures can be seen mid-root in both teeth. (**b**) Clinical picture of teeth #8 and 9. Periodontal probing depths were WNL. Marginal and attached gingiva demonstrated normal color and architecture. (**c**) and (**d**) are the sagittal views of teeth #8 and 9, respectively. Note the oblique nature of the root fractures and bone fill between the coronal and apical segments in (**d**). (**e**) 3D reconstruction demonstrating the dislocation of the fractured segments. Since the patient was asymptomatic and CBCT revealed no periradicular pathosis, a palatal splint was suggested to address the mobility, but no endodontic intervention was recommended at this time

2D nature limits the accuracy in the diagnosis of the location, severity, and extent of HRF. The risk of misdiagnosis of the location and extent of the fracture by using only 2D intraoral radiography could lead to improper treatment and an unfavorable outcome. Because of the limitations of intraoral radiography, CBCT was suggested as the preferred imaging modality for diagnosis of HRF [34].

CBCT overcomes several of the limitations of 2D imaging by providing a considerable amount of 3D information about the nature and extent of the HRF. The significant difference in the nature of HRF when assessed with 2D radiographs compared to CBCT has been reported [35]. Limited FOV CBCT imaging seems to be generally advantageous in the diagnosis, assessment of prognosis, treatment planning, and treatment follow-up of HRF cases.

In pediatric patients with TDI, it should be considered that children are at greater risk than adults from a given dose of radiation both because they are inherently more radiosensitive and because they have more remaining years of life during which a radiation-induced neoplasm could develop [36].

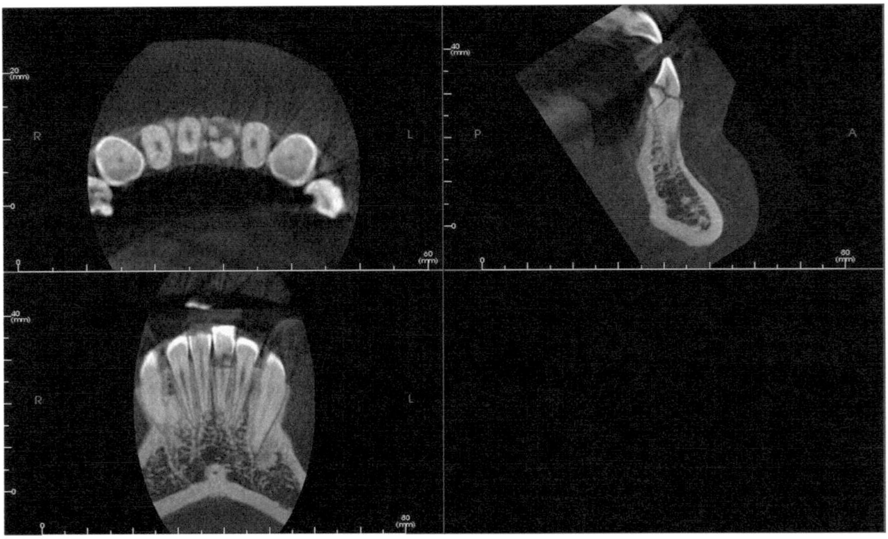

Fig. 3.28 A 13-year-old male presented approximately 2 weeks after trauma to his mandibular anterior teeth that occurred while he was playing basketball. His primary concern was the looseness of tooth #25. A CBCT scan was taken to evaluate the extent of the fracture. The original treatment plan (extraction) was modified after viewing the CBCT, since the buccal bone was very thin and likely to be lost during a surgical extraction. The treatment plan was changed to include root canal therapy, root submergence, and eventual slow extrusion of the tooth to maintain bone for a future implant

3.7 Conclusion

CBCT is a valuable adjunct to assist in the diagnosis of periapical hard tissue changes, root fractures, traumatic dental injuries, inflammatory root resorption, and orofacial pain with no clear etiology. Conventional 2D radiography and CBCT both record structural changes in bone. However, CBCT imaging has the ability to detect periapical pathosis prior to being apparent on 2D radiographs. Preoperative factors such as the presence and true size of a periapical lesion play an important role in endodontic treatment outcome. Success, when measured by radiographic criteria, is higher when teeth are endodontically treated before radiographic signs of periapical disease are detected.

According to the 2015 joint statement from the American Association of Endodontists and American Academy of Oral and Maxillofacial Radiology, CBCT is the imaging modality of choice for the following diagnostic situations:

1. Patients presenting with contradictory or nonspecific clinical signs and symptoms associated with untreated or previously endodontically treated teeth.
2. Diagnosis and management of limited dentoalveolar trauma, root fractures, luxation, and/or displacement of teeth and localized alveolar fractures, in the

absence of other maxillofacial or soft tissue injury that requires other advanced imaging modalities.
3. Localization and differentiation of external and internal resorptive defects and the determination of appropriate treatment and prognosis.
4. If clinical examination and 2D intraoral radiography are inconclusive in the detection of vertical root fracture (VRF).

References

1. Goldman M, Pearson AH, Darzenta N. Endodontic success: who's reading the radiograph? Oral Surg Oral Med Oral Pathol. 1972;33:432–7.
2. Goldman M, Pearson AH, Darzenta N. Reliability of radiographic interpretation. Oral Surg Oral Med Oral Pathol. 1974;38:287–93.
3. Tewary S, Luzzo J, Hartwell G. Endodontic radiography: who is reading the digital radiograph? J Endod. 2011;37:919–21.
4. De Paula-Silva FW, Wu MK, Leonardo MR, da Silva LA, Wesselink PR. Accuracy of periapical radiography and cone-beam computed tomography scans in diagnosing apical periodontitis using histopathological findings as a gold standard. J Endod. 2009;35(7):1009–12.
5. Patel S, Wilson R, Dawood A, Mannocci F. The detection of periapical pathosis using periapical radiography and cone beam computed tomography—part 1: preoperative status. Int Endod J. 2012;45(8):702–10.
6. Patel S, Wilson R, Dawood A, Mannocci F. The detection of periapical pathosis using periapical radiography and cone beam computed tomography—part 2: a 1-year post-treatment follow-up. Int Endod J. 2012;45(8):711–23.
7. Sogur E, Grondahl H, Bakst G, Mert A. Does a combination of two radiographs increase accuracy in detecting acid-induced periapical lesions and does it approach the accuracy of cone-beam computed tomography scanning. J Endod. 2012;38(2):131–6.
8. Patel S, Dawood A, Mannocci F, Wilson R, Pitt FT. Detection of periapical bone defects in human jaws using cone beam computed tomography and intraoral radiography. Int Endod J. 2009;42(6):507–15.
9. Pope O, Sathorn C, Parashos P. A comparative investigation of cone-beam computed tomography and periapical radiography in the diagnosis of a healthy periapex. J Endod. 2014;40(3):360–5.
10. Nixdorf D, Moana-Filho E. Persistent dento-alveolar pain disorder (PDAP): working towards a better understanding. Rev Pain. 2011;5(4):18–27.
11. Nixdorf DR, et al. Differential diagnosis for persistent pain after root canal treatment: a study in the National Dental Practice-based Reseacrh Network. J Endod. 2015;41:457–63.
12. Pigg M, List T, Petersson K, Lindh C, Petersson A. Diagnostic yield of conventional radiographic and cone-beam computed tomographic images in patients with atypical odontalgia. Int Endod J. 2011;44(12):1365–2591.
13. Hilton T, Ferracan J. Cracked Teeth Registry. National Dental PBRN Western Regional Meeting. September 28, 2013.
14. Ellis SG. Incomplete tooth fracture-proposal for a new definition. Br Dent J. 2001;190:424–8.
15. Lynch CD, McConnell RJ. The cracked tooth syndrome. J Cand Dent Assoc. 2002;68:470–5.
16. Ricucci D, Siqueira JF, Loghin S. The cracked tooth: histopathologic and histobacteriologic aspects. J Endod. 2015;41:343–52.
17. American Association of Endodontists. Cracking the cracked tooth code. Endodontics: colleague of excellence. Chicago: American Association of Endodontists; 2008.
18. Chen M, Fu K, Qiao F, et al. Predicting extension of cracks to the root from the dimensions in the crown. JADA. 2017;148:737–42.

19. AAE and AAOMR joint position statement: use of cone beam computed tomography in endodontics 2015 update. J Endod. 2015;41:1393–6.
20. Bueno M, Estrela C, Azevedo B, Diogenes A. Development of a new cone-beam computed tomography software for endodontic diagnosis. Braz Dent J. 2018;29(6):517–29.
21. Alkhalifah S, Alkandari H, Sharma NP, Moule JA. Treatment of cracked teeth. J Endod. 2017;43(9):1579–86.
22. Banerji S, Mehta B, Millar JB, Cracked tooth Syndrome. Part 2: restorative options for the management of cracked tooth syndrome. Br Dent J. 2010;208:503–14.
23. Milicich G. The compression dome concept. The restorative implications. AGD. 2017:55–60.
24. Krell KV, Rivera E. A six year evaluation of cracked teeth diagnosed with reversible pulpitis: treatment and prognosis. J Endod. 2007;33(12):1405–7.
25. Wu S, Lew H, Chen N. Incidence of pulpal complications after diagnosis of vital cracked teeth. J Endod. 2019:1–5.
26. Olivieri JG, Elmsmari F, Miro Q, Ruiz XF, Krell KV, Garcia-Font M, et al. Outcome and survival of endodontically treated cracked posterior permanent teeth: a systemic review and meta-analysis. J Endod. 2020;46:455–63.
27. Davis MC, Shariff SS. Success and survival of endodontically treated cracked teeth with radicular extensions. A 2-4-year prospective cohort. J Endod. 2019;45:848–55.
28. Sim G.B.I, Lim T, Chen N. Decision making for retention of endodontically treated posterior cracked teeth. A 5-year follow-up study. J Endod. 2016;42:225–9.
29. Fayad MI, Ashkenaz PJ, Johnson BR. Different representations of vertical root fractures detected by cone-beam volumetric tomography: a case series report. J Endod. 2012;10:1435–42.
30. Estrela C, Bueno MR, De Alencar AH, Mattar R, Valladares Neto J, Azevedo BC, De Araújo Estrela CR. Method to evaluate inflammatory root resorption by using cone beam computed tomography. J Endod. 2009;35(11):1491–7.
31. Durack C, Patel S, Davies J, Wilson R, Mannocci F. Diagnostic accuracy of small volume cone beam computed tomography and intraoral periapical radiography for the detection of simulated external inflammatory root resorption. Int Endod J. 2011;44(2):136–47.
32. Patel S, Saberi N, Pimental T, Teng P. Present status and future direction: root resorption. Int Endod J. 2022;00:1–30.
33. Diangelis AJ, Andreasen JO, Ebeleseder KA, et al. International Association of Dental Traumatology guidelines for the management of traumatic dental injuries: 1—fractures and luxations of permanent teeth. Dent Traumatol. 2012;28:2–12.
34. Contemporary management of horizontal root fractures to the permanent dentition: diagnosis—radiologic assessment to include cone-beam computed tomography. J Endod. 2013;39(3 Suppl):S20–5.
35. Iikubo M, Kobayashi K, Mishima A, et al. Accuracy of intraoral radiography, multidetector helical CT, and limited cone-beam CT for the detection of horizontal tooth root fracture. Oral Surg Oral Med Oral Pathol Oral Radiol Endod. 2009;108:e70–4.
36. Scarfe WC. All that glitters is not gold: standards for cone-beam computerized tomographic imaging. Oral Surg Oral Med Oral Pathol Oral Radiol Endod. 2011;111:402–8.

4 The Impact of Cone Beam Computed Tomography in Nonsurgical and Surgical Treatment Planning

Mohamed I. Fayad and Bradford R. Johnson

Abstract

Development of an appropriate treatment plan follows diagnosis and could be considered the foundation of a successful outcome. Until the recent introduction of cone beam computed tomography (CBCT) for dental uses, two-dimensional radiographic imaging has been the standard for dental treatment planning. In endodontics, subjective history, clinical findings, and diagnostic imaging are all essential components of the preoperative diagnosis and treatment plan (Reit C, Petersson K, Textbook of Endodontology. Wiley-Blackwell, UK, 2010). Conventional two-dimensional radiographs provide a cost-effective, high-resolution image, which continues to be the most popular method of imaging today. However, the diagnostic potential of periapical radiographs is limited. Information may be difficult to interpret, especially when the anatomy and background pattern is complex (Kundel HL, Revesz G, Am J Roentgenol 126:1233–8, 1976). Recently, CBCT has been demonstrated to be a useful tool in a number of endodontic applications. The aim of this chapter is to compare the relative value of preoperative periapical radiographs and CBCT in the decision-making process in nonsurgical and surgical endodontic treatment planning.

4.1 Introduction

Cone beam computed tomography (CBCT) is a diagnostic imaging modality which provides a three-dimensional image of the maxillofacial region and is capable of providing images at a relatively low radiation dose (please refer to Chap. 1) and with sufficient spatial resolution for applications in endodontic diagnosis and

M. I. Fayad (✉) · B. R. Johnson
Department of Endodontics, University of Illinois Chicago, Chicago, IL, USA
e-mail: mfayad1@uic.edu; bjohnson@uic.edu

M. I. Fayad, B. R. Johnson (eds.), *3D Imaging in Endodontics*,
https://doi.org/10.1007/978-3-031-32755-1_4

treatment planning. CBCT imaging has revolutionized dental and surgical diagnosis and treatment planning. The integration of CBCT and other technologies such as e-Vol DX software and navigation system interface will revolutionize the way nonsurgical and surgical endodontics will be performed. Dynamic navigation integrates surgical instrumentation and radiologic images using an optical positioning device controlled by a dedicated computerized interface. A clinical real-time interface displays and guides users to drill into the targeted position through the prefixed trace according to the output of the preoperative planning software. The guided endodontic concept has been utilized in both nonsurgical and surgical endodontics; however, they have all relied on some form of static guide. CBCT overcomes many limitations with conventional radiography such as early detection of invasive cervical resorption lesions, vertical root fractures, and three-dimensional evaluation of the root canal space and surrounding anatomy [1–10]. Diagnostic information directly influences treatment planning and clinical decisions. Accurate data leads to better treatment decisions and potentially more predictable outcomes [11]. While conventional periapical radiography has been used for many years as a diagnostic aid in endodontics, some studies now demonstrate the inferiority of periapical radiographs in detecting periradicular pathosis when compared to CBCT [12–16]. CBCT has been successfully used in endodontics, and several recent studies have demonstrated the advantages of CBCT over periapical radiographs [17–21]. The effective radiation dose when using CBCT is higher than the conventional two-dimensional radiography, and the benefit to the patient must therefore outweigh any potential risks of the additional radiation exposure. The value of CBCT for endodontic diagnosis and treatment planning should be determined on an individual basis to assure that the benefit:risk assessment supports the use of CBCT.

Ee et al. (2014) compared differences in endodontic treatment planning decisions using either CBCT or periapical radiographs [22]. Thirty endodontic cases completed in a private endodontic practice were randomly selected to be included in this study. Each case was required to have a preoperative digital periapical radiograph and a CBCT scan. Three board certified endodontists reviewed the 30 preoperative periapical radiographs. The evaluators were not involved in the initial diagnosis or treatment of these 30 cases. Two weeks later, the CBCT volumes were reviewed in random order by the same evaluators. The evaluators were asked to select a preliminary diagnosis and treatment plan based solely on interpretation of the periapical and CBCT images. Diagnosis and treatment planning choices were then compared to determine if there was a change in decision-making from viewing just the periapical radiograph to the CBCT scan. In addition, both decisions were compared to the reference standard (known diagnosis confirmed during nonsurgical treatment and/or surgical exploration or extraction). A difference in treatment plan between the two imaging modalities was recorded in 19 out of 30 cases (63.3%) ($P = 0.001$) for examiner #1, 17 out of 30 cases (56.6%) ($P = 0.012$) for examiner #2, and 20 out of 30 cases (66.7%) ($P = 0.008$) for examiner #3 (Fig. 4.1). The problem of incorrect, delayed, or inadequate endodontic diagnosis and treatment planning places the patient at risk and could result in unnecessary or inappropriate treatment.

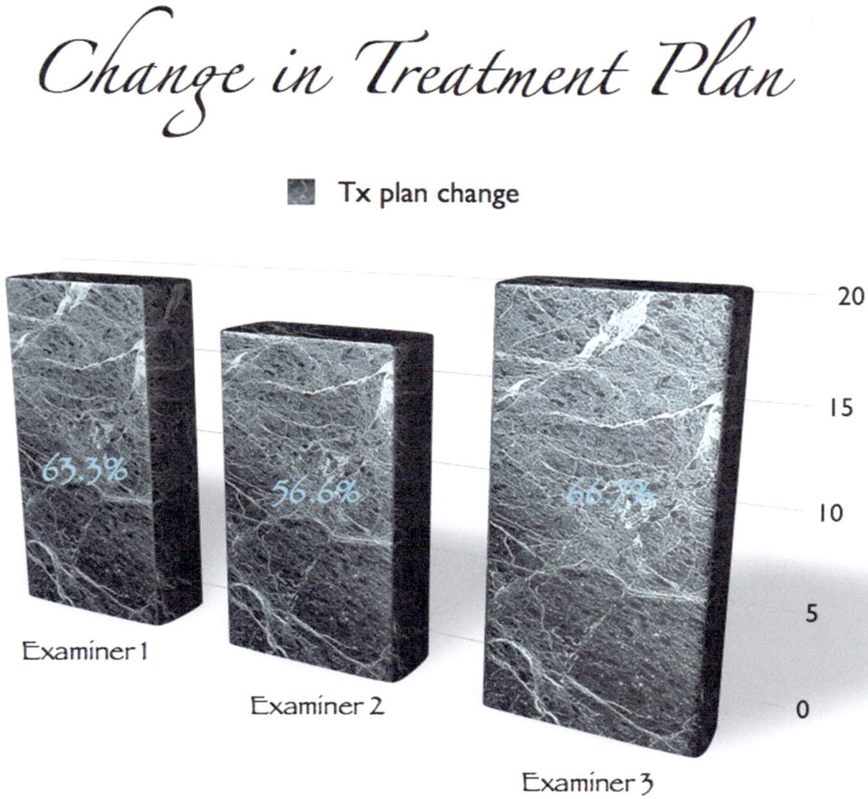

Fig. 4.1 Percentage of treatment plans changed by each of the three examiners after reviewing the CBCT

4.2 Implications for Clinical Practice

Under the conditions of the previous study [22], CBCT was a more accurate imaging modality for diagnosis of tooth anatomy and periradicular pathosis when compared to diagnosis using only periapical radiographs. An accurate diagnosis was reached in 36.6% to 40% of the cases when using periapical radiographs compared to an accurate diagnosis in 76.6% to 83.3% of the cases when using CBCT (Fig. 4.2). This high level of misdiagnosis is potentially clinically relevant, especially in cases of invasive cervical root resorption and vertical root fracture where a lack of early detection could lead to unsuccessful treatment and tooth loss. The previous study also demonstrates that the treatment plan may be directly influenced by information gained from a CBCT scan as the examiners altered their treatment plan after viewing the CBCT scan in 62.2% of the cases overall (range from 56.6% to 66.7%). This high number indicates that CBCT had a significant influence on the examiners' treatment plan.

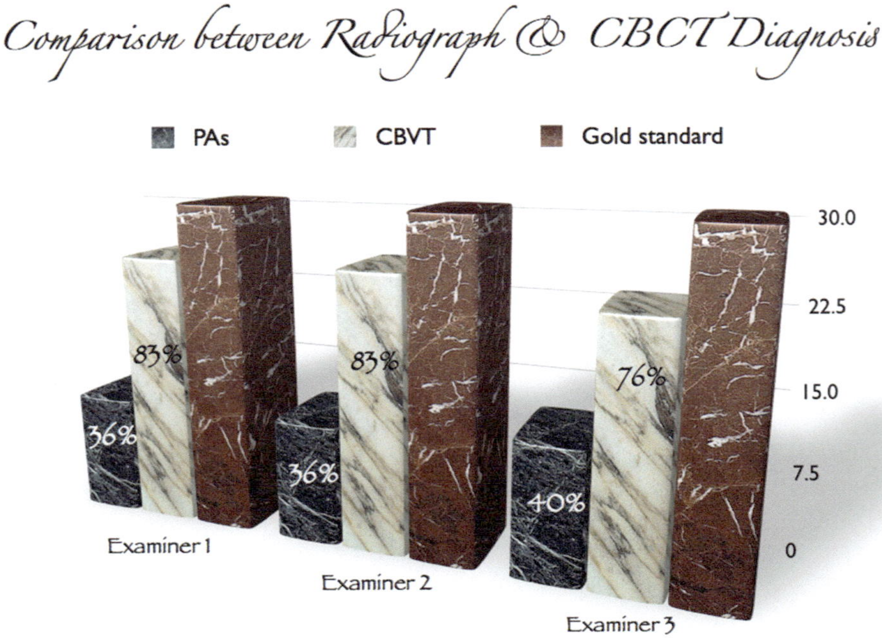

Fig. 4.2 Comparison between diagnosis after viewing a periapical radiograph vs. diagnosis after viewing CBCT for examiners 1, 2, and 3

Rodriguez et al. evaluated the influence of CBCT imaging on clinical decision-making choices among different specialists (prosthodontists, endodontists, oral surgeons, and periodontists) in endodontic treatment planning [23]. A secondary objective was to assess the self-reported level of difficulty in making a treatment choice before and after viewing a preoperative CBCT scan. CBCT scans only had a significant influence on the treatment plan when the endodontic case was classified as high difficulty ($P < 0.05$). The level of difficulty in choosing a treatment choice was significantly more difficult after viewing a preoperative CBCT scan ($P < 0.05$), with the exception of the endodontists ($P = 0.033$). After viewing the CBCT scan, the extraction option increased significantly ($P < 0.05$). It was concluded that CBCT imaging has a substantial impact on endodontic decision-making among specialists, particularly in high-difficulty cases.

Bhatt et al. compared conventional radiographic and CBCT findings with reference to the American Association of Endodontists and American Academy of Oral and Maxillofacial Radiology (AAE/AAOMR) joint position statement and to determine the effect of the CBCT on the initial diagnoses and treatment plans in a single-center postgraduate endodontic program [24].

CBCT scans of patients referred for treatment at the Endodontics Department of the University of British Columbia were reviewed and compared with the corresponding radiographs. The features considered were periapical lesions, missed/

extra canals, root fractures, complex anatomy, calcified canals, and root resorption of tooth/teeth in question. Reasons for the CBCT prescriptions were assigned to three groups: to formulate the primary diagnosis, to confirm the diagnosis achieved by clinical examination and conventional radiographs, and to assist in treatment planning. Variables were compared statistically using chi-square and McNemar tests. A total of 128 CBCT examinations were performed on 110 patients. Overall, 76% of CBCT examinations were performed on previously root-filled teeth. CBCT images revealed a significantly higher incidence of periapical lesions ($P = 0.002$), missed canals ($P < 0.001$), vertical root fractures ($P = 0.004$), and complex anatomy ($P = 0.008$) than periapical radiographs. CBCT was prescribed most frequently to assist surgical treatment planning (62%) rather than for generating a diagnosis (9%) or confirming diagnoses (29%). Both the diagnosis ($P = 0.001$) and the treatment plan ($P = 0.005$) initially made by examining periapical radiographs were altered significantly by the subsequent CBCT examination by revealing information such as new periapical lesions, missed canals, or involvement of buccal or lingual cortical bone. It was concluded that CBCT examinations were prescribed mainly to assist treatment planning rather than for diagnosis. The majority of CBCT examinations were performed on previously root-filled teeth. The additional information obtained from CBCT scans resulted in the alteration of the initial diagnoses as well as subsequent treatment plans in 59 out of 128 cases.

It was concluded that a preoperative CBCT scan provides more diagnostic information than a preoperative periapical radiograph and that this information can directly influence a clinician's treatment plan. Although imaging is a very important diagnostic tool in endodontics, it should always be used as an adjunct to the clinical exam. The addition of subjective and objective clinical findings to CBCT should allow for an even more accurate clinical diagnosis and appropriate treatment plan.

4.3 Conclusion

Cone beam computed tomography overcomes many of the limitations of periapical radiography. The increased diagnostic information provided by the CBCT scan should result in more accurate diagnosis and improved decision-making for the management of complex endodontic problems. CBCT is a desirable addition to the endodontist's armamentarium. Examples of cases where CBCT made a significant difference in the treatment planning process are presented in Figs. 4.3, 4.4, 4.5, 4.6, 4.7, 4.8, 4.9, 4.10, 4.11, 4.12, 4.13, 4.14, 4.15 and 4.16. Figures 4.17, 4.18, 4.19, 4.20, 4.21, 4.22, 4.23, 4.24, 4.25 and 4.26 demonstrate the utilization of CBCT as a scaffold for additional technologies such as e-Vol DX software and Navident dynamic navigation. The CBCT DICOM images imported into e-Vol DX software allow clinicians to utilize the task-specific rendering filters for diagnosis and treatment planning. The CBCT DICOM images imported into Navident software for treatment planning allow real-time navigation of calcified canals and greater precision in endodontic microsurgery.

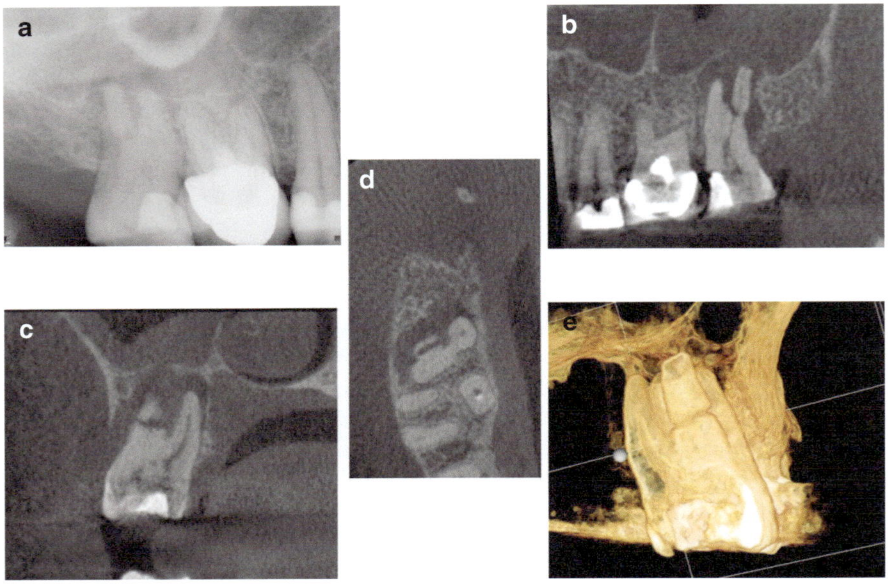

Fig. 4.3 (**a**) Periapical radiograph of tooth #2. The patient was referred to nonsurgical root canal treatment with a diagnosis of pulp necrosis and asymptomatic apical periodontitis. (**b**) Sagittal view showing the distobuccal root fracture. (**c**) Coronal view showing the unusual horizontal fracture of the distobuccal root. (**d**) Axial view of the apical one-third showing a vertical buccopalatal root fracture. (**e**) 3D reconstruction showing the extent of the distobuccal root fracture

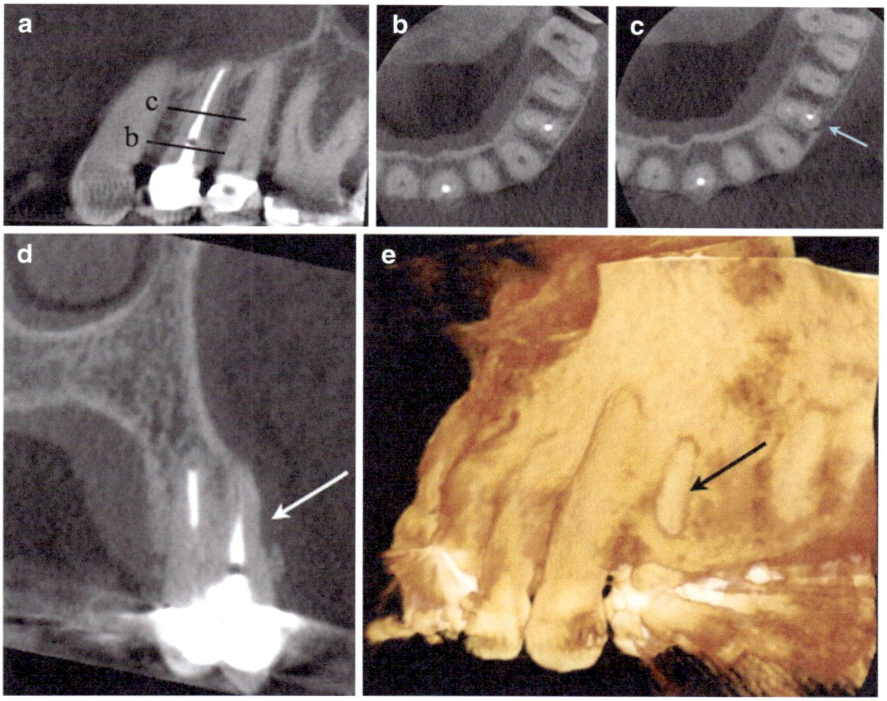

Fig. 4.4 Patient was referred for evaluation of pain to biting related to tooth #12. Tooth # 12 had a previous root canal treatment. Periodontal probing depths were WNL. The two lines (**b** and **c**) correspond to the axial section views in (**a**). (**c**) demonstrates buccal loss of bone mid-root which is a pattern of bone loss (blue arrow) that is suggestive of VRF. (**d**) Coronal view of tooth #12 demonstrating mid-root buccal bone loss (black arrow). The intact collar of marginal bone has a tight periodontal fiber attachment, which explains why many roots with VRF do not probe in the early stages. (**e**) 3D reconstruction demonstrating the intact marginal bone and loss of buccal bone (black arrow). The buccal bone loss is usually adjacent to the VRF site

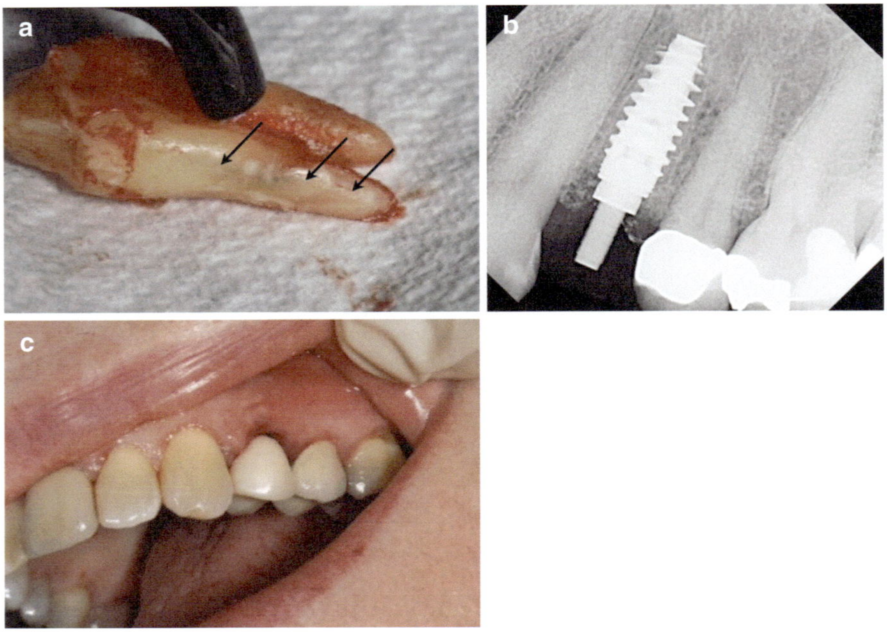

Fig. 4.5 Continuation of the case in Fig. 4.4: (**a**) Tooth #12 after surgical extraction. The black arrows are the VRF which corresponds to the area of buccal bone loss in the CBCT. (**b**) An immediate implant was placed after the extraction. (**c**) Temporary restoration in place without loading the implant

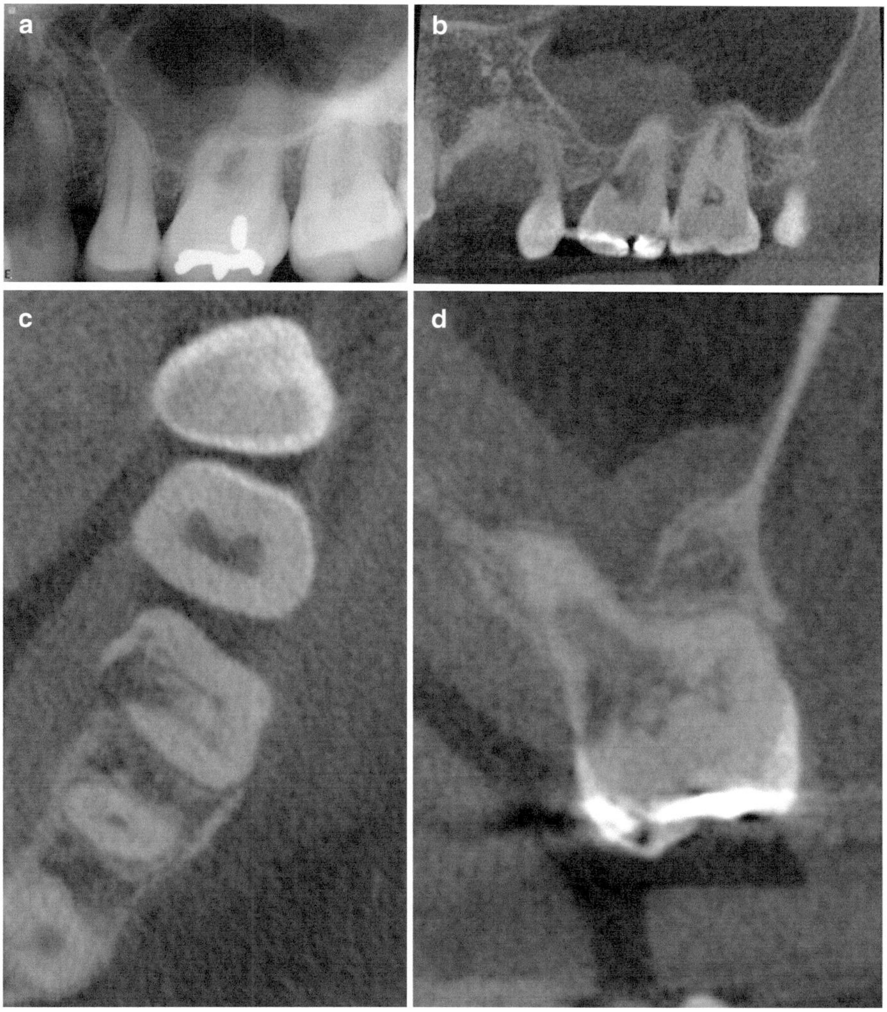

Fig. 4.6 (**a**) Periapical radiograph of tooth #14. Symptoms included spontaneous pain and abnormal sensitivity to cold. After clinical examination and testing, the diagnosis was symptomatic irreversible pulpitis with symptomatic apical periodontitis. (**b**) CBCT sagittal view of tooth #14 showing an invasive cervical resorptive defect (ICR—Heithersay Class IV) that cannot be detected on the periapical radiograph. (**c**) Axial view demonstrating the palatal and mesial location of the defect. (**d**) Coronal view demonstrating the internal aspect of the ICR defect, rendering tooth #14 non-restorable. A change in treatment plan was made and the patient was referred for extraction

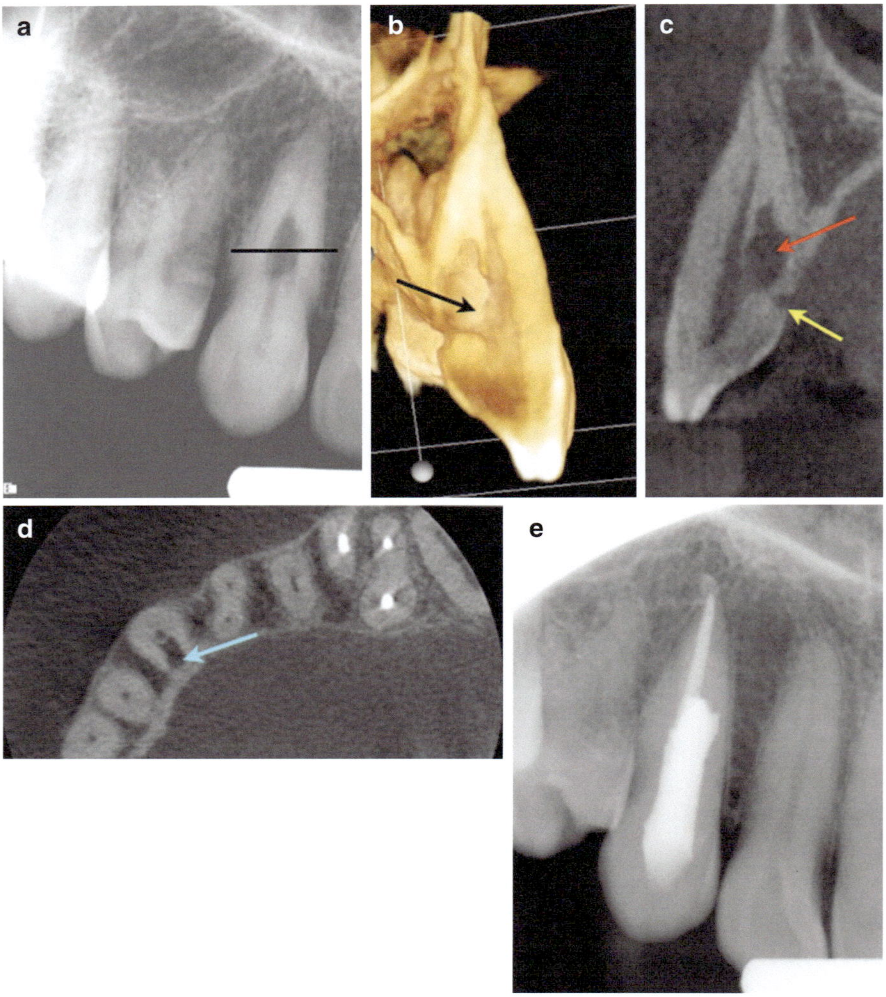

Fig. 4.7 (**a**) Periapical radiograph of tooth #6. The patient was referred for evaluation and treatment of an internal resorptive defect. The line corresponds to the axial section view in (**d**). (**b**) 3D reconstruction of the resorptive defect (black arrow). (**c**) Sagittal view of tooth #6 demonstrating the internal resorptive defect (red arrow), and confirming that the defect is an external ICR defect with initial entry at the cemento–enamel junction (yellow arrow). (**d**) Axial view demonstrating the ICR nature of the defect. Note in (c and d) that the pulp was not involved. (**e**) Postoperative radiograph of tooth #6 after root canal therapy and repair of the resorptive defect

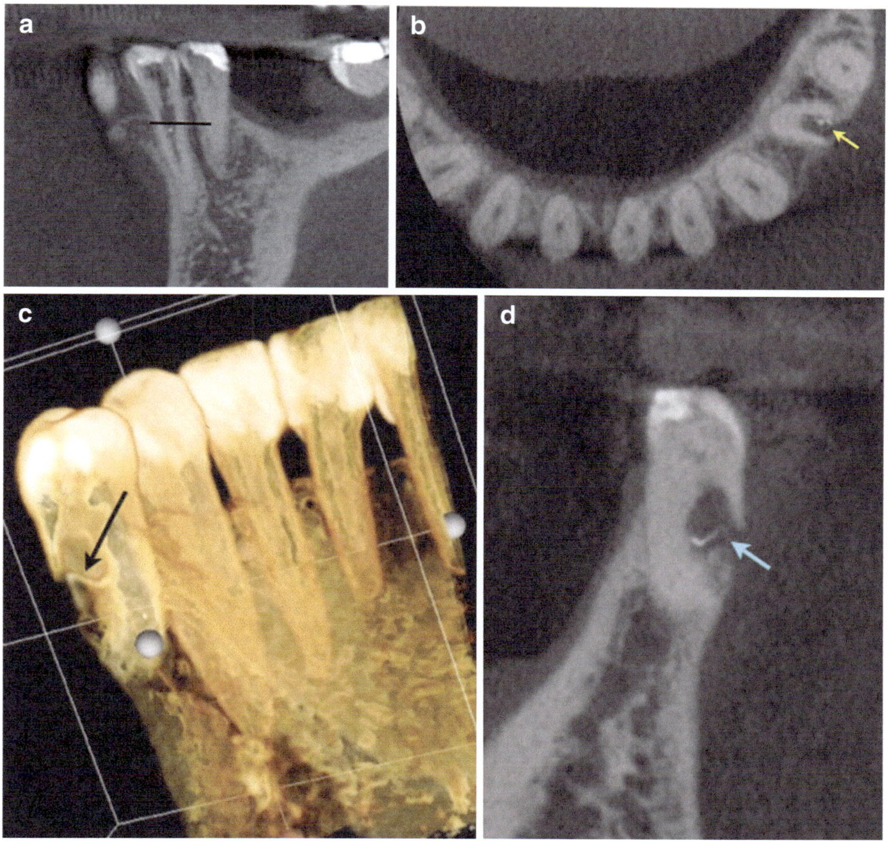

Fig. 4.8 (**a**) Periapical radiograph of tooth #21. The patient was referred for evaluation and treatment of an internal resorptive defect. The line corresponds to the axial section view in (**b**). (**b**) Axial view demonstrating the ICR nature of the defect (yellow arrow). (**c**) 3D reconstruction of the resorptive defect (black arrow). (**d**) Coronal view of tooth #21 demonstrating the external/internal resorptive defect (blue arrow). Note in (**b**, **c**, and **d**) the perforated root on the buccal aspect renders tooth #21 non-restorable. The treatment plan changed after reviewing the CBCT images

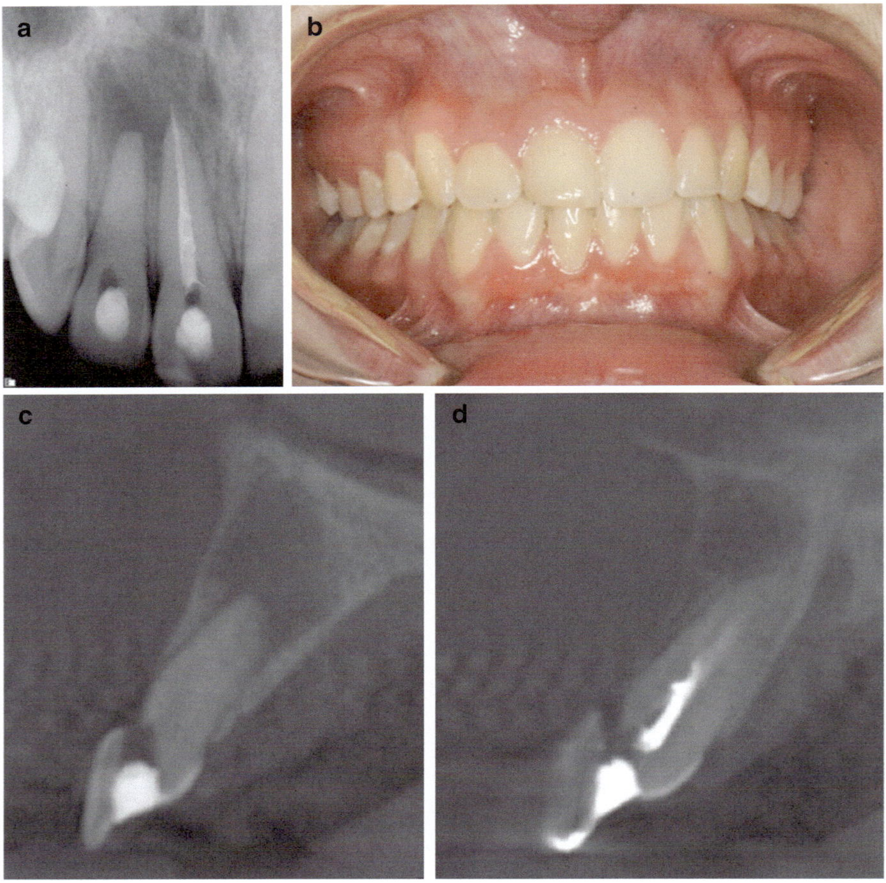

Fig. 4.9 (**a**) Periapical radiograph of teeth #7 and 8. Treatment was initiated on both teeth before referral to an endodontist. (**b**) Clinical picture showing normal soft tissue color and architecture. (**c**) and (**d**) are sagittal CBCT images showing facial perforations on teeth #7 and 8, respectively

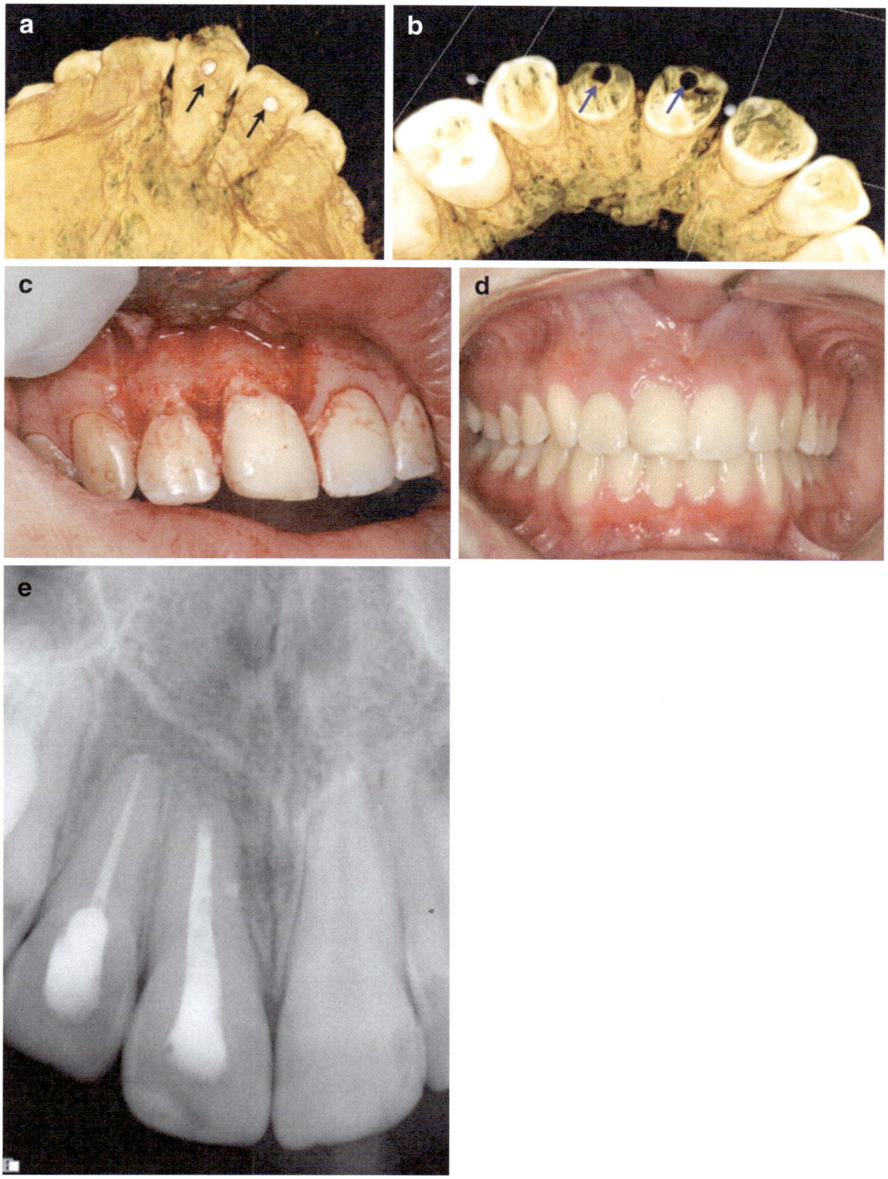

Fig. 4.10 Continuation of case in Fig. 4.9. (**a**) and (**b**) are 3D reconstructions showing the facial perforations on teeth #7 and 8. (**c**) Reflection of a full-thickness mucoperiosteal flap confirmed the presence of perforations on both teeth. The perforations were repaired with Geristore™ (DenMat, Lompoc, CA). Both teeth were then treated via an orthograde approach with subsequent surgical root-end resection and filling of tooth #8. (**d**, **e**) One-year recall radiograph demonstrating soft and hard tissue healing

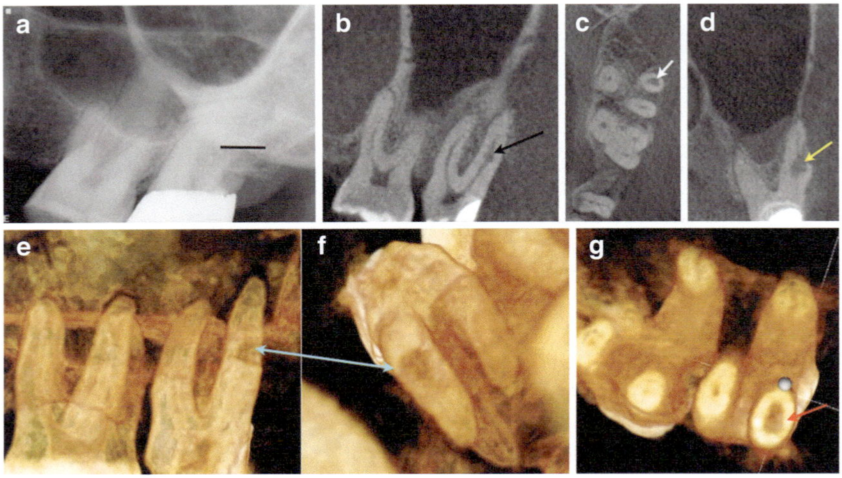

Fig. 4.11 (**a**) Periapical radiograph of tooth #15. The line corresponds to the axial section view in (**c**). Tooth #15 presented with pain on biting. The tooth was non-responsive to cold and periodontal probing depths were WNL. A diagnosis of necrotic pulp and symptomatic apical periodontitis was established. (**b**) Sagittal view of tooth #15 demonstrating an internal resorptive defect in mid-root of the distobuccal root (black arrow). (**c**) Axial view demonstrating the internal resorptive defect (white arrow). (**d**) Sagittal view demonstrating the internal resorptive defect and distobuccal root fracture (yellow arrow). (**e**, **f**, **g**) are 3D reconstructions of tooth #15 demonstrating the internal resorptive defect from different views (blue and red arrows)

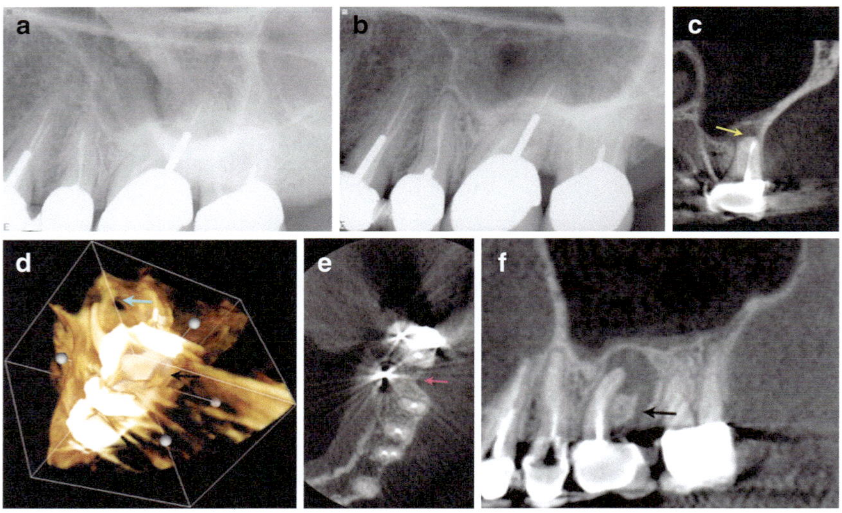

Fig. 4.12 Patient was referred for consultation and treatment of a previously treated tooth #14. Patient presented with a sinus tract related to tooth #14. (**a**, **b**) Periapical radiographs of tooth #14, mesial and distal angles, respectively. (**c**) Coronal view of the mesiobuccal root showing a missed mesiobuccal canal (yellow arrow). (**d**) 3D reconstruction showing a crestal bony defect (blue arrow). (**e**) Axial view showing a previous distobuccal root amputation site (purple arrow) that was not obvious on the periapical radiographs. (**f**) Sagittal CBCT view showing the crestal defect communicating with the periapical lesion (black arrow) and elevating the floor of the maxillary sinus with no evidence of sinus perforation

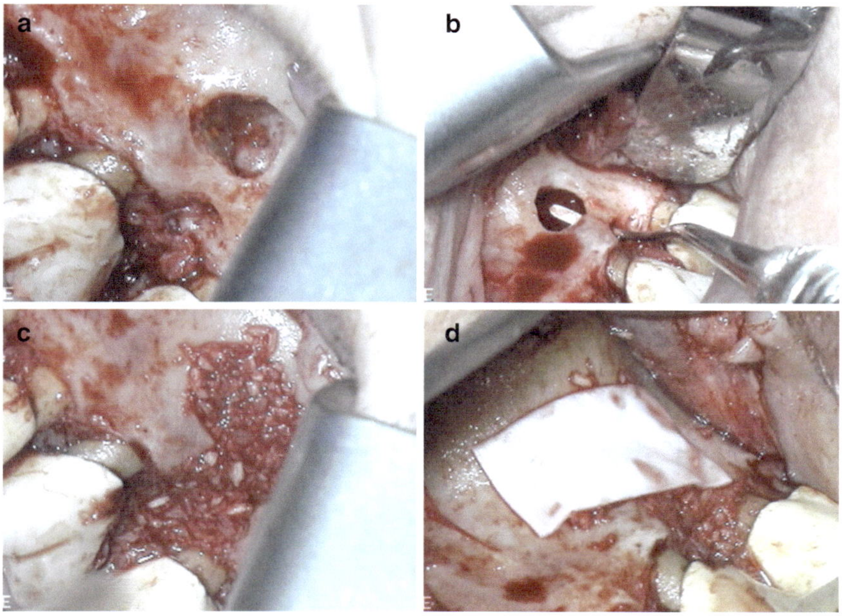

Fig. 4.13 Continuation of case in Fig. 4.12 (**a**) Clinical picture after flap reflection showing both crestal and periapical lesions. (**b**) Communication between both defects. (**c**) Both defects grafted with an EnCore™ combination allograft (Osteogenics Biomedical, Lubbock, TX). (**d**) CopiOs pericardium membrane (Zimmer, Warsaw, IN)

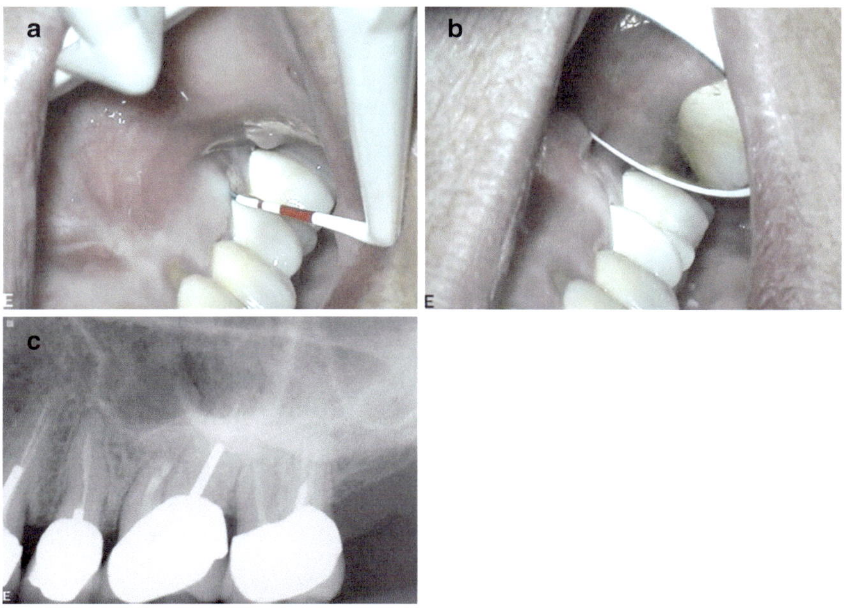

Fig. 4.14 Continuation of case in Figs. 4.12 and 4.13. (**a**, **b**) are clinical images of soft tissue healing after 1 year recall. (**c**) One-year recall radiograph

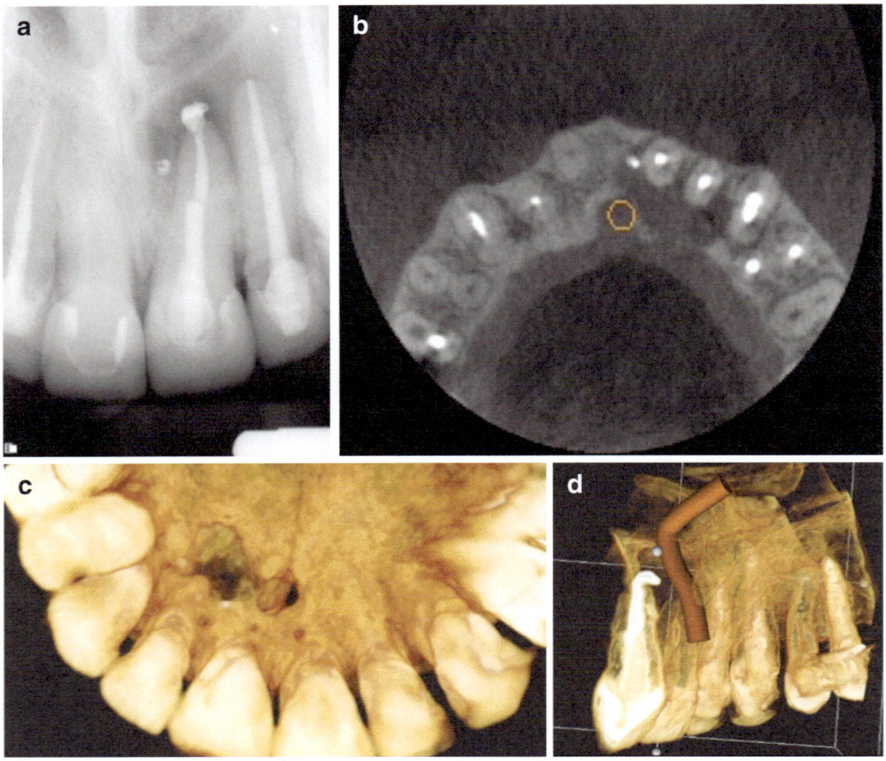

Fig. 4.15 (**a**) Periapical radiograph of the maxillary anterior region showing a periapical lesion associated with tooth #9. (**b**) Axial view showing the extent of the lesion, palatal plate perforation, and relationship of the nasopalatine neurovascular bundle to the periapical lesion. (**c**) Palatal view of the 3D reconstruction showing perforation of the palatal plate. (**d**) 3D reconstruction showing the nasopalatine bundle

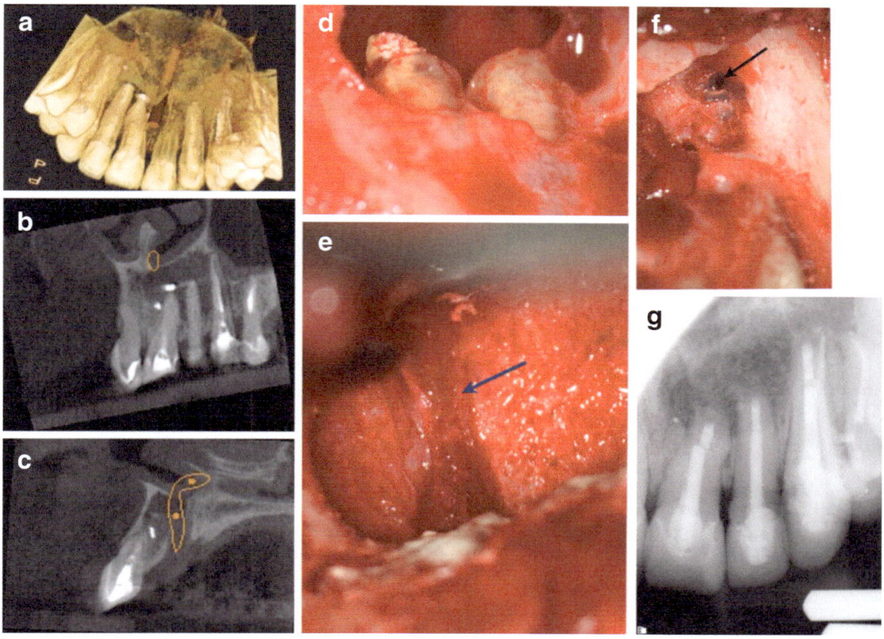

Fig. 4.16 Continuation of case in Fig. 4.15. (**a**) Palatal view CBCT reconstruction showing the exit of the nasopalatine bundle from the incisive canal. (**b**) Sagittal view showing periapical radiolucency involving teeth #9, 10, and 11. (**c**) Coronal view of the exit of the nasopalatine bundle from the incisive canal. (**d**) Periapical defect after degranulation showing the apices of teeth #9 and 10 before resection. (**e**) Clinical picture of the intact nasopalatine neurovascular bundle after degranulation (blue arrow). (**f**) Lateral wall of the maxillary sinus distal to tooth #11 (black arrow). (**g**) An immediate postoperative radiograph after grafting the through-and-through defect with Puros™ allograft (Zimmer Dental, Warsaw, IN) material and CopiOs™ membrane

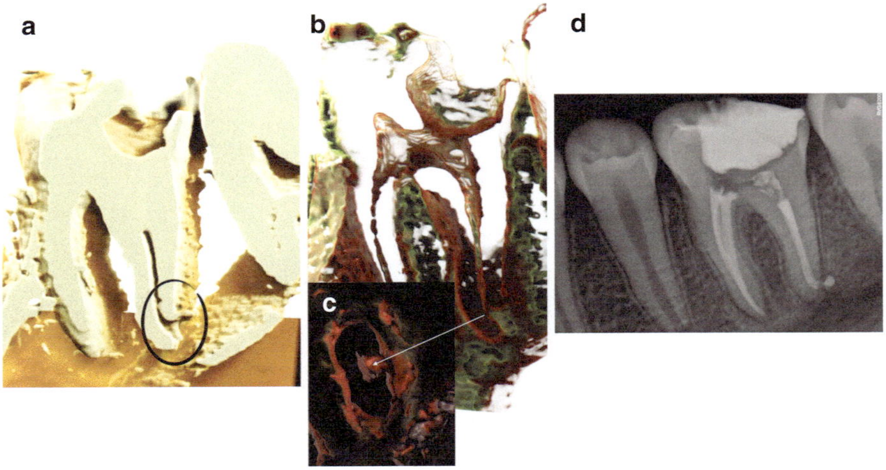

Fig. 4.17 Tooth #19 presented with distal caries and pulpal exposure. (**a**) e-VOLDx task-specific realistic rendering utilizing the canal anatomy filter. The apical resorption of the distal root can be noted as well as the lateral exit of the distal canal toward the distal aspect of the root. Utilizing the pulp filter in (**b**) and (**c**) the pulp exiting the lateral aspect of the distal root can be visualized. (**d**) the final obturation of tooth #19. The obturation coincides with the anatomy on the e-VOLDx images

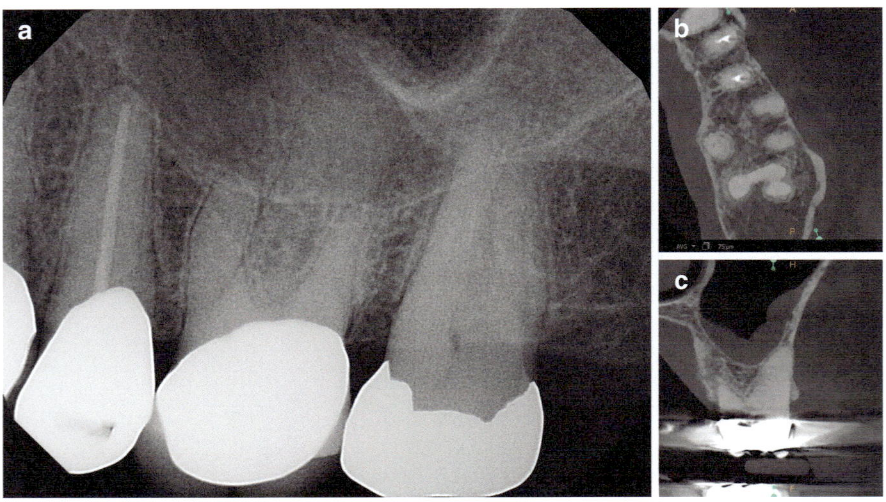

Fig. 4.18 A 80-year-old patient presenting for root canal therapy for tooth #14. (**a**) A periapical digital radiograph of tooth #14 demonstrating the pulp and root canal calcification. (**b**, **c**) are axial and coronal views of tooth #14. A trace of the canal can be seen in the apical one-third

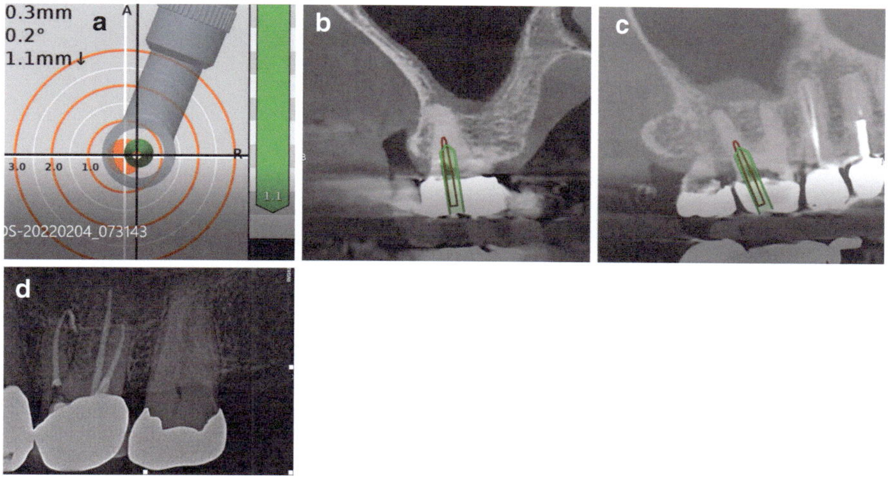

Fig. 4.19 Continuation of Fig. 4.18. The CBCT DICOM images were imported into Navident software. Treatment planning and troughing were performed in real time (**a**, **b**, **c**). The distance from the drill tip and to the center of the virtual guide, depth, and angular deviation can be monitored in real time during the access preparation. The final obturation was completed (**d**). Conservative access and canals were located with minimal removal of tooth structure guided by dynamic navigation

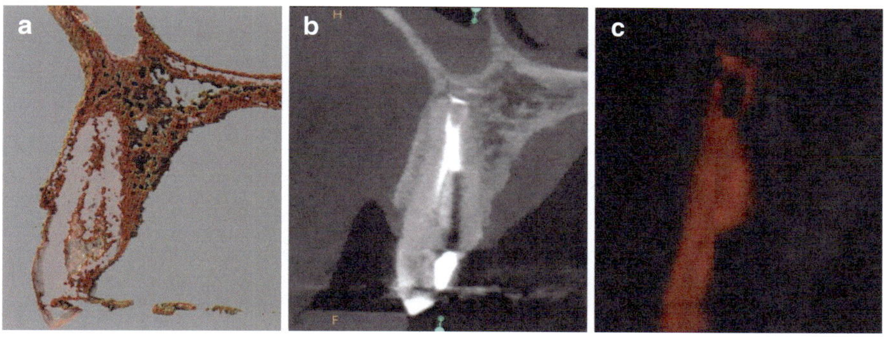

Fig. 4.20 A 57-year-old male presented for evaluation of treatment of tooth #4. Tooth #4 had a palatal cusp fracture. (**a**) CBCT DICOM images were imported into e-VOLDx software and the proximity of the palatal pulp horn to the palatal cusp fracture can be noted. The complex anatomy of the root system can be visualized utilizing the pulp realistic rendering filter. The apical delta can be noted at the apical one-third. (**b**, **c**) Coronal view of the final obturation demonstrating the correlation between the preoperative anatomy on the e-VOLDx and final obturation. (**c**) id the coronal view applying the fill filter

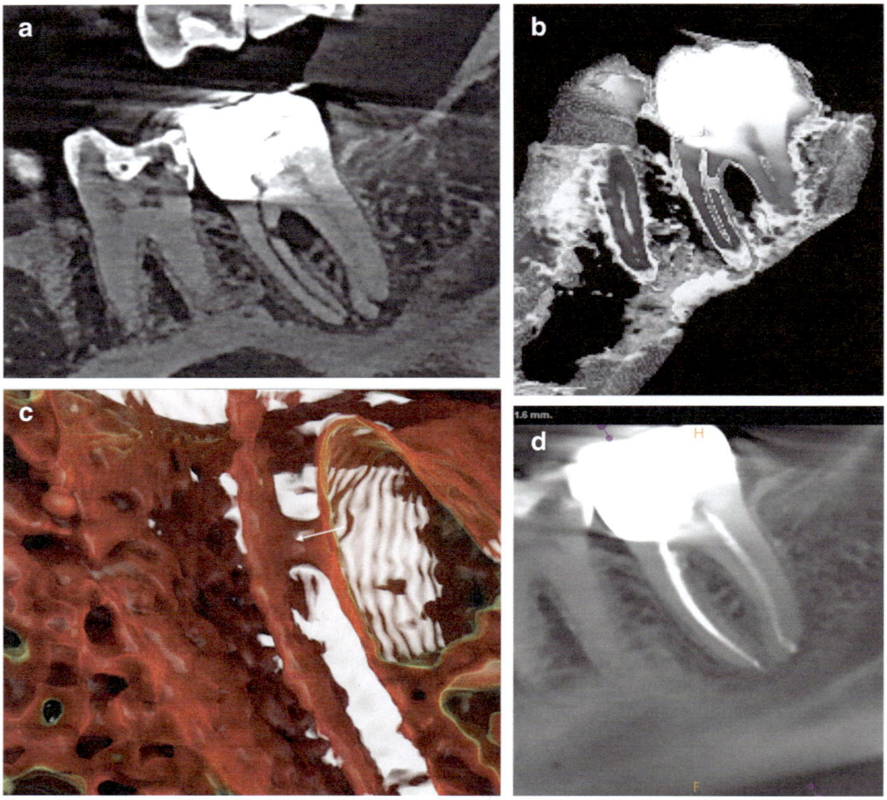

Fig. 4.21 (**a**) Sagittal view of tooth #18 presented with a low-density area in the furcation. Distal root presented with apical resorption and lateral exit of the apical foramen. A lateral canal can be noted in the coronal one-third of the mesial root. (**b**) CBCT DICOM images imported into e-VOLDx software utilizing the pulp filter. The pulp in the mesial canal can be visualized as well as the lateral canal (white arrow). (**c**) e-VOLDx anatomy filter demonstrating the mesial lateral canal and the furcation bone loss. (**d**) One year recall showing the mesial canal as well as the lateral canal obturated. Complete bone remodeling in the furcation can be noted. The final obturation CBCT sagittal view correlates to the pre-operative anatomy evaluated with e-VOLDx

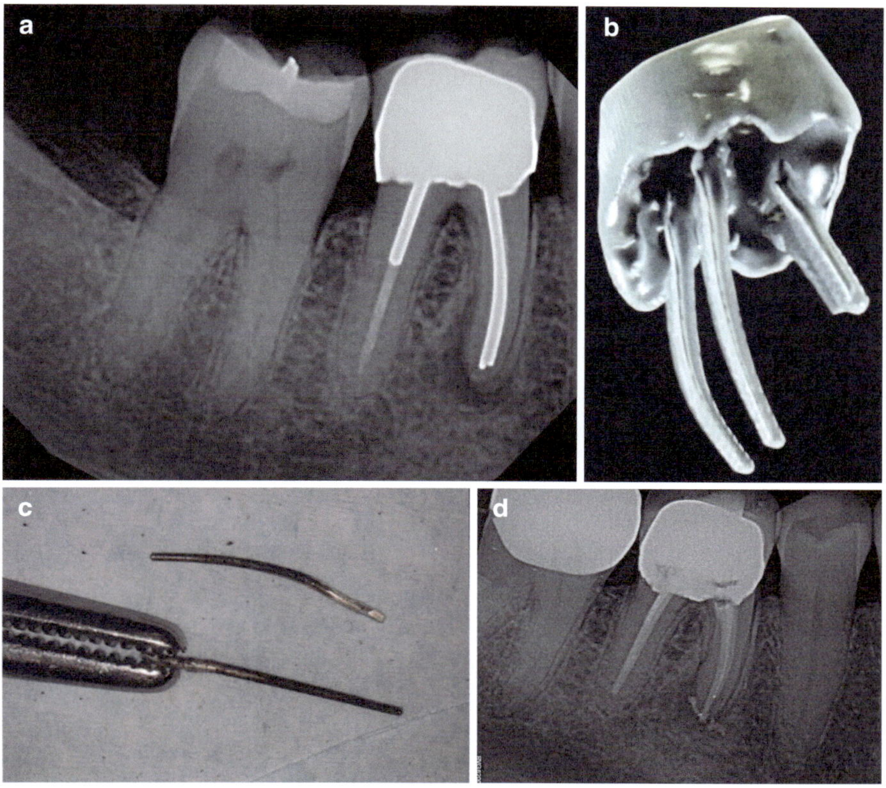

Fig. 4.22 (**a**) A digital periapical radiograph of a 69-year-old female that was referred for nonsurgical retreatment of tooth #30. A low-density area related to the mesial root can be noted. The periapical radiograph revealed 2 silver cones in the mesial root and a post in the distal root. (**b**) CBCT DICOM images were imported into e-VOLDx software and the implant filter was applied to evaluate the coronal extent of the silver cones and post in the pulp chamber. It sounds strange, but is correct in this context. The "implant filter" is used to mask/eliminate unwanted tooth structure is eliminated and 3D visualization of the extension of the sliver cones and well as the post height in relation to the crown. (**c**) Clinical picture of the retrieved silver cones from the mesial canal. (**d**) Final obturation of tooth #30. The patient is asymptomatic

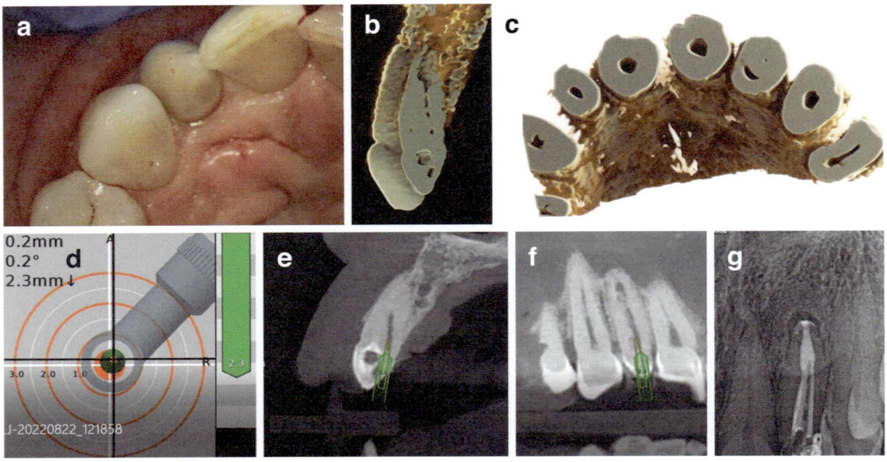

Fig. 4.23 (**a**) A clinical picture of tooth #7. Tooth #7 presented with dens in dente. (**b**, **c**) e-VOLDx images with the realistic rendering with task-specific anatomy filter. CBCT DICOM images were imported into Navident (ClaroNav). (**d**, **e**, **f**) is the workflow, planning, and troughing for the 2 canals utilizing the dynamic navigation system. (**f**) Postoperative periapical radiograph. Note the conservative access and the correlation of the pre- and postoperative anatomy (**g**)

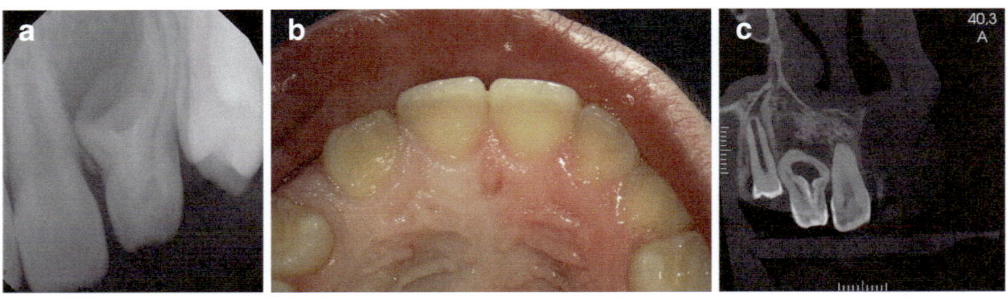

Fig. 4.24 (**a**) A periapical radiograph of tooth #10 presenting with gemination. (**b**) Clinical picture of tooth #10. (**c**) CBCT view of tooth #10 demonstrating the gemination and complexity of anatomy. CBCT DICOM image demonstrates the invagination between the 2 roots with little margin of error during access preparation

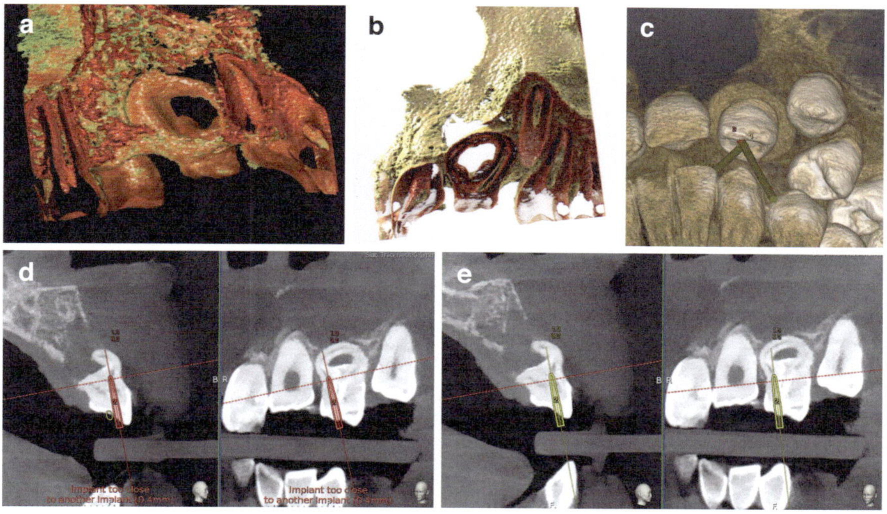

Fig. 4.25 Continuation of case in Fig. 4.24. CBCT DICOM images were imported into e-VOLDx software and applied the task-specific realistic rendering filters for anatomy and pulp. Note the complexity of the anatomy and gemination of tooth #10 (**a**, **b**). CBCT Dicom images imported into Navident software and analysis demonstrated in (**c**, **d**, **e**) and treatment planning of the 2 separate access preparation. The treatment planning allows the clinician to establish a real-time guided conservative access preparation

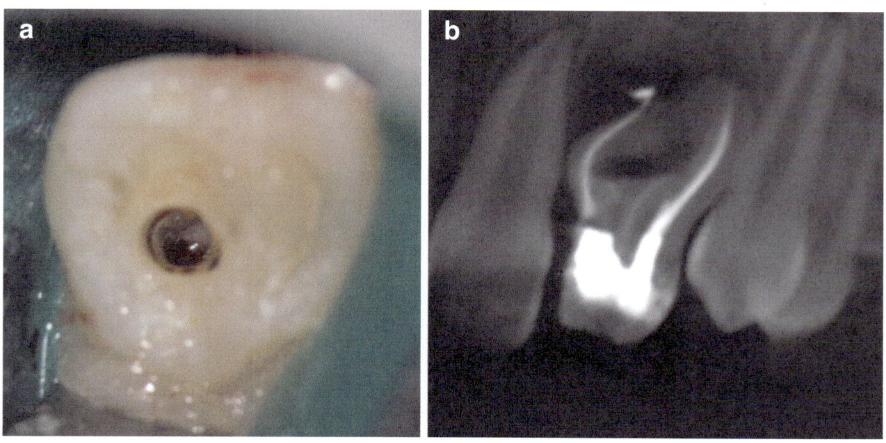

Fig. 4.26 Continuation of Fig. 4.25. (**a**) Clinical picture of the first access performed utilizing guided dynamic navigation. (**b**) Final postoperative radiograph of the obturation of tooth #10

References

1. Reit C, Petersson K. Diagnosis of pulpal and periradicular disease. In: Bergenholtz G, Horsted-Bindslev P, Reit C, editors. Textbook of endodontology. 2nd ed. UK: Wiley-Blackwell; 2010. p. 235–53.
2. Kundel HL, Revesz G. Lesion conspicuity, structured noise, and film reader error. Am J Roentgenol. 1976;126:1233–8.
3. Maini A, Durning P, Drage N. Resorption: within or without? The benefit of cone-beam computed tomography when diagnosing a case of an internal/external resorption defect. Br Dent J. 2008;9:135–7.
4. Patel S, Ricucci D, Durak C, Tay F. Internal root resorption: a review. J Endod. 2010;36:1107–21.
5. Estrela C, Bueno M, De Alencar AH, et al. Method to evaluate inflammatory root resorption by using cone beam computed tomography. J Endod. 2009;35:1491–7.
6. Hassan B, Metska ME, Ozok AR, et al. Detection of vertical root fractures in endodontically treated teeth by a cone beam computed tomography scan. J Endod. 2009;35:719–22.
7. Bernardes RA, de Moraes IG, Húngaro Duarte MA, et al. Use of cone-beam volumetric tomography in the diagnosis of root fractures. Oral Surg Oral Med Oral Pathol Oral Radiol Endod. 2009;108:270–7.
8. Edlund M, Nair MK, Nair UP. Detection of vertical root fractures by using cone-beam computed tomography: a clinical study. J Endod. 2011;37:768–72.
9. Fayad MI, Ashkenaz PJ, Johnson BR. Different representations of vertical root fractures detected by cone-beam volumetric tomography: a case series report. J Endod. 2012;38:1435–42.
10. Michetti J, Maret D, Mallet JP, Diemer F. Validation of cone beam computed tomography as a tool to explore root canal anatomy. J Endod. 2010;36:1187–90.
11. Liang YH, Li G, Wesselink PR, Wu MK. Endodontic outcome predictors identified with periapical radiographs and cone-beam computed tomography scans. J Endod. 2011;37:326–31.
12. de Paula-Silva FW, Wu MK, Leonardo MR, et al. Accuracy of periapical radiography and cone-beam computed tomography scans in diagnosing apical periodontitis using histopathological findings as a gold standard. J Endod. 2009;35:1009–12.
13. Velvart P, Hecker H, Tillinger G. Detection of the apical lesion and the mandibular canal in conventional radiography and computed tomography. Oral Surg Oral Med Oral Pathol Oral Radiol Endod. 2001;92:682–8.
14. Stavropoulos A, Wenzel A. Accuracy of cone beam dental CT, intraoral digital and conventional film radiography for the detection of periapical lesions: an ex vivo study in pig jaws. Clin Oral Investig. 2007;11:101–6.
15. Nakata K, Naitoh M, Izumi M, et al. Effectiveness of dental computed tomography in diagnostic imaging of periradicular lesion of each root of a multirooted tooth: a case report. J Endod. 2006;32:583–7.
16. Lofthag-Hansen S, Huumonen S, Grondahl K, Grondahl HG. Limited cone-bean CT and intraoral radiography for the diagnosis of periapical pathology. Oral Surg Oral Med Oral Pathol Oral Radiol Endod. 2007;103:114–9.
17. Cotton TP, Geisler TM, Holden DT, et al. Endodontic applications of cone-beam volumetric tomography. J Endod. 2007;33:1121–32.
18. Patel S, Dawood A, Whaites E, Pitt FT. New dimensions in endodontic imaging: part 1. Conventional and alternative radiographic systems. Int Endod J. 2009;42:447–62.
19. Patel S. New dimensions in endodontic imaging: part 2. Cone beam computed tomography. Int Endod J. 2009;42:463–75.
20. Scarfe WC, Farman AG, Sukovic P. Clinical applications of cone-beam computed tomography in dental practice. J Can Dent Assoc. 2006;72:75–80.
21. Nair MK, Nair UP. Digital and advanced imaging in endodontics: a review. J Endod. 2007;33:1–6.
22. Ee J, Fayad MI, Johnson BR. Comparison of endodontic diagnosis and treatment planning decisions using cone-beam volumetric tomography versus periapical radiography. J Endod. 2014;40:910–6.

23. Rodriguez G, Abella F, Duran-Sindreu F, Patel S, Roig M. Influence of cone-beam computed tomography in clinical decision making among specialists. J Endod. 2017;43:194–9.
24. Bhatt M, Coil J, Chehroudi B, Esteves A, Aleksejuniene J, MacDonald D. Clinical decision-making and importance of the AAE/AAOMR position statement for CBCT examination in endodontic cases. Int Endod J. 2021;54:26–37.

Three-Dimensional Evaluation of Internal Tooth Anatomy

5

William J. Nudera

Abstract

The study of human tooth anatomy is fundamental to clinical endodontics. Several histologic methods used to evaluate tooth anatomy have been described for the purpose of identification and categorization of various root and root canal types. In addition, multiple publications have attempted to classify root and root canal configuration as it relates to tooth type, tooth location, root type, gender, geographic location, and ethnic background. For decades, two-dimensional radiography (captured at various angulations) has been the primary method for evaluating tooth anatomy before endodontic treatment. Attempting to assess multidimensional anatomy from planar imaging has significant limitations. Technological advancements in three-dimensional tomographic imaging have given rise to a more accurate method for the preoperative clinical evaluation of tooth anatomy. Cone beam computed tomography (CBCT) provides a non-destructive real-time capture of three-dimensional anatomic and morphologic information. A short acquisition time and a level of detail equivalent to that of in vitro tooth sectioning make CBCT imaging the first and currently only practical method available for the accurate, undistorted, chair-side evaluation of tooth anatomy in three spatial planes prior to initiating root canal treatment.

William J. Nudera: Author of NUENDO ReThinking Endodontics, A Systematic Approach to Diagnosis and Case Selection, Published by EDRA

W. J. Nudera (✉)
Department of Endodontics, University of Illinois at Chicago, Chicago, IL, USA

Private Practice, Specailized Endodontic Solutions, Bloomingdale, IL, USA

M. I. Fayad, B. R. Johnson (eds.), *3D Imaging in Endodontics*,
https://doi.org/10.1007/978-3-031-32755-1_5

5.1 Introduction

The non-surgical endodontic treatment model is simple—eliminate as much of the tooth's internal contents as possible and create a favorable environment to prevent or heal periapical disease. Although a simple concept, many complex steps are involved, and several uncontrollable variables exist. A prerequisite for predictable endodontic treatment begins with establishing a thorough knowledge of the tooth's anatomy and morphology. Ignorance of this knowledge ranks second only to errors in diagnosis and treatment planning as a cause of persistent apical pathosis [1].

The complexity of the root canal system has been well documented over the last century (Fig. 5.1). A detailed description of these complex anatomical structures first appeared in the German dental literature in 1917 and was later translated for republication in the *Journal of the American Dental Association* in 1921. Dr. Walter Hess was the first to describe the relationship of the dental pulp and its conformity with the external roots, suggesting a wide variety in the number and form of root canal systems, "thus complicating the picture greatly" [2].

The clinical application of CBCT technology has impacted every aspect of dentistry, with endodontics being a significant beneficiary. CBCT imaging has allowed clinicians to fully grasp the complexity of root anatomy and morphology, thus eliminating the variable of two-dimensional radiographic speculation. Adopting a

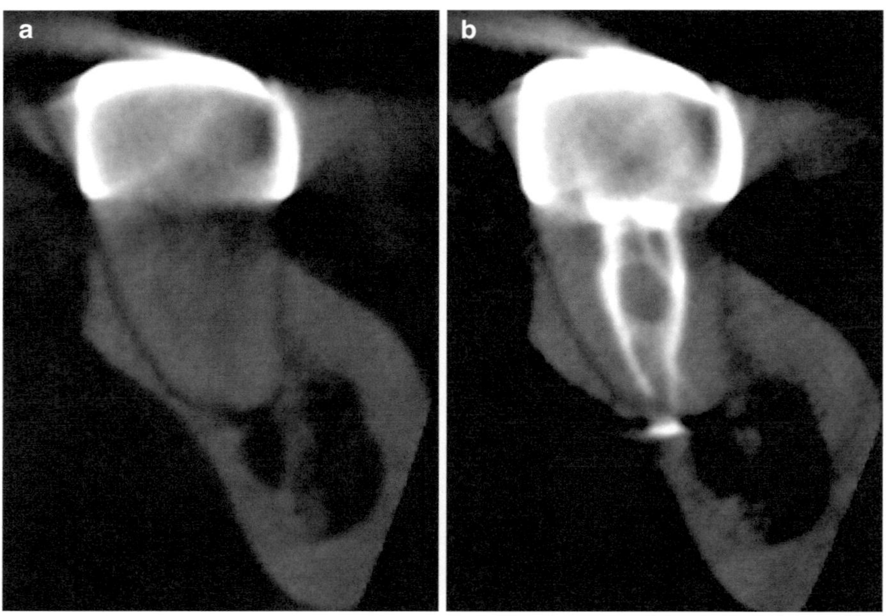

Fig. 5.1 Coronal CBCT section of the mesial root of a mandibular first molar (**a**) and the post-endodontic coronal CBCT section (**b**) demonstrating the complex nature of the root canal system

preoperative radiographic protocol that includes a CBCT scan has significantly enhanced the clinician's ability to execute the non-surgical endodontic treatment model more predictably and efficiently.

5.2 Methods for Studying Tooth Anatomy

The methods used to study tooth anatomy can be categorized as in vitro or in vivo. In vitro techniques allow for detailed microscopic and histologic examination of teeth in all dimensions and include demineralization, clearing, sectioning, modeling, scanning electron microscopy, and micro-computed tomography [3]. In vivo approaches have more clinical implications and consist of traditional radiography, various types of tomographic imaging, ultrasound, and magnetic resonance imaging. In vitro histologic evaluation via canal staining and tooth clearing represents the gold standard for evaluating root canal anatomy and morphology [4, 5]. However, in vitro methods are destructive and limited to bench top examination only.

CBCT scanning has been reported to be equivalent to that of histologic sectioning and staining with respect to accuracy when identifying canals and unusual anatomy. A study directly comparing tomographic scans to the histologic sectioning of 152 maxillary molar teeth found identical canal configurations using the two methods [6]. A 2010 study of 233 tooth sections found a "strong to very strong correlation" between CBCT imaging and histologic sections [7]. Neelakantan et al. compared the efficacy of six different imaging methods to that of canal staining and clearing. CBCT scanning was reported to be as accurate in identifying root canal systems as the modified staining and clearing techniques and significantly more accurate than conventional radiographic methods [8]. In another study comparing traditional radiographic techniques to that of CBCT scanning and clinical sectioning, Blattner et al. reported that CBCT scanning was a reliable method for canal detection and represents a highly accurate in vivo method for the evaluation of tooth anatomy equivalent to that of the histologic gold standard [9] (Fig. 5.2).

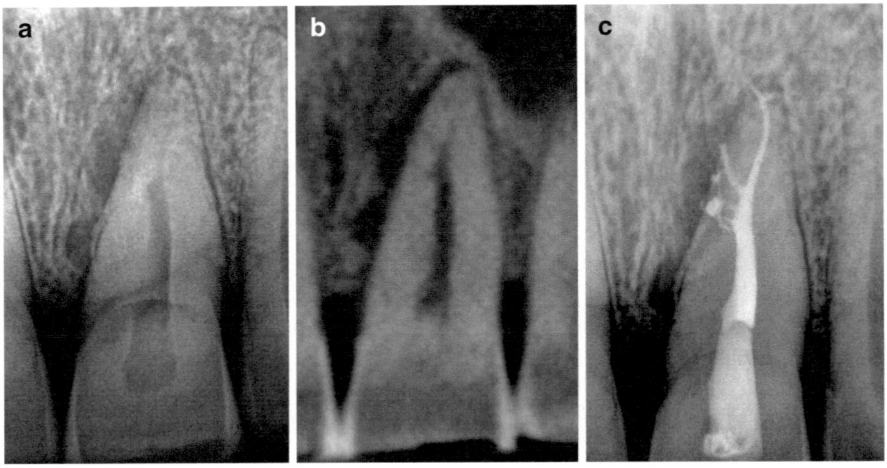

Fig. 5.2 Periapical radiograph of a maxillary left central incisor (**a**), with a corresponding coronal CBCT section (**b**) demonstrating visible complex internal anatomy. Post-endodontic periapical radiograph (**c**) shows accurate clinical management of the complex anatomy

5.3 Clinical Methods for the Evaluation of Tooth Anatomy

Methods used for the chair-side evaluation of a tooth's anatomy and morphology prior to endodontic treatment are traditionally limited to direct clinical analysis and multiple two-dimensional projection radiographs captured at various angulations. This immediate radiographic information is used in conjunction with the collective insight gained from numerous anatomic and morphologic studies, the knowledge of common root variations, and the individual clinician's experience. This approach introduces subjectivity and is influenced by the competence of the treating clinician [10]; confirmation of the true anatomical configuration can only be realized following completion of an irreversible endodontic access.

The current body of endodontic literature cites average statistics for permanent human teeth with respect to type and location as well as common canal arrangements. In addition, several works have classified various canal configurations identified within a single root [3, 11]. Population studies have attempted to identify common morphologic and anatomic features of roots and root canal systems relating to gender, ethnicity, and geographic location [12, 13]. In their classic study evaluating the pulp chambers of 500 molars, Krasner and Rankow proposed several "anatomic laws," suggesting that the cement-enamel junction represents the most reproducible and predictable clinical landmark to assist in the identification of root canal anatomy during endodontic treatment [14].

Studies attempting to categorize tooth anatomy and morphology can only provide clinical treatment recommendations and guidelines related to generalizations. These guidelines are based on weighted averages and broad observations. Averages

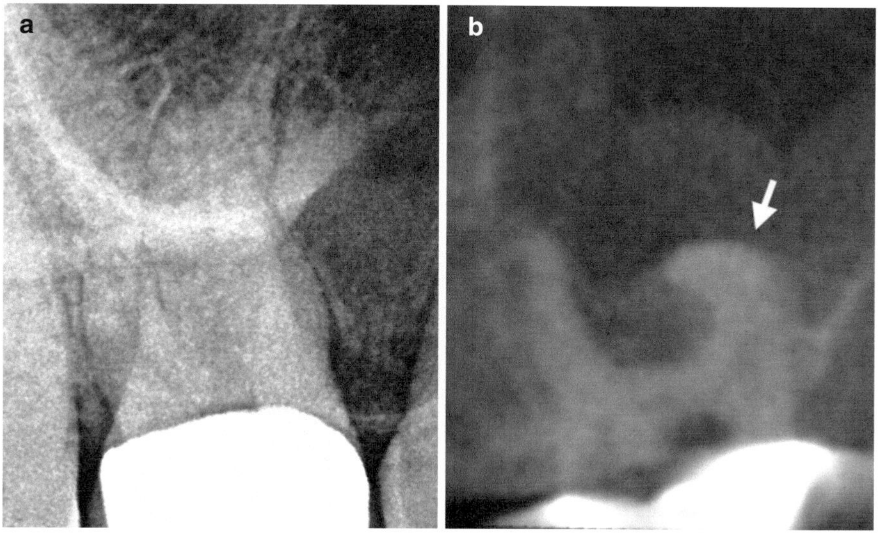

Fig. 5.3 Periapical radiograph of a maxillary right first molar (**a**) with a corresponding coronal CBCT section (**b**) demonstrating a significant curvature of the mesiobuccal root in the buccal-palatal orientation (arrow)

are helpful when studying populations' characteristics, but have limited predictive value for treating the individual patient. The application of a preoperative CBCT scan provides real-time, chair-side anatomic, and morphologic data for the actual tooth being treated at the time of treatment, eliminating the variable of subjectivity and rendering the traditional methods moot.

CBCT imaging overcomes several limitations found with conventional radiographic methods. Dimensionally accurate image acquisition and viewing in all three spatial planes eliminates the superimposition of multiple roots and surrounding anatomic structures and provides more sensitivity with respect to the detection of periradicular pathosis, root resorption, and root fractures [15]. Visualizing multidimensional root curvature allows for precise treatment planning and predictable canal management [16] (Fig. 5.3). Geometrically accurate measurement capabilities assist in the determination of root length as well as establish precise intra- and inter-canal distance relationships [17] (Fig. 5.4). Additionally, information obtained from a cone beam scan before endodontic treatment has been reported to improve diagnostic capabilities and prompt endodontic treatment plan changes [18, 19].

A preoperative CBCT scan provides an undistorted reconstruction of a tooth's internal and external morphologic features, providing the ability to detect more roots and root canals with greater accuracy and higher frequency [20]. (Fig. 5.5). Figure 5.6 represents the periapical radiographs of two different maxillary second molars and their corresponding axial CBCT slices. Although both teeth appear radiographically similar, the corresponding axial CBCT slices reveal two very different anatomic root features and canal configurations.

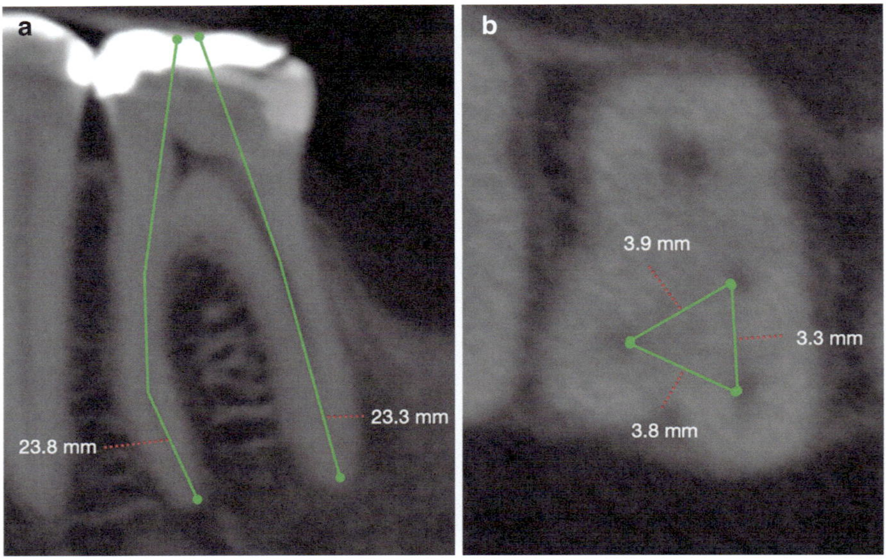

Fig. 5.4 Sagittal CBCT section of a mandibular first molar (**a**) demonstrating accurate working length measurements made prior to initiating endodontic treatment. Axial CBCT section of a maxillary right first molar (**b**) demonstrating inter-canal distance measurements made to aid in the identification of the second mesiobuccal canal orifice during treatment

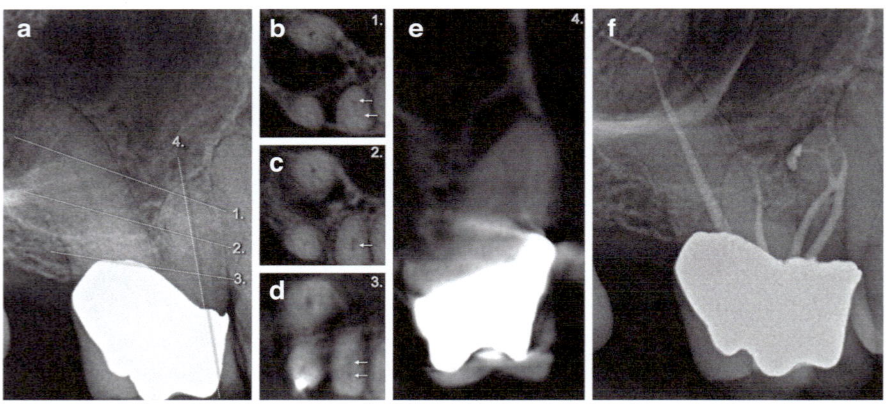

Fig. 5.5 Periapical radiograph of a maxillary right first molar (**a**), with axial CBCT sections 1, 2, and 3 (**b**, **c**, **d**), coronal CBCT section 4 (**e**), and post-endodontic periapical radiograph (**f**), demonstrating an undistorted reproduction of the root's internal morphologic features. Note the mid-root confluence followed by the apical bifidity in the axial sections (arrows) *(Case courtesy of Dr. Kyung Choi, Specialized Endodontic Solutions, Bloomingdale, IL)*

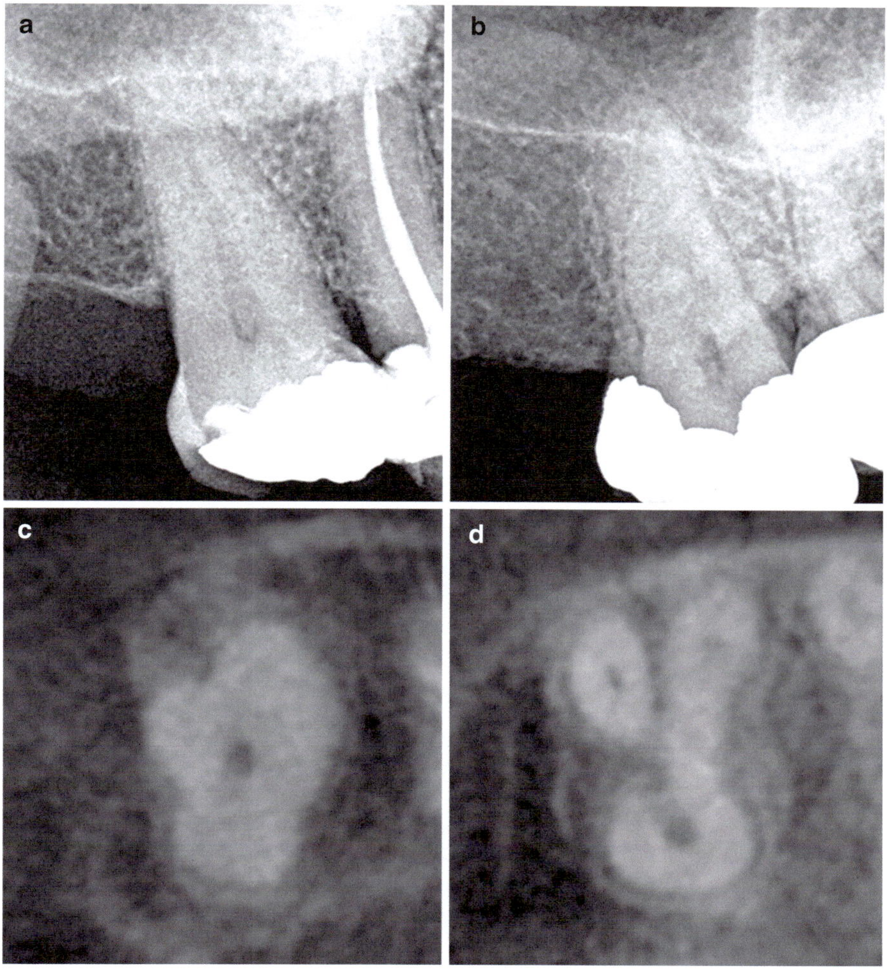

Fig. 5.6 Periapical radiographs of two similar right maxillary second molars with conically shaped roots (**a**, **b**), and their corresponding axial CBCT sections below (**c**, **d**), demonstrating different external root forms and different internal canal configurations

5.4 Preoperative Assessment of Complex Anatomy

In endodontics, complexity is the norm; many variations in tooth anatomy exist within the global population [12, 13, 21, 22]. As such, any tooth has the potential to present with an anatomic configuration that lies beyond the boundaries of the documented models (Fig. 5.7). An array of complex anatomic variations related to tooth, root, and canal type, as well as detailed descriptions of atypical root development, fill the pages of the academic journals. In addition, characteristics associated with

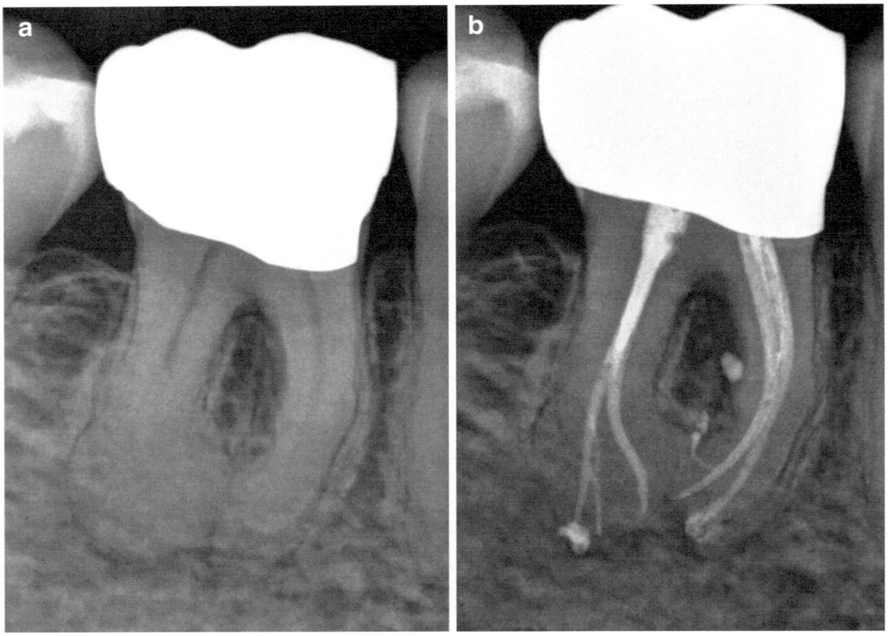

Fig. 5.7 Periapical radiograph of a mandibular left first molar (**a**) and post-endodontic periapical radiograph (**b**) depicting an undocumented canal configuration

root canal systems, in general, may be present and can potentially increase the anatomic complexity of root canal treatment.

Although well documented, it is impossible to completely understand each tooth's unique internal and external anatomical relationship when considering the limitations of two-dimensional projection radiography. Multiple case reports have demonstrated significant advantages when using CBCT scanning over traditional radiographic imaging techniques to detect and manage more complex tooth, root, and canal variations [23–25]. Therefore, the only way to fully appreciate the anatomic diversity of roots and their root canal systems before endodontic treatment is by acquiring a preoperative CBCT scan.

5.5 Maxillary Molar Teeth

5.5.1 The Mesiobuccal Root Complex

The mesiobuccal root complex of the maxillary first molar is one of the endodontic literature's most well-documented (and studied) root canal systems. It is generally broad buccolingually with prominent depressions on the mesial and distal surfaces and usually contains two canals. One ex vivo study reported the presence of two mesiobuccal canals in the coronal half of maxillary first molars to be as high as

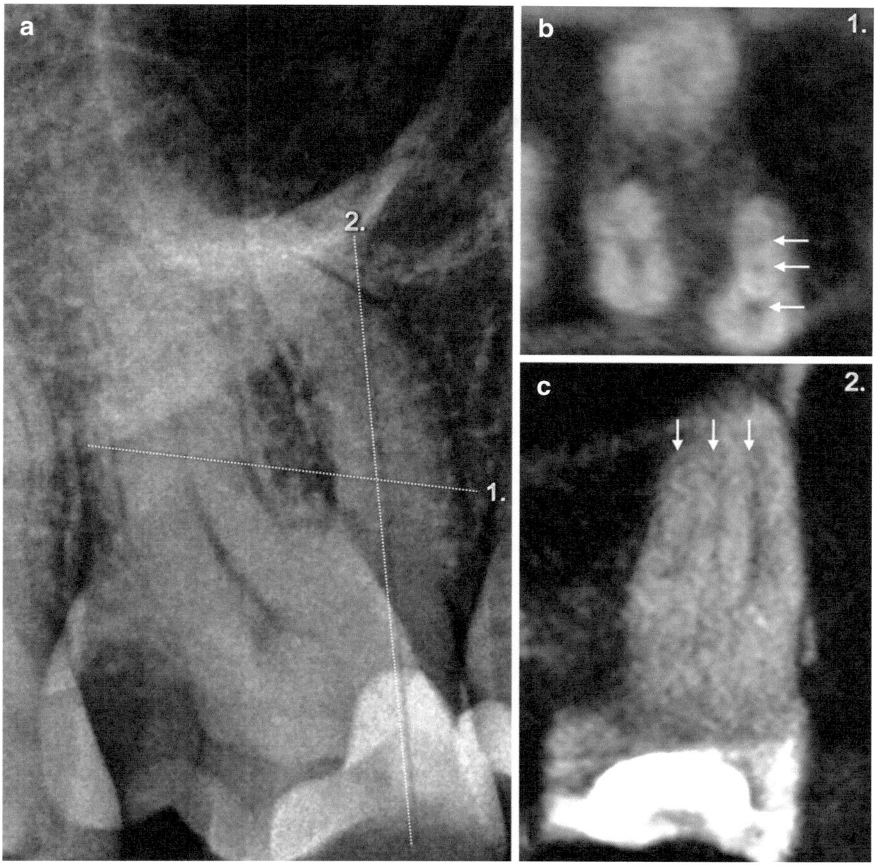

Fig. 5.8 Periapical radiograph of a maxillary right first molar (**a**), with corresponding mid-root axial CBCT Section 1 (**b**) and coronal CBCT Section 2 (**c**) demonstrating mesiobuccal root anatomy with three distinct root canal systems (arrows)

95.2%, with 71% having separate apical portals of exit [26]. Similar variations occur in the maxillary second molars with less reported frequency. The acquisition of a CBCT scan can enhance the detection and treatment of multiple mesiobuccal canals [27] (Figs. 5.8 and 5.9). Observing the mesiobuccal root complex in the axial and coronal planes can often detect the exact number of canals, as well as the configuration. (Fig. 5.10).

5.5.2 Fused Roots

With a reported frequency of approximately 42% in specific populations [28], the prevalence of fused roots has been noted to be four times higher in maxillary second

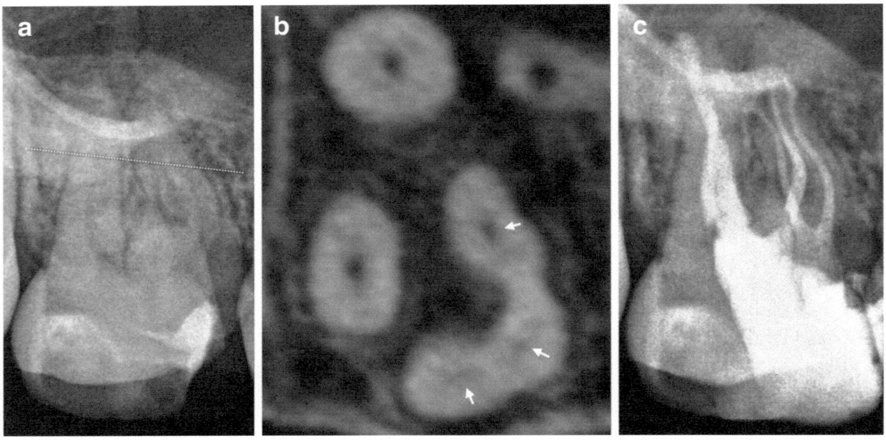

Fig. 5.9 Periapical radiograph of a maxillary right first molar (**a**), with corresponding axial CBCT section from the apical third (**b**) demonstrating a mesiobuccal root with an unusual morphologic root form and three distinct root canal systems (arrows). Post-endodontic periapical radiograph (**c**) shows the accurate clinical management of this complex anatomy (*Case courtesy of Dr. Hong Chon, Specialized Endodontic Solutions, Bloomingdale, IL)*

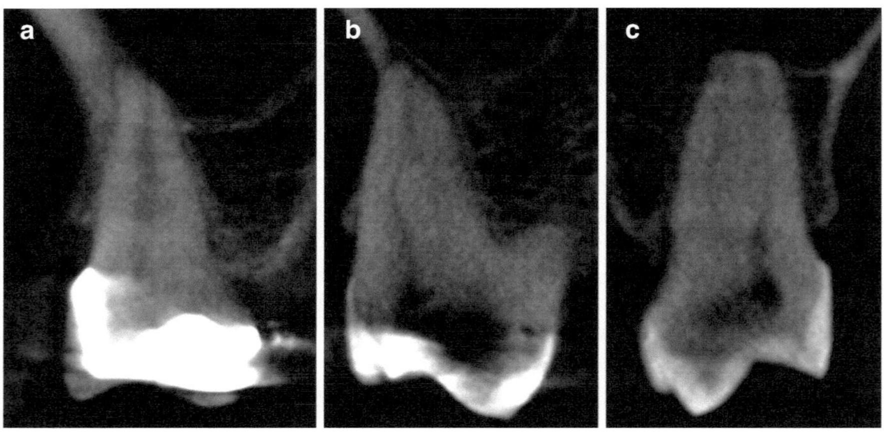

Fig. 5.10 Coronal CBCT sections of three mesiobuccal root complexes demonstrating three different internal root canal configurations—a single canal with one portal of exit (**a**), two canals with a single portal of exit (**b**), and two canals with two separate portals of exit (**c**)

molars when compared to maxillary first molars [29]. Root fusion can occur between the mesiobuccal and distobuccal roots (Fig. 5.11), mesiobuccal and palatal roots (Fig. 5.12), distobuccal and palatal roots (Fig. 5.13), or all three roots, resulting in a "C-shaped" root configuration (Fig. 5.14). In addition, fused roots often contain isthmuses or additional root canal systems that connect some (or all) of the roots [30]—a relationship that can only be fully appreciated by studying the axial plane of the preoperative CBCT scan (Fig. 5.15).

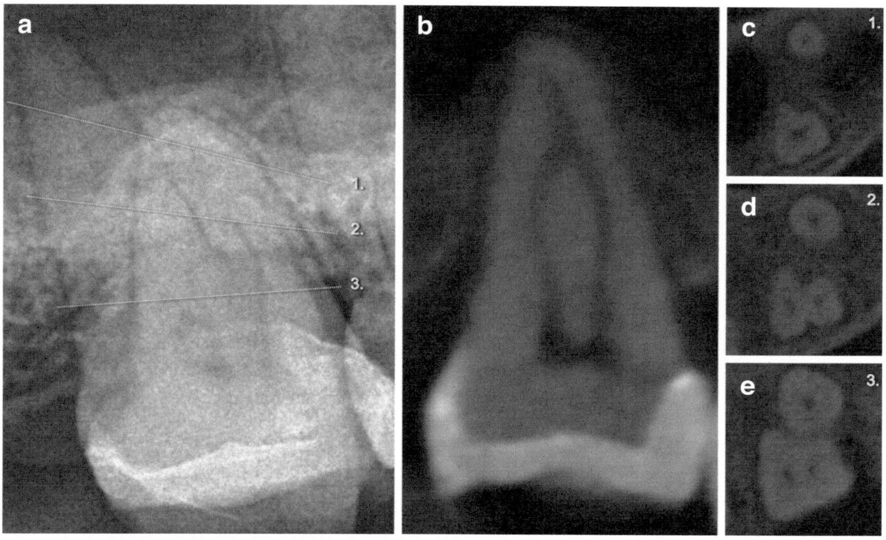

Fig. 5.11 Periapical radiograph of a maxillary right second molar (**a**), with a corresponding sagittal CBCT section through the buccal roots (**b**), and axial CBCT Sections 1, 2, and 3 (**c**, **d**, **e**)—showing fusion and canal confluence of the mesiobuccal and distobuccal roots

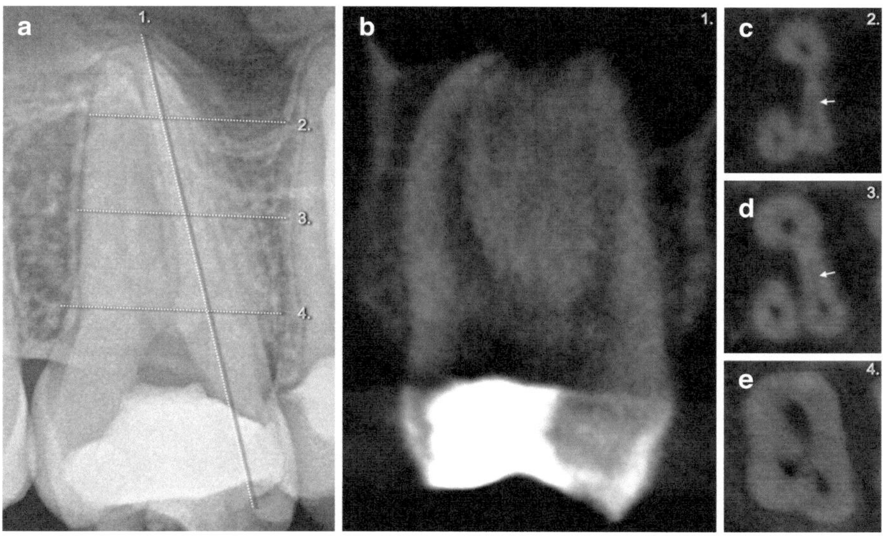

Fig. 5.12 Periapical radiograph of a maxillary right second molar (**a**), with a corresponding coronal CBCT Section 1 (**b**), and axial CBCT Sections 2, 3, and 4 (**c**, **d**, **e**)—showing fusion of the mesiobuccal and palatal roots. Note the isthmus space projecting from the mesiobuccal canal (arrows)

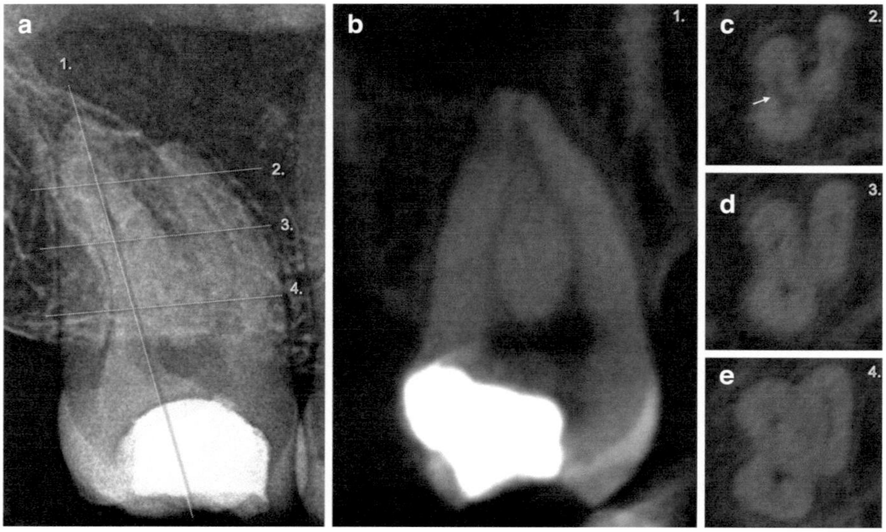

Fig. 5.13 Periapical radiograph of a maxillary right second molar (**a**), with a corresponding coronal CBCT Section 1 (**b**), and axial CBCT Sections 2, 3, and 4 (**c**, **d**, **e**)—showing fusion and canal confluence of the distobuccal and palatal roots (arrow)

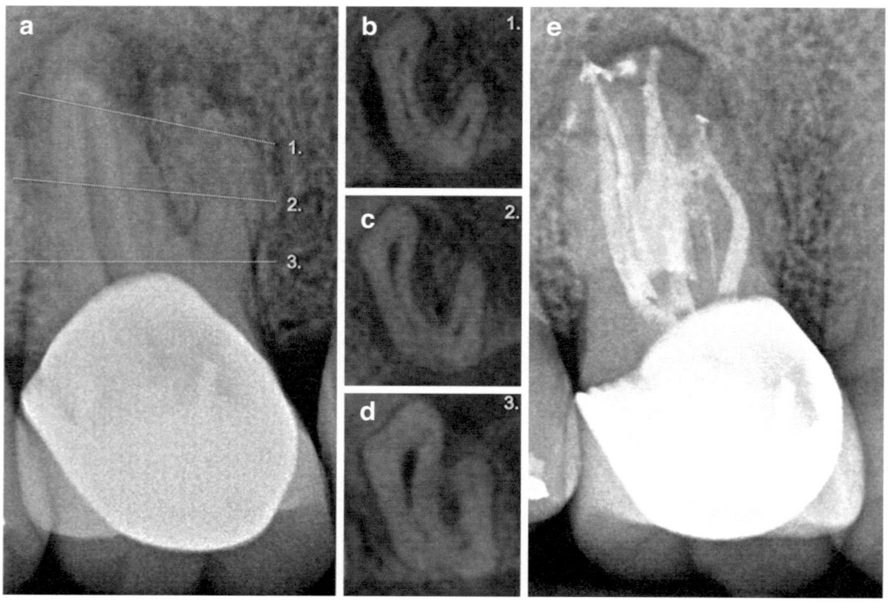

Fig. 5.14 Periapical radiograph of a maxillary right second molar (**a**) with corresponding axial CBCT Sections 1, 2, and 3 (**b**, **c**, **d**)—showing total root fusion and multiple levels of canal confluence. Post-endodontic periapical radiograph (**e**), depicting the accurate clinical management of this complex anatomy (*Case courtesy of Dr. Hong Chon, Specialized Endodontic Solutions, Bloomingdale, IL)*

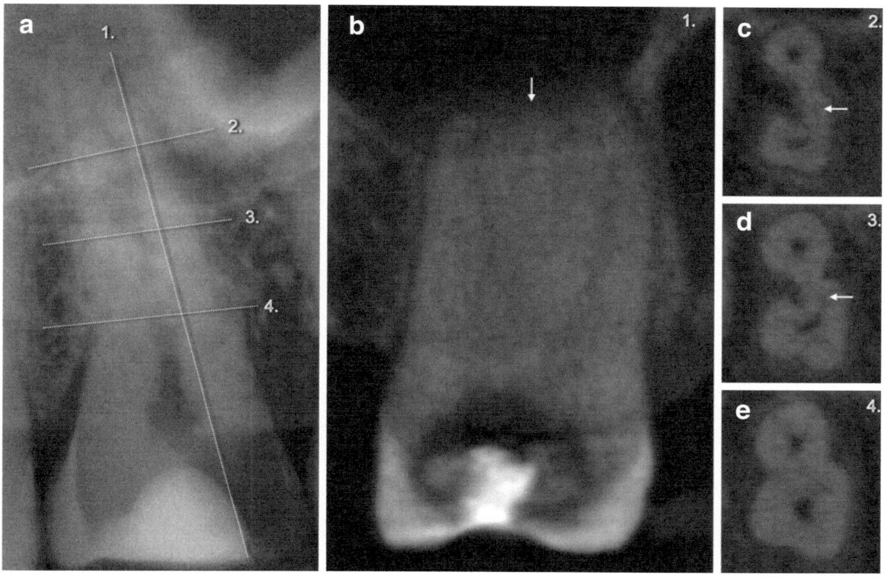

Fig. 5.15 Periapical radiograph of a maxillary right second molar (**a**), with a corresponding coronal CBCT Section 1 (**b**), and axial CBCT Sections 2, 3, and 4 (**c**, **d**, **e**)—showing the presence of a separate canal (arrows) within the fused dentin of the mesiobuccal and palatal roots

5.5.3 Double Palatal Roots and Canals

The presence of an additional palatal root or canal has been described in the literature. With an ex vivo frequency ranging between 1.2% and 33.3% (within a specific population) [31, 32], this anatomic variation is much less common than the aforementioned maxillary molar configurations. Due to its infrequency and the superimposition of multiple roots, this canal arrangement may not be readily visible (or observed) using two-dimensional radiographic imaging. However, this unique configuration becomes apparent with the aid of three-dimensional volumetric analysis . A preoperative CBCT scan can readily identify this rare anatomical arrangement and determine the exact location of the additional canal orifice for maximum conservation of tooth structure during endodontic treatment (Fig. 5.16).

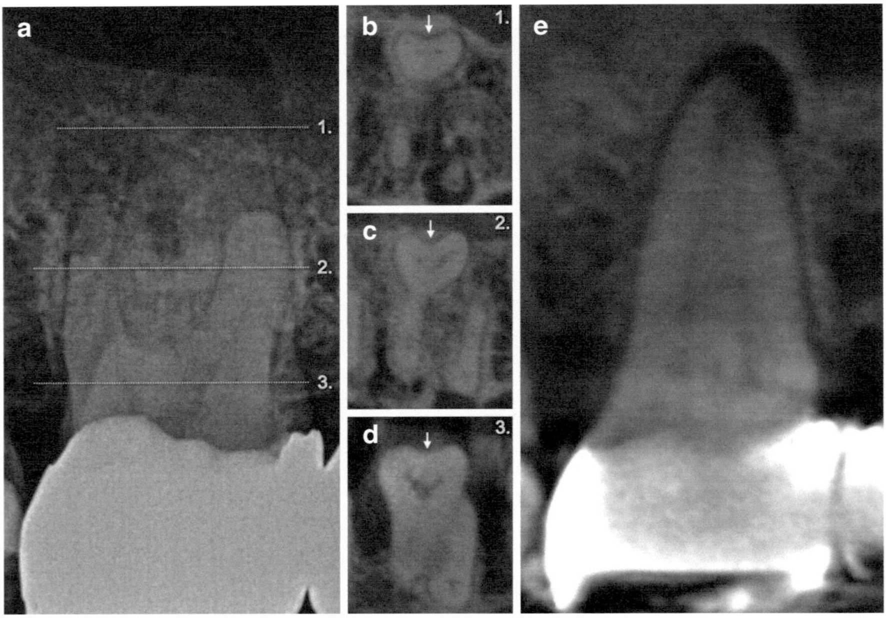

Fig. 5.16 Periapical radiograph of a maxillary right first molar (**a**), with corresponding axial CBCT Sections 1, 2, and 3 (**b**, **c**, **d**), and sagittal CBCT section through the palatal root (**e**), depicting two distinct canals within a single palatal root form. Note the developmental depression in the axial sections (arrows) extending along the entire length of the palatal root

5.6 Maxillary Premolar Teeth

Maxillary premolar teeth are generally broad buccolingually and narrow mesiodistally. They can present with two separate roots containing one canal per root or one broad root containing one or multiple canals. When one broad root is present, the corresponding internal anatomy can consist of a single ribbon-shaped canal or one of several documented canal classifications consisting of multiple canal divisions [33]. Occasionally, these teeth can present with a third root or third root canal. The frequency for this anatomic variation has an overall incidence of 1.7% in maxillary first premolars [34] and 2.6% in maxillary second premolars [35] (Fig. 5.17). The addition of a CBCT scan can help determine the class of canal division, as well as the exact level at which the canal division(s) occurs.

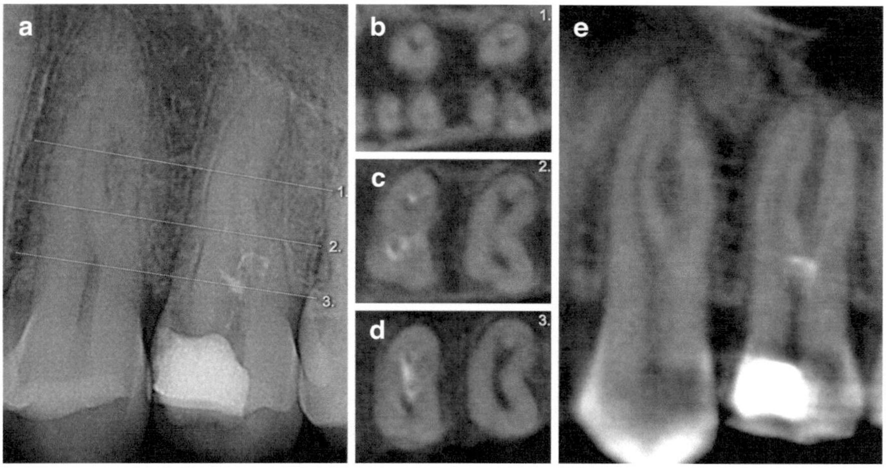

Fig. 5.17 Periapical radiograph (**a**), with corresponding axial CBCT Sections 1, 2, and 3 (**b**, **c**, **d**), and sagittal CBCT section through the buccal roots (**e**), depicting of a maxillary first and second premolar, both with a mid-root trifidity and three independent roots

5.7 Mandibular Molar Teeth

5.7.1 Radix Entomolaris and Radix Paramolaris

Mandibular molars will occasionally present with an additional separate root located either to the lingual (radix entomolaris) or to the buccal (radix paramolaris). The literature suggests the highest incidence of these morphologic variations is present in populations with Mongoloid ancestry (such as Asian, Eskimo, and Native Americans) and occurs at a frequency of 5–40% [36]. Although traditional two-dimensional imaging at various angles can reveal clues as to the presence of these additional roots (Fig. 5.18), uncovering their anatomic location during endodontic access can pose a clinical challenge. Therefore, a CBCT scan will not only confirm the presence of these extra roots but assist in determining the exact location of the canal orifice so that a proper access design can be planned (Fig. 5.19).

5.7.2 C-Shaped Roots

"C-shaped" anatomy is considered to be a variation in root morphology that causes the root to take on the shape of the letter "C" when viewed in cross-section (Fig. 5.20). This morphological configuration has been documented in several tooth types but is most common in mandibular second molars [37]. C-shaped canal configurations vary significantly among different ethnicities and have been reported to be as high as 44% among individuals of Asian descent [38]. The preoperative

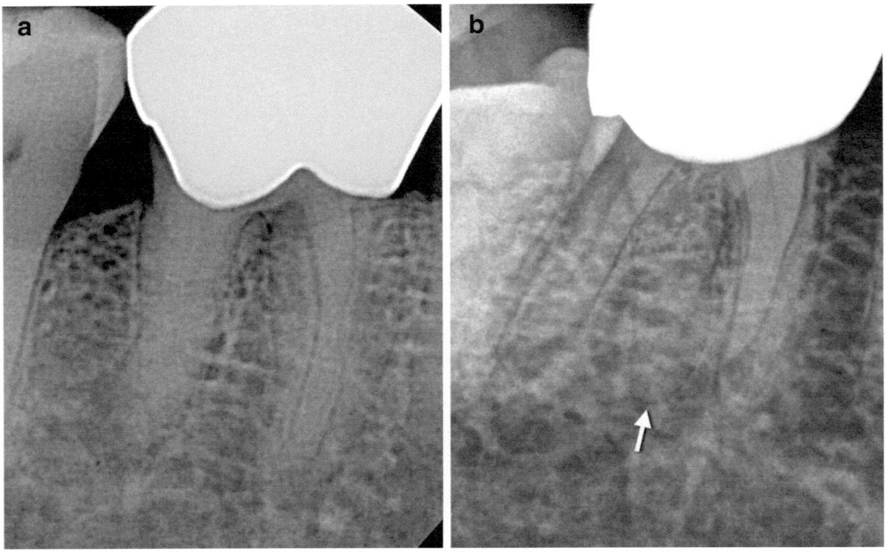

Fig. 5.18 Parallel periapical radiograph of a mandibular right first molar (**a**) and a corresponding distal cone shift radiograph (**b**) revealing the presence of an additional root (arrow), consistent with that of a radix endomolaris

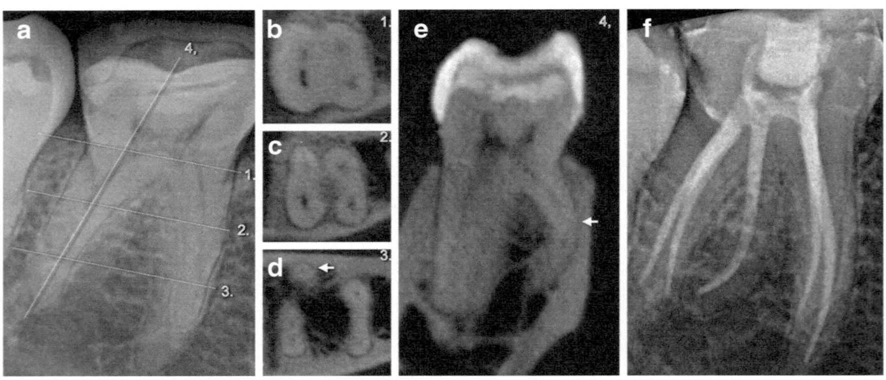

Fig. 5.19 Periapical radiograph of a mandibular right first molar (**a**), with corresponding axial CBCT Sections 1, 2, and 3 (**b**, **c**, **d**), and coronal CBCT section 4 (**e**), through the distal root, depicting an anatomical presentation of a radix endomolaris. Note the additional root positioned to the lingual (arrows). Post-endodontic periapical radiograph (**f**), shows the accurate clinical management of this complex anatomy *(Case courtesy of Dr. Hong Chon, Specialized Endodontic Solutions, Bloomingdale, IL)*

determination of C-shaped morphology using two-dimensional radiographic techniques is impossible and often not realized until after the endodontic access has been created. However, volumetric analysis of the axial plane on a preoperative CBCT scan will predictably identify these challenging root configurations before any irreversible treatment is rendered (Fig. 5.21).

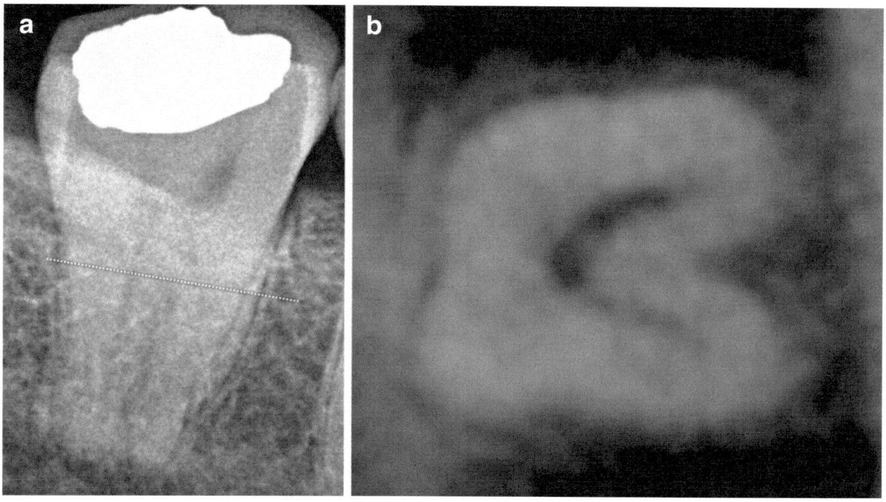

Fig. 5.20 Periapical radiograph of a mandibular second molar (**a**) and a corresponding mid-root axial CBCT section at the mid-root level (**b**) showing the internal and external root anatomy taking the form of a letter "C"

5.7.3 Isthmus Canals

An isthmus is often present between the buccal and lingual canals in mesial or distal roots of mandibular molar teeth. Occasionally, an additional canal (or root) can be identified and treated within this isthmus space. These canals are referred to (and labeled as) "middle mesial" or "middle distal" canals, respectively. Isthmus canals can be classified into three categories: fin (Fig. 5.22), confluent (Fig. 5.23), or independent (Fig. 5.24) [39]. The current literature reports a frequency of middle mesial canals ranging from 16% to 46% [40, 41]. The incidence of a middle distal canal is suggested to be much less, with the highest frequency reported at 3% (Fig. 5.25). It is possible to identify isthmus canals on preoperative CBCT scans. The usefulness of CBCT imaging in identifying and managing such canals has been well documented [42, 43]. Navigating the axial and coronal plane of the preoperative CBCT scan represents the most practical method to screen for potential isthmus canals.

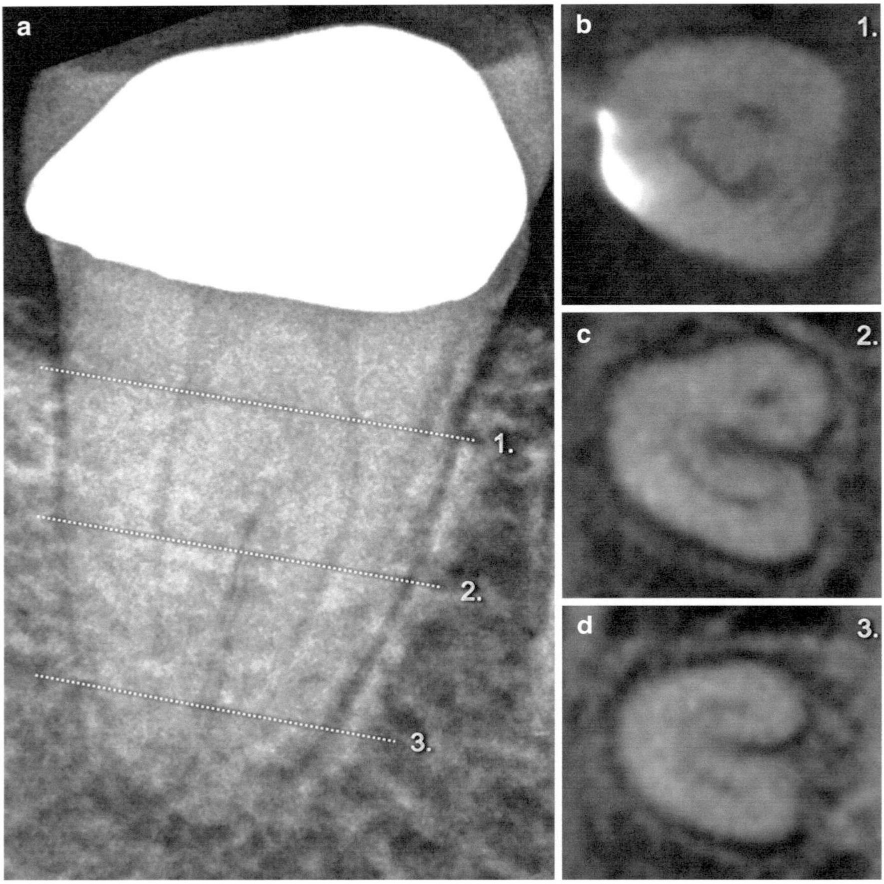

Fig. 5.21 Periapical radiograph (**a**) and corresponding axial CBCT Sections 1, 2, and 3 (**b**, **c**, **d**) of a C-shaped mandibular right second molar. Note the total canal confluence in axial CBCT Section 3 (**d**)

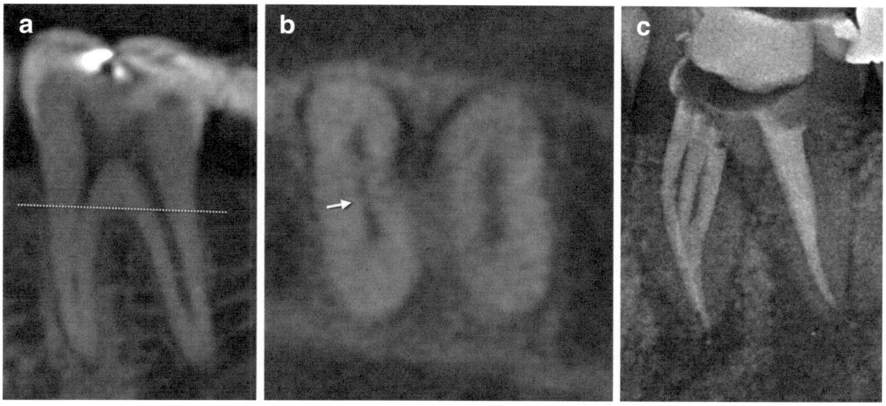

Fig. 5.22 Sagittal CBCT section (**a**) and corresponding mid-root axial CBCT section (**b**) depicting a "fin" isthmus canal type (arrow). Post-endodontic periapical radiograph (**c**) demonstrates the accurate clinical management of this canal configuration

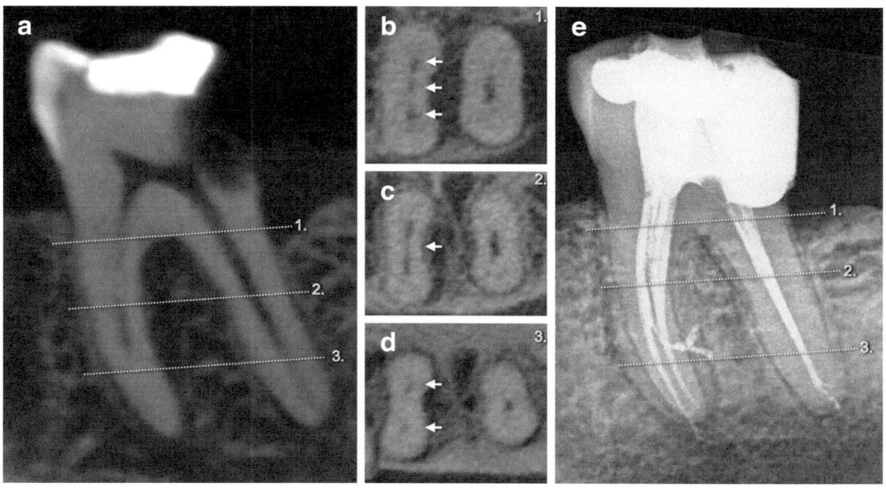

Fig. 5.23 Sagittal CBCT section (**a**) and corresponding axial CBCT Sections 1, 2, and 3 (**b**, **c**, **d**) depicting a "confluent" isthmus canal type. Note the three independent canals in the coronal section (**b**), the canal confluence in the mid-root section (**c**), and the bifidity in the apical section (**d**) (arrows). Post-endodontic periapical radiograph (**e**) demonstrates the accurate clinical management of this canal configuration

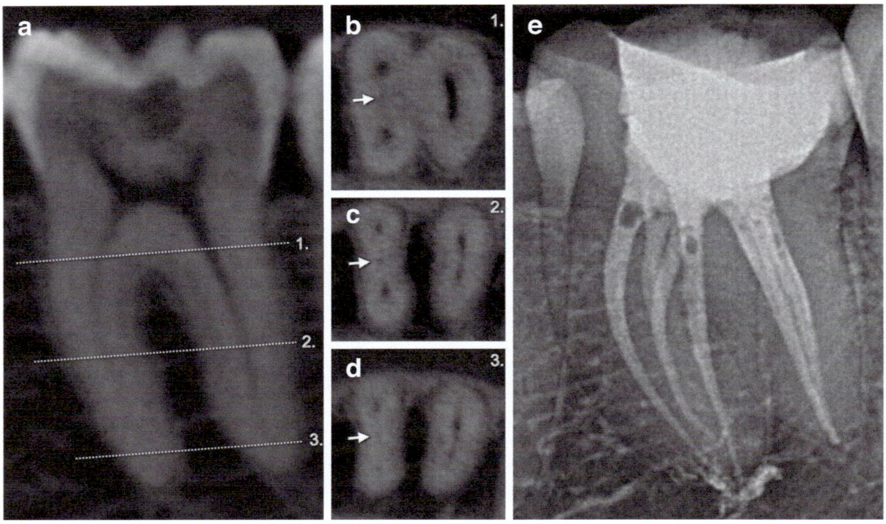

Fig. 5.24 Sagittal CBCT section (**a**) and corresponding axial CBCT Sections 1, 2, and 3 (**b**, **c**, **d**) depicting an "independent" isthmus canal type. Note three distinct canals present at all levels of the root canal system (arrows). Post-endodontic periapical radiograph (**e**) demonstrates the accurate clinical management of this canal configuration (*Case courtesy of Dr. Hong Chon, Specialized Endodontic Solutions, Bloomingdale, IL)*

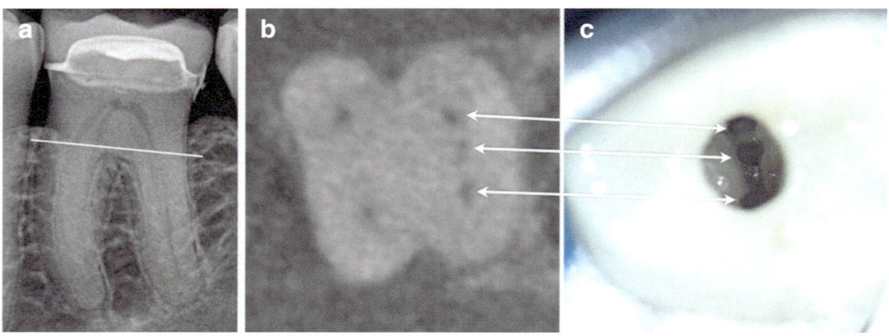

Fig. 5.25 Preoperative periapical radiograph of a left mandibular first molar (**a**) and corresponding axial CBCT section (**b**) demonstrating three identifiable distal canals. Corresponding clinical photo (**c**) demonstrating three instrumented distal canals through a conservative access design in the exact location as shown in the preoperative axial CBCT section (arrows)

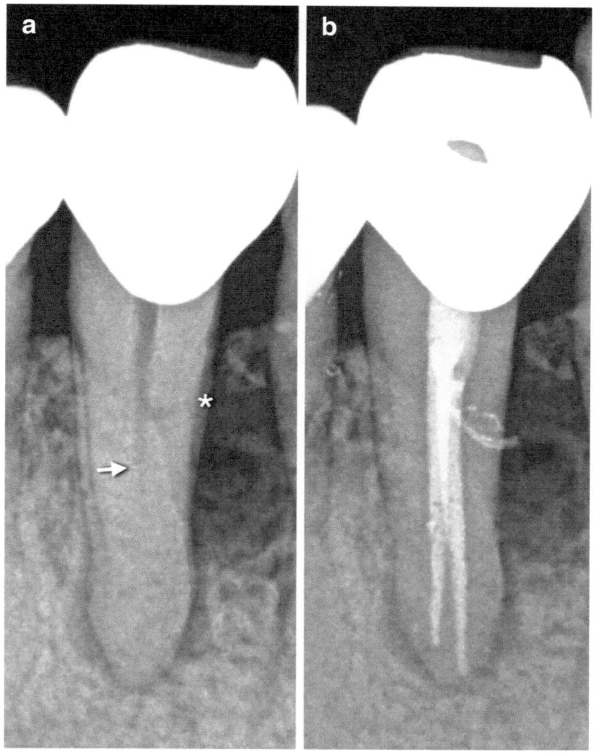

Fig. 5.26 Periapical radiographic of a mandibular right first premolar demonstrating the presence of a "fast break" (**a**). Note the abrupt absence of a visible canal at the mid-root level (arrow). Post-endodontic periapical radiograph (**b**) captured at nearly the same angulation, demonstrating the treatment of two separate root canal systems. Note the visible accessory anatomy (*) and its relationship to the lateral radiolucency

5.8 Mandibular Premolar Teeth

First and second mandibular premolars are reported to have one canal most of the time. However, when more than one canal exists, this additional anatomic feature is most often present on the lingual. The worldwide prevalence of a lingual canal in mandibular first premolars is close to 24% and just above 5% in mandibular second premolars [22]. The two-dimensional radiographic appearance of a "fast break" generally indicates a canal division [44] (Fig. 5.26); the buccal object rule is then used to interpret the position of the additional canal(s). Acquiring a preoperative CBCT scan will definitively determine the presence of an additional canal(s) (Fig. 5.27). In addition, CBCT imaging can accurately measure the distance to the canal division (Fig. 5.28) and reveal its exact spatial orientation, rendering the buccal object rule obsolete.

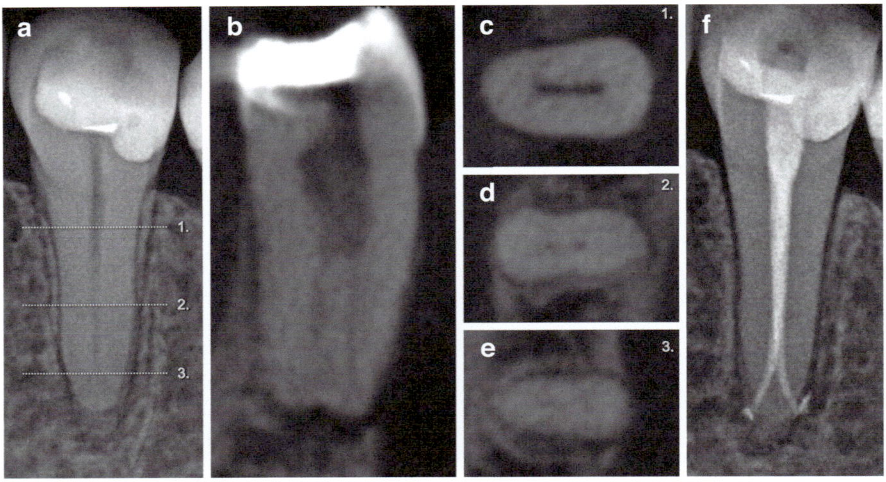

Fig. 5.27 Periapical radiograph of a mandibular left second premolar (**a**), with corresponding coronal CBCT section (**b**) demonstrating a mid-root division of the root canal system. Axial CBCT Sections 1, 2, and 3 (**c**, **d**, **e**) demonstrate a single canal bifurcating into two separate canals within a single root. Post-endodontic periapical radiograph (**f**) demonstrates the accurate clinical management of this canal configuration

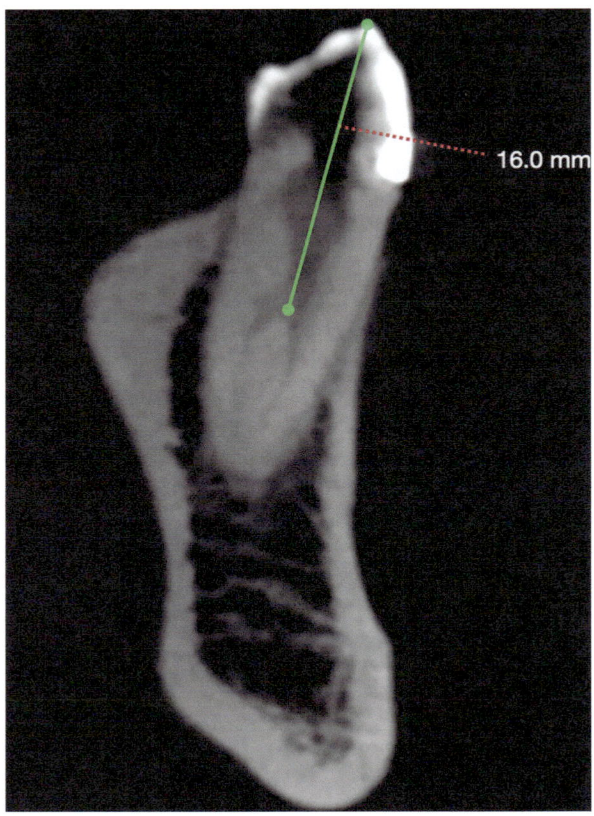

Fig. 5.28 Coronal CBCT section of a bifid mandibular first premolar demonstrates an accurate distance measurement to the exact level at which the canal division occurs

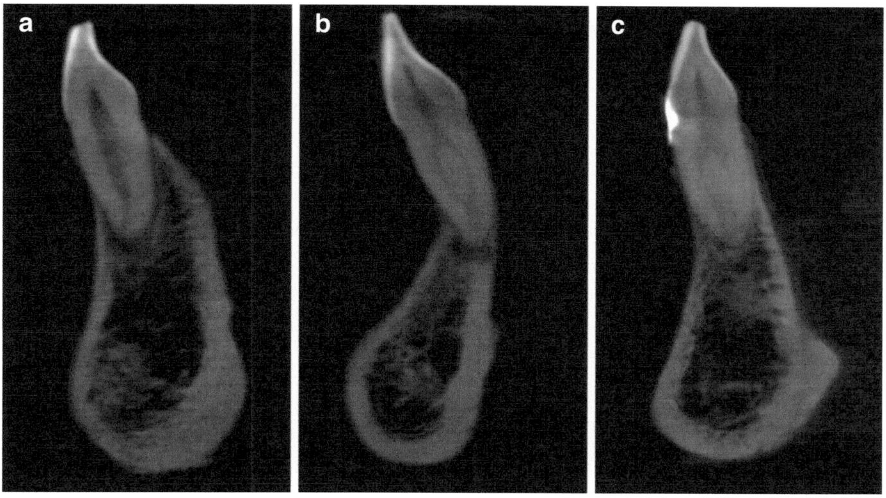

Fig. 5.29 Sagittal CBCT sections of three mandibular incisors demonstrating three different internal root canal configurations—a single canal with one portal of exit (**a**), two canals with a single portal of exit (**b**), and two canals with two separate portals of exit (**c**)

5.9 Mandibular Incisor Teeth

Mandibular central and lateral incisors are narrow mesiodistally and broad buccolingually, with corresponding ribbon-shaped root canal systems. Although most mandibular incisors are reported to have one canal, a dentinal bridge is often present, which can divide the pulp chamber into two separate canals. It is common for these two canals to rejoin into a single canal before reaching the apex, but it is also possible that each canal may lead to a separate portal of exit. The incidence of two canals has been reported to range from 12.4% to 53%, with 1.3% of these canals having separate foramina [45]. A more recent publication noted the frequency of multiple canals in mandibular central and lateral incisors to be 50% and 62%, respectively [46]. The sagittal and axial plane of a preoperative cone beam scan can determine the presence (or absence) of an additional canal and aid in creating an endodontic access designed for maximum visualization and conservation of tooth structure (Fig. 5.29).

5.10 Complex Canal Features

5.10.1 Accessory Canals

Multiple communications exist between the dental pulp and the surrounding periodontium via the apical foramen and accessory (lateral) canals. The distribution of accessory canals has been documented to occur at various levels throughout the root canal system as well as the floor of the pulp chamber, with the most significant number of accessory canals concentrated in the apical third of the root [3]. Occasionally, accessory canals can be identified on a CBCT scan. The verifiable

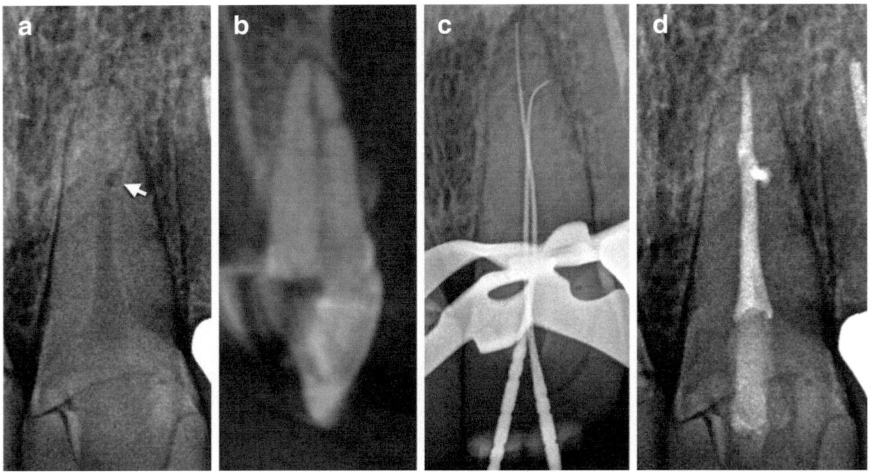

Fig. 5.30 Periapical radiograph of a maxillary left central incisor (**a**). Note the radiolucent area superimposed on the root in the apical third (arrow). The sagittal CBCT section (**b**) demonstrates the presence of an accessory canal with a buccal portal of exit. A mid-treatment periapical radiograph (**c**) demonstrates an endodontic file placed in the main root canal system, as well as the accessory anatomy. Post-endodontic periapical radiograph (**d**) demonstrates proper management of both the main root canal system, as well as the accessory anatomy

presence of these canals and the ability to measure their exact location can facilitate the successful treatment of such intricate ancillary anatomy (Fig. 5.30).

5.10.2 Canal Confluence

When two canals leave the pulp chamber and merge along the length of the root, the canals are considered confluent. The confluent canals can remain as a single canal, leading to one common portal of exit, or they may diverge—giving rise to multiple portals of exit. In addition, unions and divisions of canal space may occur numerous times throughout the length of the root canal system, creating multiple points of canal confluence. With the exception of severely rotated teeth, it is impossible to appreciate canal confluence using two-dimensional radiography. However, a CBCT scan viewed in the coronal and axial planes for posterior teeth or the sagittal and axial planes for anterior teeth provides an opportunity to identify the presence of canal confluence and the level at which the unions and divisions occur (Fig. 5.31).

5.10.3 Position of the Apical Foramen

The main anatomical opening of the root, through which nerves and blood vessels pass, represents the apical foramen. This anatomic landmark (generally positioned at or close to the root apex) represents the recommended level for which root canal instrumentation and obturation should terminate. It is not uncommon for the apical foramen to present in a coronal position relative to the radiographic apex [47].

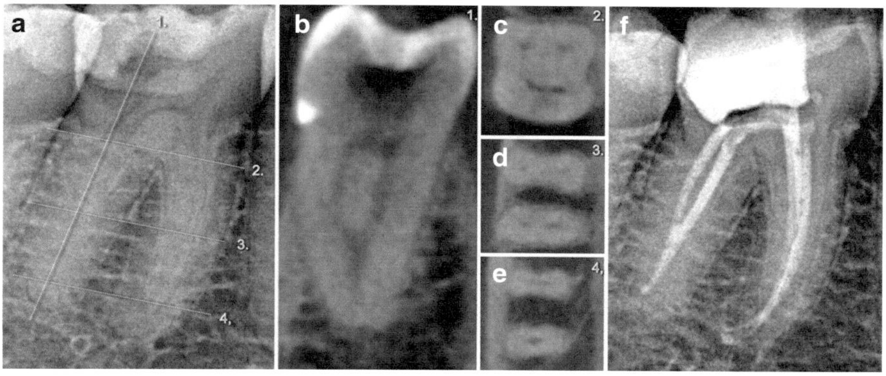

Fig. 5.31 Preoperative periapical radiograph of a right mandibular first molar (**a**), with corresponding coronal CBCT Section 1 of the distal root (**b**) demonstrating canal confluence of the root canal system in the apical third. Axial CBCT Sections 2, 3, and 4 (**c**, **d**, **e**) demonstrate canal confluence in both the mesial and distal root canal systems. Post-endodontic periapical radiograph (**f**) shows he accurate clinical management of this anatomy

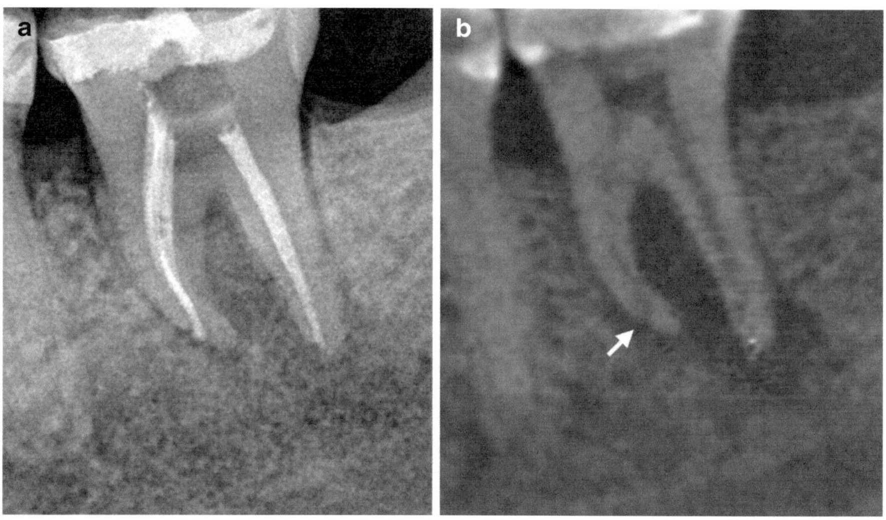

Fig. 5.32 Post-endodontic periapical radiograph of a left mandibular second molar (**a**) demonstrating a coronal position apical foramen on the mesial root, mimicking mismanaged root canal treatment in the apical third. The sagittal CBCT section (**b**) demonstrates a coronally positioned apical foramen in relation to the anatomic root apex (arrow), verifying accurate canal management

However, when this relationship is exaggerated, two-dimensional radiographs following endodontic treatment create an illusion of clinically inadequate, incomplete, or inappropriate canal management. A preoperative CBCT scan can reveal the actual position of the apical foramen as it relates to the anatomic root apex, therefore confirming (and validating) the proper treatment of these unique anatomic scenarios (Fig. 5.32).

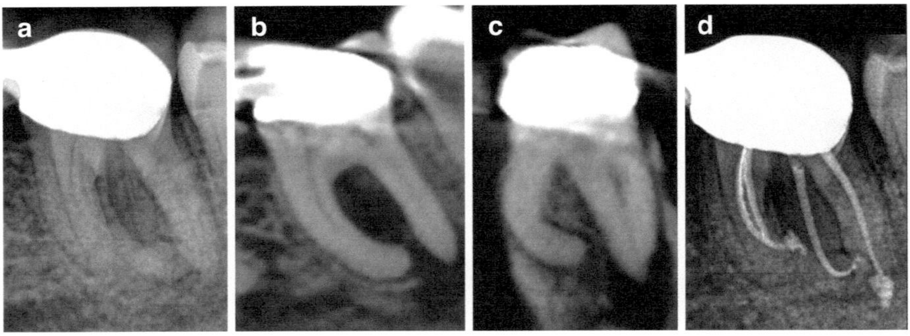

Fig. 5.33 Periapical radiograph of a mandibular left first molar (**a**), with apparent root curvature in the mesiodistal spacial plane. Sagittal CBCT section (**b**) confirms the mesiodistal curvature. The coronal CBCT section (**c**) reveals a significant curvature in the buccoligual spacial plane. Post-endodontic periapical radiograph (**d**) shows the accurate clinical management of this complex anatomy

5.10.4 Multi-Planar Root Curvature

The presence of root curvature has been shown to influence root canal instrumentation—the greater the curvature, the greater the risk for an iatrogenic error [48]. Root curvature does not occur linearly, as it may appear on a two-dimensional radiograph; it can be present in all three spatial planes, sometimes simultaneously. Therefore, the acquisition of a preoperative CBCT scan can be used to identify multi-planar root curvature before initiating root canal treatment (Fig. 5.33). Understanding the location, degree, and relationship of root curvature in all three planes can help avoid (or minimize) the likelihood of iatrogenic errors during root canal treatment.

5.10.5 Dens Invaginatus

Dens invaginatus has been suggested to be one of the most prevalent developmental tooth anomalies clinically observed, occurring at a reported frequency between 1% and 10% [49]. It results from an infolding of the enamel organ into the dental papilla during tooth development before the calcification process. Dens invaginatus mostly affects maxillary lateral incisors but has also been reported in maxillary central incisors, canines, and premolars [50]. These developmental anomalies present with varying degrees of complexity and cannot be fully appreciated with two-dimensional radiographic imaging. The acquisition of a preoperative CBCT scan will reveal, in detail, the intricacies of these convoluted anatomic challenges. When the internal anatomy of these developmental anomalies can be viewed and studied in all three spatial planes, the clinical treatment approach can be more predictable (Fig. 5.34).

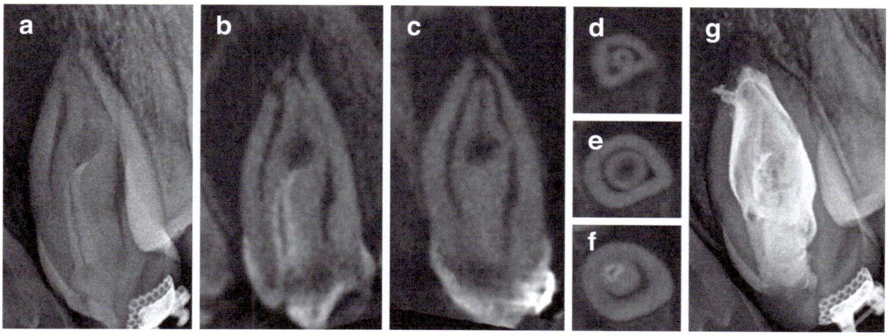

Fig. 5.34 Periapical radiograph (**a**) of a maxillary left lateral incisor presenting with dens invaginatus. Coronal and sagittal CBCT sections (**b**, **c**), as well as axial CBCT sections captured from the apical third (**d**), mid-root (**e**), and coronal third (**f**), demonstrate the complex anatomical configuration of the developmental anomaly. Post-endodontic periapical radiograph (**g**), shows the accurate clinical management of this complex anatomy (*Case courtesy of Dr. Hong Chon, Specialized Endodontic Solutions, Bloomingdale, IL)*

5.11 Conclusion

Different root shapes may appear at any level within a single root. Two-dimensional radiographs make the root canal system appear uniform and consistent in shape, and aberrant canal configurations are not generally visible. The more CBCT volumes that are viewed, the more the realization that unconventional anatomy should be considered the norm rather than the exception.

Proper knowledge of root canal anatomy and morphology will cue the astute clinician to look for canal orifices in typically observed locations. However, canals are not always readily apparent or easily identified. Cone beam imaging has introduced an accurate, non-destructive, real-time method for clinical chair-side evaluation of tooth anatomy and morphology—comparable to the histologic gold standard. Incorporating a preoperative CBCT scan into the mainstream radiographic imaging protocol can significantly enhance the clinician's ability to manage complex root anatomy.

References

1. Walton WE, Vertucci FJ. Internal anatomy. In: Walton WE, Torabinejad M, editors. Principles and practice of endodontics. 3rd ed. Philadelphia: Saunders; 2002. p. 176–81.
2. Hess W. Formation of root canals in human teeth II. J Nat Dental Assoc. 1921;8:790–832.
3. Gutmann JL, Fan B. Tooth morphology, isolation, and access. In: Hargreaves KM, Berman LH, editors. Cohen's pathways of the pulp. 11th ed. St. Louis: Elsevier; 2016. p. 130–208.
4. Grover C, Shetty N. Methods to study root canal morphology: a review. In: Bonaccorso A, Chong BS, Schafer E, van der Sluis L, editors. ENDO—endodontic practice today. 2012; 6(3):171–188.

5. Gomes BP, Rodrigues H, Tancredo N. The use of modeling technique to investigate the root canal morphology of mandibular incisors. Int Endod J. 1996;29:29–36.
6. Eder A, Kantor M, Moser T, Gahleitner A, Schedle A, Sperr W. Root canal system in the mesiobuccal root of the maxillary first molar: and in vitro comparison study of computer tomography and histology. Dentinomax Radiol. 2006;35:175–7.
7. Michetti J, Maret D, Mallet JP, Diemer F. Validation of come beam computed tomography as a tool to explore root canal anatomy. J Endod. 2010;36:1187–90.
8. Neelakantan P, Subbarao C, Subbarao CV. Comparative evaluation of modified canal clearing technique, cone beam computed tomography, peripheral quantitative computed tomography, spiral computed tomography, and plain and contrast medium-enhances digital radiography in studying root canal morphology. J Endod. 2010;36:1547–51.
9. Blattner TC, George N, Lee CC, Kumar V, Yelton DJ. Efficacy of cone beam computed tomography as a modality to accurately identify the presence of second mesiobuccal canals in maxillary first and second molars: a pilot study. J Endod. 2010;36:867–79.
10. Teary S, Luzon J, Hartwell G. Endodontic radiography: who is reading the digital radiograph? J Endod. 2011;37:919–21.
11. Weine FS, Healey HJ, Gerstein H, Evanson L. Canal configuration in the mesiobuccal root of the maxillary first molar and its endodontic significance. Oral Surg Oral Med Oral Pathol. 1969;28:419–25.
12. Gulabivala K, Aung TH, Ng YL. Root and canal morphology of Burmese mandibular molars. Int Endod J. 2001;34(5):359–70.
13. Sert S, Bayiril GS. Evaluation of root canal configurations of the mandibular and maxillary permanent teeth by gender in the Turkish population. J Endod. 2004;30:391–8.
14. Krasner P, Rankow HJ. Anatomy of the pulp chamber floor. J Endod. 2004;30:5–16.
15. Patel S, Dawood A, Whaites E, Pitt FT. New dimensions in endodontic imaging: part 1: conventional and alternative radiographic systems. Int Endod J. 2009;42:447–62.
16. Estrela C, Bueno MR, Sousa-Neto MD, Pecora JD. Method for determination of root curvature radius using cone-beam computed tomography images. Braz Dent J. 2008;19:114–8.
17. Scarfe WC, Farman AG, Sukovic P. Clinical applications if cone-beam computed tomography in dental practice. J Can Dent Assoc. 2006;72:75–80.
18. Ee J, Fayad MI, Johnson BR. Comparison of endodontic diagnosis and treatment planning decisions using cone-beam volumetric tomography versus periapical radiography. J Endod. 2014;40:910–6.
19. Rodriguez G, Abella F, Duran-Sindreu F, Patel S, Roig M. Influence of cone-beam computed tomography in clinical decision making among specialists. J Endod. 2017;43:194–9.
20. Vizzotto MB, Silveira PF, Arus NA, Montagner F, Gomes BO, da Silveira HE. CBCT for the assessment of second mesiobuccal (MB2) canals in maxillary molar teeth: effect of voxel size and presence of root filling. Int Endod J. 2013;46:870–6.
21. von Zuben M, Martins JN, Berti L, et al. Worldwide prevalence of mandibular second molar C- shaped morphologies evaluated by cone-beam computed tomography. J Endod. 2017;43:1442–7.
22. Martins JNR, et al. Worldwide prevalence of a lingual canal in mandibular premolars: a multicenter cross-sectional study with meta-analysis. J Endod. 2021;47:1253–64.
23. Kotoor J, Velmurugan N, Sudha R, Hemamalathi S. Maxillary first molar with seven root canals diagnosed with cone-beam computed tomography: a case report. J Endod. 2010;36:915–21.
24. Zoya-Farook A, Abhishek P, Shahabadi A. Cone-beam computed tomographic evaluation and endodontic management of a mandibular first premolar with type IX canal configuration: case report. J Endod. 2017;43:1207–13.
25. Ring J, Ring KC. Rare root canal configuration of mandibular second premolar using cone-beam computed tomographic scanning. J Endod. 2017;43:1897–900.
26. Kulild JC, Peters DD. Incidence and configuration of canal systems in the mesiobuccal root of maxillary first and second molars. J Endod. 1990;16:311–6.
27. Martins JNR, et al. Worldwide analyses of maxillary first molar second mesiobuccal prevalence: a multicenter cone-beam computed tomographic study. J Endod. 2018;44:1641–9.

28. Zhang Q, Chen H, Fan B, Fan W, Gutmann J. Root and root canal morphologies in maxillary second molar with fused root from a native Chinese population. J Endod. 2014;40:871–85.
29. Martins JNR, Mata A, Marques D, Carames J. Prevalence of root fusions and main root canal merging inhuman upper and lower molars—a CBCT in vivo study. J Endod. 2016;42:900–8.
30. Ordinola-Zapata R, Martins JNR, Bramante CM, Villas-Boas MH, Duarte MH, Versiani MA. Morphological evaluation of maxillary second molars with fused roots: a micro-CT study. Int Endod J. 2017;50:1–9.
31. Al Shalabi RM, Omer OE, Glennon J, et al. Root canal anatomy of maxillary first and second permanent molars. Int Endod J. 2000;33:405–14.
32. Wasti F, Shearer AC, Wilson NH. Root canal systems of the mandibular and maxillary first permanent molar teeth of south Asian Pakistanis. Int Endod J. 2001;34:263–6.
33. Kartal N, Ozcelik B, Cimilli H. Root canal morphology of maxillary premolars. J Endod. 1998;24:417–9.
34. Beltes P, Kalaitzoglou ME, Kantilieraki E, Beltes C, Angelopoulos C. 3-rooted maxillary first premolars: and *ex vivo* study of external and internal morphologies. J Endod. 2017;43:1267–72.
35. Wolf TG, Kozaczek C, Campus G, Paque F, Wierichs RJ. Root canal morphology of 116 maxillary second premolars by micro-computed tomography in a mixed Swiss-German population with systematic review. J Endod. 2020;46:1639–47.
36. De Moor R, Deroose C, Calberson F. The radix entomolaris in mandibular first molars: an endodontic challenge. Int Endod J. 2004;37:789–99.
37. Jin GC, Lee SJ, Roh BD. Anatomical study of C-shaped canals in mandibular second molars by analysis of computed tomography. J Endod. 2006;32:10–3.
38. Chai WL, Thong YL. Cross sectional morphology and minimum canal wall widths in c-shaped roots of mandibular molars. J Endod. 2004;30:509–12.
39. Weinberg EM, Pedra AE, Khurana S, Lotikar PP, Falcon C, Hirschberg C. Incidence of middle mesial canals based on distance between mesial canal orifices in mandibular molars: a clinical and cone-beam computed tomographic analysis. J Endod. 2020;46:40–3.
40. Tahmasbi M, Jalali P, Nair MK, Bargham S, Nair UP. Prevalence of middle mesial canals and isthmi in the mesial root of mandibular molars: and *in vivo* cone-beam computed tomographic study. J Endod. 2017;43:1080–3.
41. Azim AA, Deutsch AS, Solomon CS. Prevalence of middle mesial canals in mandibular molars after guided troughing under high magnification: an in vivo investigation. J Endod. 2015;41:164–8.
42. Ahmed HA, Abubakr NH, Yahia NA, Ibrahim YE. Root and canal morphology of permanent mandibular molars in a Sudanese population. Int Endod J. 2007;40:766–71.
43. La SH, Jung DH, Kim EC, Min KS. Identification of independent middle mesial canal in mandibular first molar using cone-beam computed tomography imaging. J Endod. 2010;237:1–4.
44. Slowey RR. Radiographic aids in the detection of extra root canals. Oral Surg Oral Med Oral Pathol. 1974;37:762–72.
45. Boruah LC, Bhuyan AC. Morphologic characteristics of root canal of mandibular incisors in North-East Indian population: an in vitro study. J Conserv Dent. 2011;14:346–50.
46. Leoni GB, Versiani MA, Pecora JD, de Sousa-Neto MD. Micro-computed tomographic analysis of the root canal morphology of mandibular incisors. J Endod. 2014;40:710–6.
47. Souza RA, Figueiredo JAP, Colombo S, Dantas JCP, Lago M, Pecora JD. Location of the apical foramen and its relationship with foramina file size. Dental Press Endod. 2011;1:64–8.
48. van der Vyver PJ, Vorster M, Palerker F, de Wet FA. Errors in root canal preparation: a review of the literature and clinical case reports. SADJ. 2019;74:246–54.
49. Alani A, Bishop K. Dens invaginatus: part 1—classification, prevalence and aetiology. Int Endod J. 2008;41:1123–36.
50. Siqueria JF, Rocas IN, Hernandez SR, Brissin-Suarez K, Baasch AC, Perez AR, Alvez FRF. Dens invaginatus: clinical implications and antimicrobial endodontic treatment considerations. J Endod. 2022;48:161–70.

Non-surgical Retreatment Utilizing Cone Beam Computed Tomography

6

Stephen P. Niemczyk

Abstract

Successful discovery and localization of all roots and potential canal spaces are critical to favorable endodontic outcomes and therapies. This is especially challenging in the retreatment environment, where the native anatomy within the chamber has been altered or destroyed, and conventional radiographs are inconclusive. The use of the Cone Beam Computed Tomography (CBCT) has proven indispensable in these instances, focusing any excavation in the proper dimension and direction to facilitate a more thorough treatment delivery. The exceptional analysis of these difficult presentations afforded by the use of this technology is illustrated using various clinical case scenarios, including anomalous root morphologies, additional canal spaces, and insights into eccentric periapical pathologies.

The primary tenet for conventional endodontic therapy is the negotiation, debridement, and disinfection of the affected and infected canal spaces [1, 2]. Advances in instrumentation notwithstanding, successful outcomes have been enhanced through the widespread utilization, at the specialist level, of the surgical operating microscope (SOM). It has proven itself indispensable in locating canals [3], identifying the location of MB_2 [4–6], removing separated instruments [7], perforation repair [8], and generally enhancing the delivery of quality care [9]. The mantra for its use, especially in the surgical environment, is "if you can see it better, you can do it

S. P. Niemczyk (✉)
Albert Einstein Medical Center, Dental Department in Philadelphia, Philadelphia, PA, USA

Walter Reed National Medical Center in Bethesda, Bethesda, MD, USA

U. S. Army Endodontic Residency Program in Fort Gordon, Fort Gordon, GA, USA

M. I. Fayad, B. R. Johnson (eds.), *3D Imaging in Endodontics*,
https://doi.org/10.1007/978-3-031-32755-1_6

better." While this holds true for structures readily apparent, what is our recourse for those anatomical variants that are not so easily disclosed or discovered? The corollary then becomes "you can only treat what you can see" especially when evaluating the patient in the pretreatment phase of the procedure. Clinicians have long relied on varied resources for the basis of their preoperative assessments. The classic India-ink perfusions by Hess [10] provided insights into the variation and complexity of the canal spaces in extracted teeth but, along with other observations in extracted teeth [5, 11], furnished only postmortem evidence about canal morphology. There are numerous reports of clinical observations employing radiographs [12, 13] or using various methods of magnification for canal discovery [14]. Empiricism also plays a significant role, but experience cannot be taught or contained in a textbook. An important element to consider with all these methodologies is that they are not patient-specific and may not be an accurate representation of an anatomical variant that submits for clinical treatment.

It is in this regard that the cone beam computed tomography (CBCT) has proven invaluable and, in terms of its impact on the discipline of endodontics, could be regarded as the surgical operating microscope of the twenty-first century. The ability to view the selected field from an infinite number of angles, coupled with a 3-D rendered perspective of the jaw segment, enables the clinician to perform a "Virtual Surgery"© [15] in the selected field that is patient specific and non-destructive. The ability to discern the size, number, and location of canals using the CBCT is statistically superior when compared to conventional imaging [16–18]. It is especially advantageous when employing this technology as an inter-treatment survey for the location of undisclosed canals that may be atypically placed or dystrophically obscured [19]. A critical assessment as to the location and depth of the missing canal relative to known anatomical landmarks within the root is paramount to the successful acquisition in teeth that have been prosthetically altered. The margin for error can be miniscule when considering the available width and fragility of the root form undergoing treatment. An example of this challenge is presented in the first clinical case (Sect. 6.1, Case #1). An appreciation for the number and curvature of the roots is reinforced when surveying the cone beam scan that is absent in a two-dimensional assessment of the same tooth [20–23], especially in light of geographic diversity and variations. The presence of periapical disease can be masked in the uniplanar image because of the overlying structures; a scan of the same site often reveals obvious pathology coincident with the patient's signs and symptoms [24, 25]. Collectively, this expansion of available data expedites a focused and patient-centric treatment decision tree, where options and pitfalls can be disclosed with a greater degree of confidence and accomplished without subjecting the patient to unnecessary procedures or empirical guesswork. This is especially germane when a retreatment is being considered, where oftentimes the internal anatomy may be obliterated, and the accompanying visual cues to certain structures are altered or nonexistent.

Case 1: #5 Calcified Access

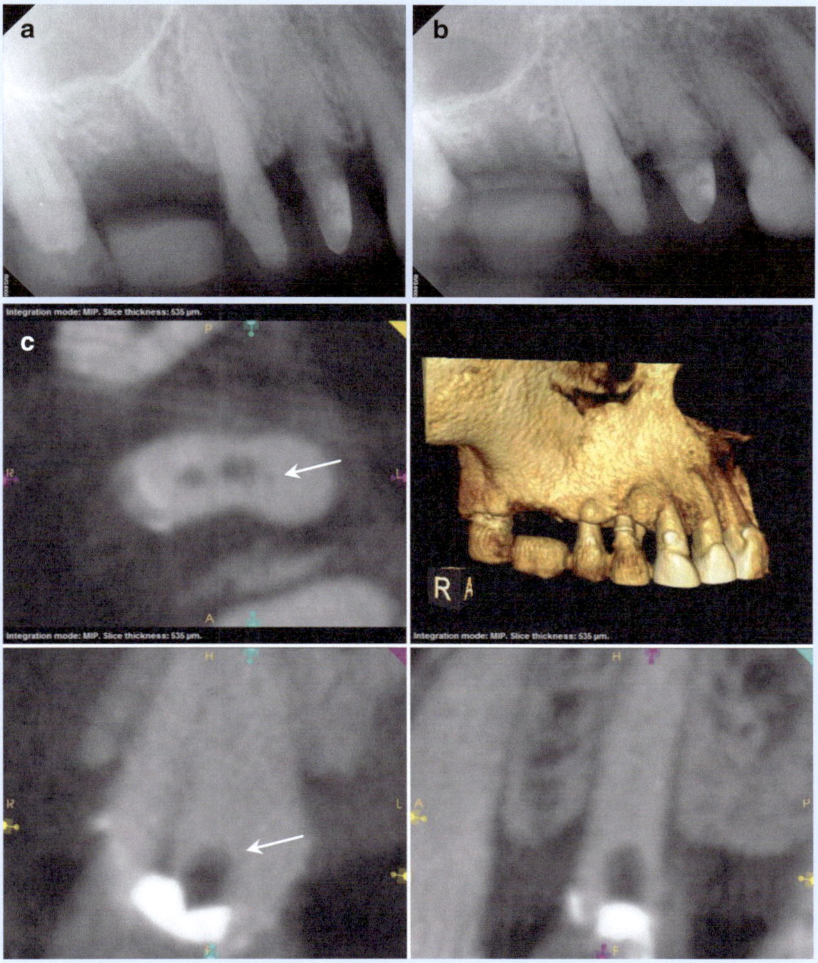

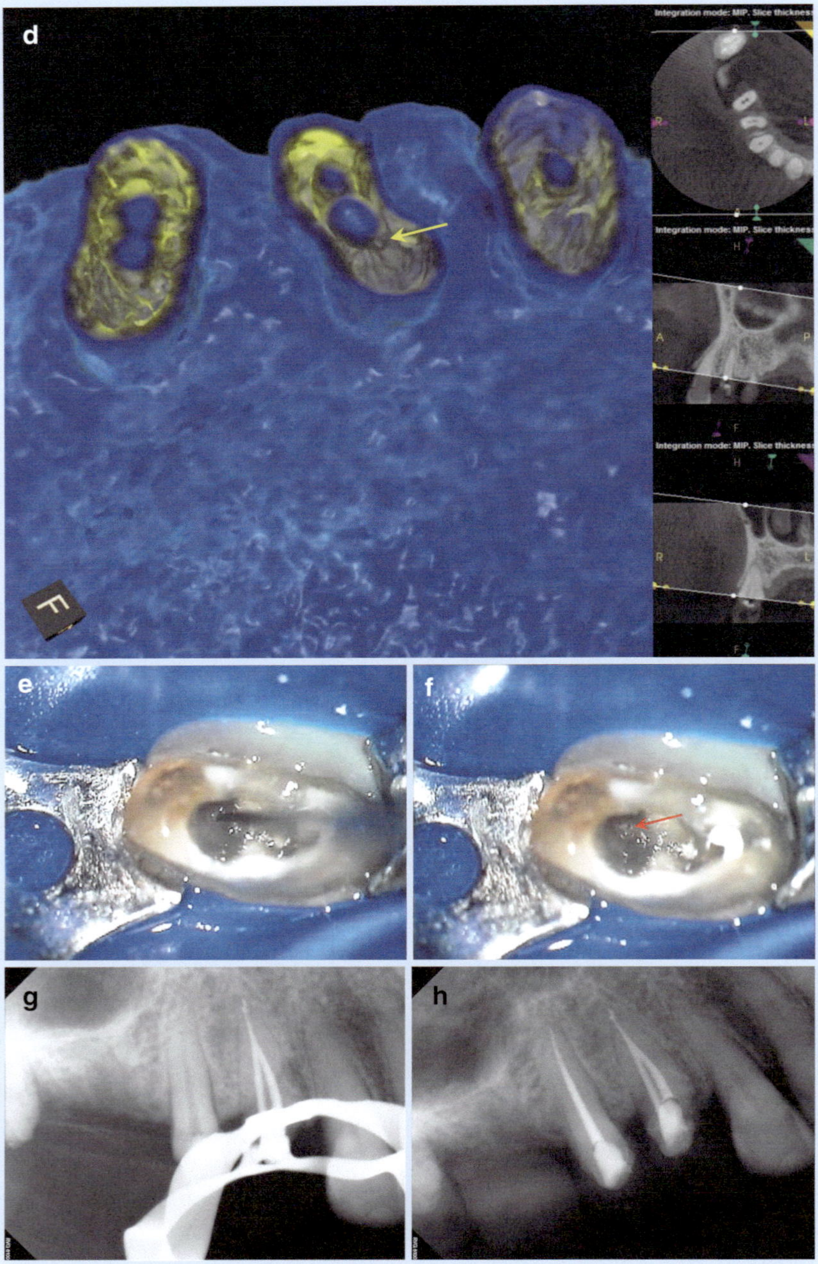
d
F
e
f
g
h

Case 1 Description: The patient presents for intentional treatment of #4/5 for prosthetic reasons.

1 a,b: Preoperative radiographs reveal dystrophic obliteration of the canal spaces in tooth #5. Access and instrumentation was performed on #4, but only the buccal canal in #5 could be located.

1 c: An intra-treatment CBCT disclosed the location of the palatal canal 1 mm palatal and mesial to the area of ultrasonic excavation (white arrow). Note the kidney bean shape and mesial invagination of the root form not appreciated on the 2-D image.

1 d: A colorized axial section of the 3-D model demonstrates the instrumented canal diameters of #4, and the location of the palatal canal (yellow arrow) in #5.

1 e,f: Using a NiTi D-11T spreader as an explorer, the palatal canal space is engaged, and the orifice uncovered (red arrow). A small file will be inserted into the canal for verification and working length measurement.

1 g,h: Mid-obturation and final radiographs. Precise triangulation and accurate measurements guided the conservative excavation and location of this "calcified" canal in a critical abutment.

It is this arena of retreatment, or "revision" of an endodontically treated tooth that is failing, that has garnered the majority of attention and case reports in the literature involving CBCT. One retrospective study [26] reported that missed canal anatomy was responsible for 48% of the unsuccessful initial therapies in molars, with the preponderance being the mesiobuccal root of maxillary first molars. The authors, in their concluding statements, made the following observation: "Given that failure to locate all canal systems of a tooth contributes significantly to unsuccessful endodontic treatment, all measures available to the clinician to maximize canal identification should be used." While it is not an outright endorsement of the technology, it presents a compelling argument for cone beam scanning of not only teeth requiring retreatment, but also any tooth that demonstrates an "other than normal" initial radiographic appearance. Although not currently promoted for initial therapy, prudent scanning of selected cases can maximize the operators' understanding of the underlying morphology and allow them to confidently address the anatomy. Although not guaranteeing success, it is a significant step toward enhancing the outcome and reducing the likelihood of future treatment interventions.

An appropriate introduction to the non-surgical use of CBCT would be with the simplest of all retreatments and one that is illustrative of the teeth in the above referenced study: missed canal anatomy in the mesiobuccal roots of maxillary molars

(Sect. 6.2, Case #2). The patient had received treatment for both teeth within the previous 14 months and had remained symptomatic for much of that time. Conventional radiographs failed to disclose any significant clues as to the etiology, and the patient was presenting for consultation. Unfortunately, this clinical scenario is not that unusual, and it is frustrating for the patient who is often told that "nothing is showing up in the X-rays."

Case 2: #2,3 Retreatment: Undiagnosed MB_2 canal

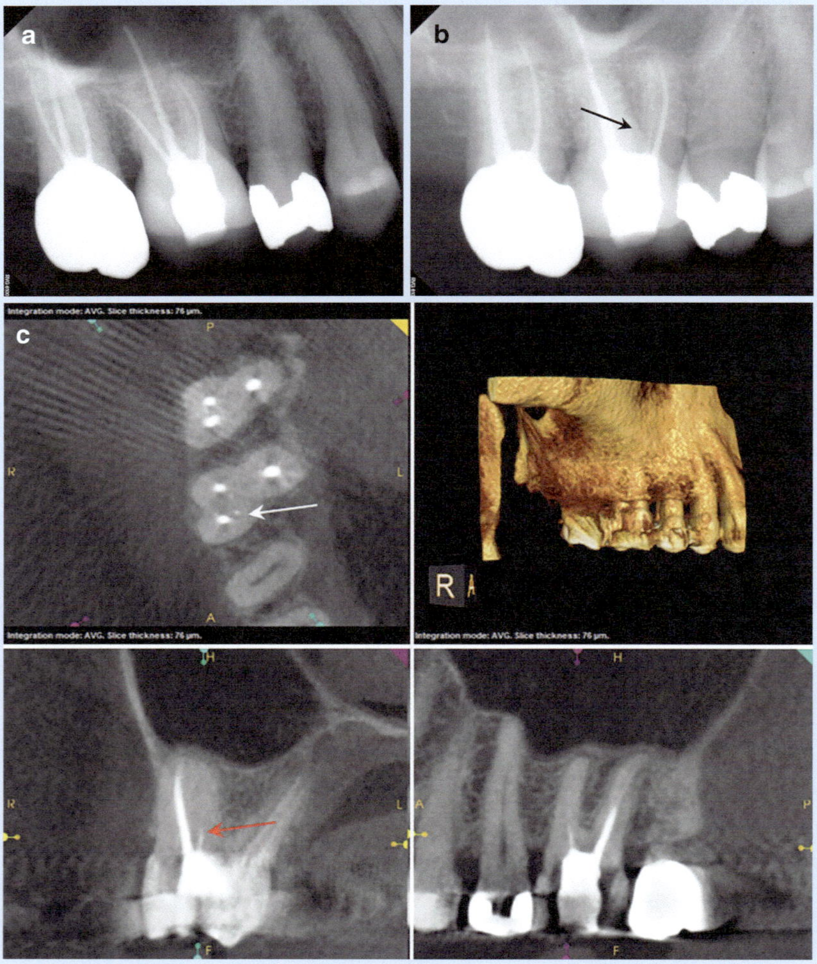

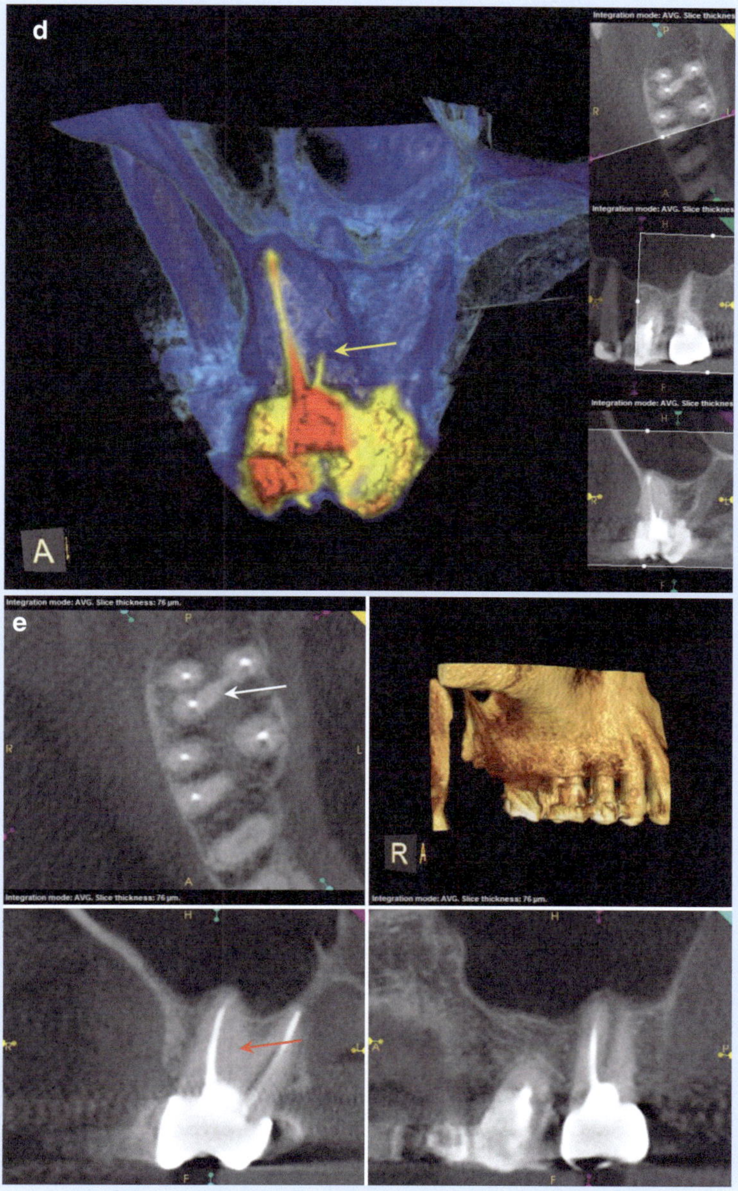
d
e
A
R
Integration mode: AVG. Slice thickness: 76 µm.
P
R
L
A
H
F

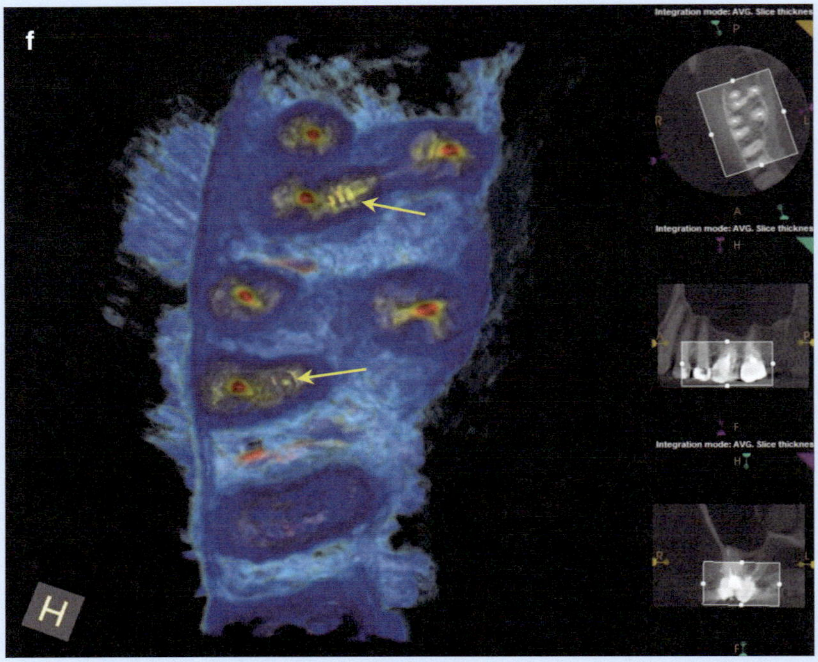

Case 2 Description: The patient had RCT in teeth #2/3 approximately 14 months ago; both teeth have remained symptomatic. She is presenting for consultation.

2 a,b: Preoperative radiographs disclose no obvious periapical pathology, but the obturation of the MB root in #3 appears to be off-center, and a thin radio-opaque line is evident slightly distal to the filled MB canal (black arrow).

2 c: The axial section of #3 reveals a small high-density dot palatal to the MB_1 canal (white arrow). The location as well as the configuration relative to the MB_1 (red arrow) is suggestive of a sealer tract in the uninstrumented MB_2 canal.

2 d: The colorized 3-D coronal section highlights the presence of the sealer in MB_2, with a similar density to the root canal filling material (yellow arrow).

2 e: The axial section of #2 demonstrates a broad fusion of the MB and palatal roots (white arrow), while the coronal section reveals a low-density line that is suggestive of MB_2 (red arrow).
2 f: The colorized 3-D axial section discloses the sealer tract in #3 and an area of dentin density in the MB root of #2 that may contain the MB_2 canal (yellow arrows).

The CBCT of posterior segment revealed the presence of MB_2 in teeth #2 and #3, with slight edema at the respective apices. Axial sections demonstrated the typical asymmetrically located obturations, with evidence of the MB_2 either as a sealer streak (#3) or a radiolucent dot. These features are even more evident when examining the coronal sections of the MB root. Especially interesting is the colorized coronal section of #3, with the MB_2 canal orifice clearly patent enough to accept the sealer.

A more subtle example of a missed canal is shown in the next case (Sect. 6.3, Case #3) involving tooth #18. The patient presented with similar signs and symptoms, with the past dental history of treatment and subsequent retreatment without resolution. The tooth was diagnosed as "fractured" and was presenting for consultation prior to extraction. The typical signs of fracture were not present in the preoperative exam or radiographs (deep isolated probing depths, vertical bone defects), but the multiple radiographic angles did accentuate the asymmetry of the obturation in the seemingly fused root form. A seasoned practitioner would observe this asymmetry and suspect an additional canal, but two principal questions remain: where would you commence the excavation, and in what direction? Careful examination of the axial sections, slice by slice, disclosed a minute sealer streak 4 mm from the floor of the chamber and inclined toward the mesiolingual line angle of the root. Coincidentally, the root is also slightly more bulbous in the same area: further evidence of an additional canal. Colorized versions of the axial and coronal sections illustrated the extent and angle of this streak, enhancing the three-dimensional comprehension preoperatively. Careful measurements and directional landmarks simplified the discovery of the mesiolingual canal after the filling materials were harvested, allowing for negotiation and debridement of the missing canal. The patient was asymptomatic after 1 week and has remained so since.

Case #3: #18 Retreatment: Undiagnosed ML canal

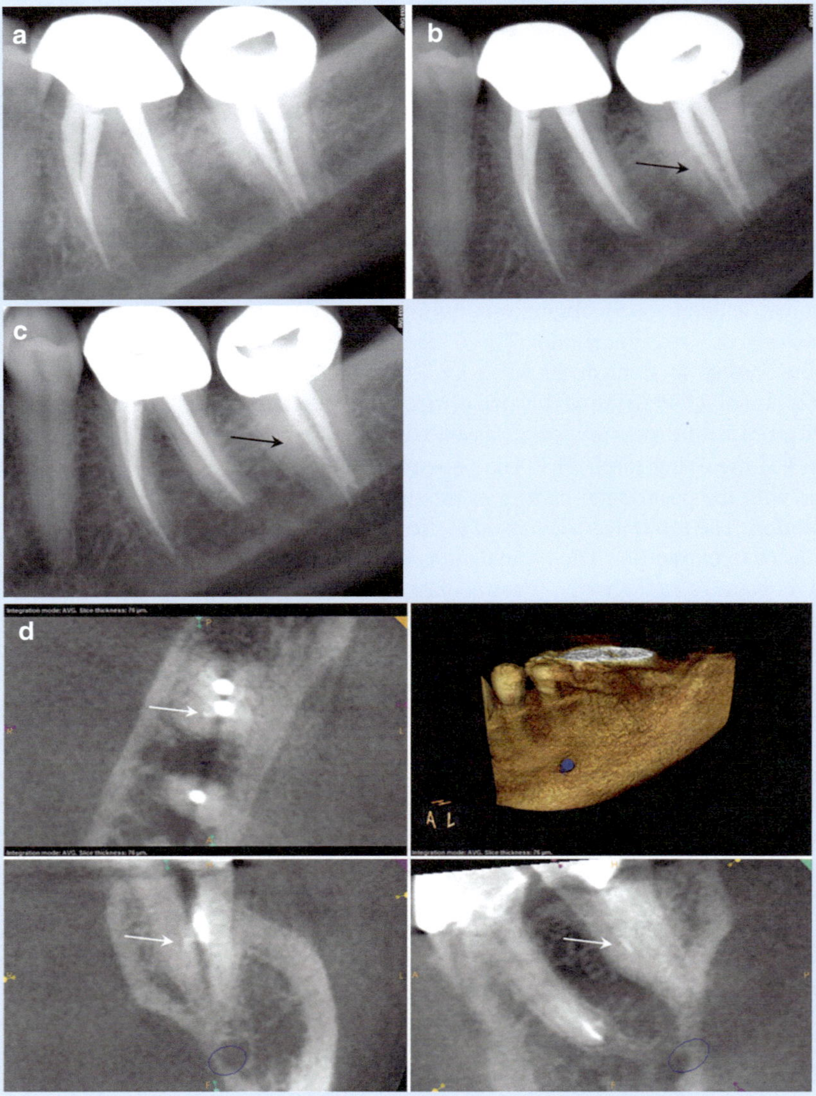

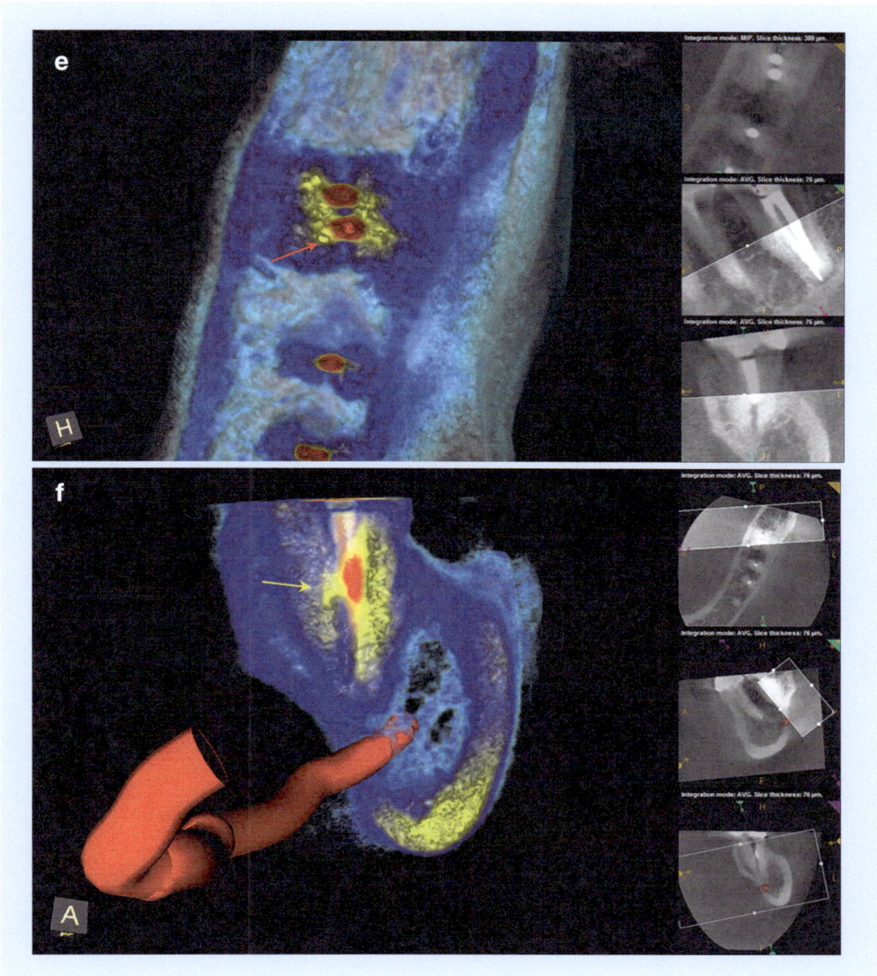

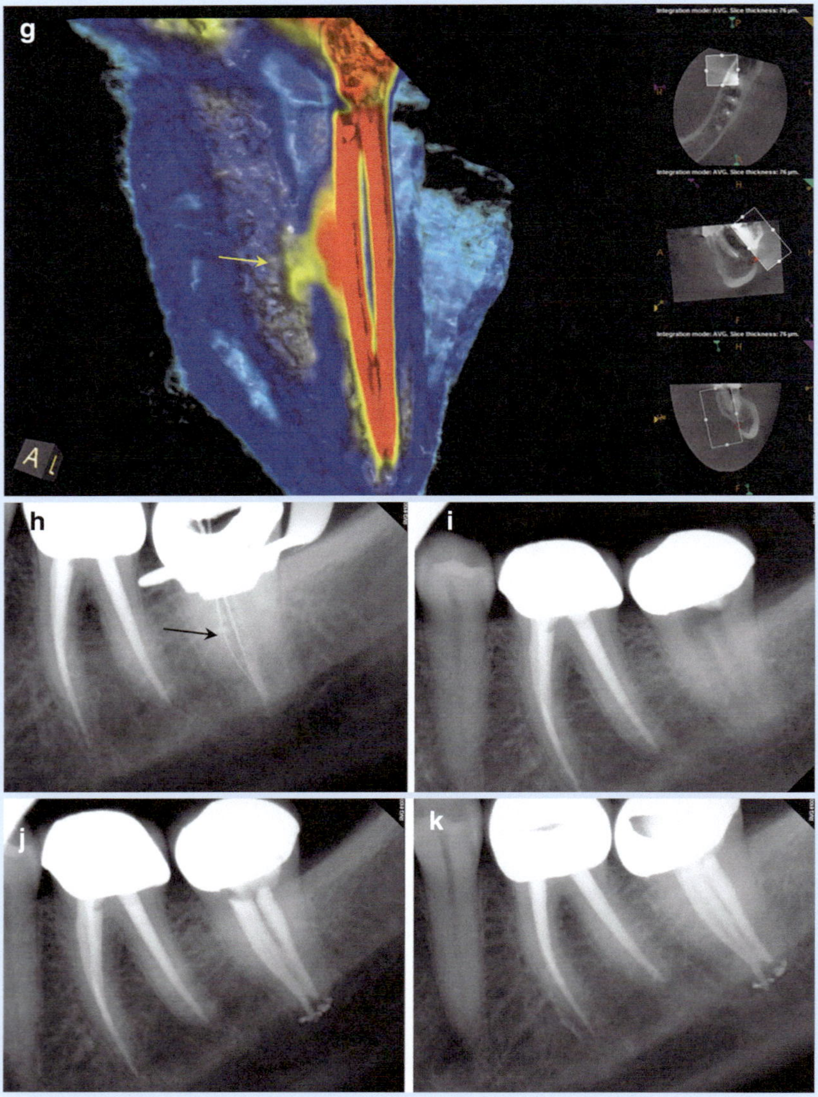

Case 3 Description: The patient received RCT in tooth #18 approximately 3 years ago; the tooth was retreated 12 months prior to presentation. The patient has been symptomatic for the previous 2 years, and recently reported a diagnosis of fractured tooth. The patient desires a second opinion.

3 a–c: Preoperative radiographs from several different angulations fail to disclose a definitive diagnosis. However, closer examination of the magnified image suggests a thin radio-opaque line from the mesial canal in two of the

images (black arrows). The obturation is also off-center, again suggestive of additional canal spaces within the root.
3 d: The axial, coronal, and sagittal sections of the CBCT scan reveal a high-density dot or line, highly suggestive of sealer extruded into the uninstrumented ML canal space (white arrows).
3 e: The colorized 3-D axial section highlights the high-density object adjacent to the MB canal; the direction is on a line from the ML canal to the ML line angle of the root surface (red arrow).
3 f: The colorized 3-D coronal section reveals the bifurcation of the main canal, with sealer streaming into the lingual aspect of the bifurcation (yellow arrow).
3 g: A magnified view of the colorized coronal section with part of the sagittal aspect of the root removed. The detail of the bifurcation is displayed, and accurate measurements regarding depth can be obtained. It was ascertained from the scan that the depth from the floor of the chamber to the bifurcation entrance was 4 mm, on an angle towards the ML line angle of the mesial root.
3 h,i: The root canal filling (RCF) was harvested from the canal spaces, and the ML canal was located and negotiated (black arrow). A periapical radiograph was exposed to verify the complete removal of the RCF material. The canals were treated with $Ca(OH)2$ for 3 weeks; the patients symptoms subsided in 1 week, and were absent at the completion appointment.
3 j,k: Right-angle and off-angle radiographs of the completed case, demonstrating the presence of three canals with multiple anastomoses between them.

A variation of an extra canal is represented by Sect. 6.4, Case #4. The patient was asymptomatic, but presented with a sinus tract tracing to the mesial root apex. Multiple radiographic angles failed to disclose what the axial sections of the CBCT indicate with clarity: the presence of a middle mesial (MM) canal. A study in extracted teeth [27] correlated intercanal distances between the mesiobuccal and mesiolingual canals with the likelihood of these roots containing a middle mesial canal. Measurement of the isthmus in the axial section exceeded the mean dimension of 3.0 mm, strongly indicative of a patent MM canal space. Conservative treatment of this canal and retreatment of all the remaining spaces effectively addressed the etiology, as evidenced by the resolution of the sinus tract within 1 week. Examination of the axial and coronal sections in a postoperative scan demonstrates a Type VIII canal configuration of the mesial root according to Torres [22].

Case #4: #30 Retreatment: Middle Mesial canal (MMes)

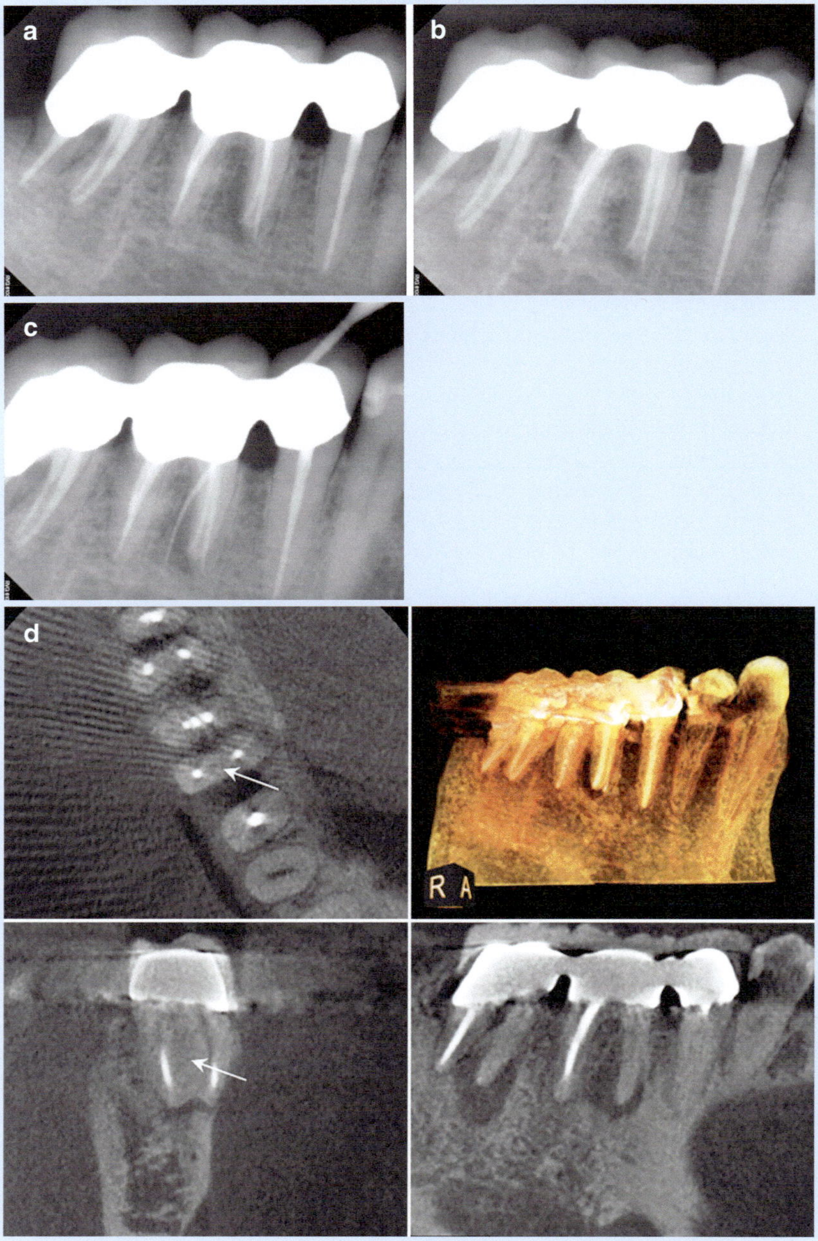

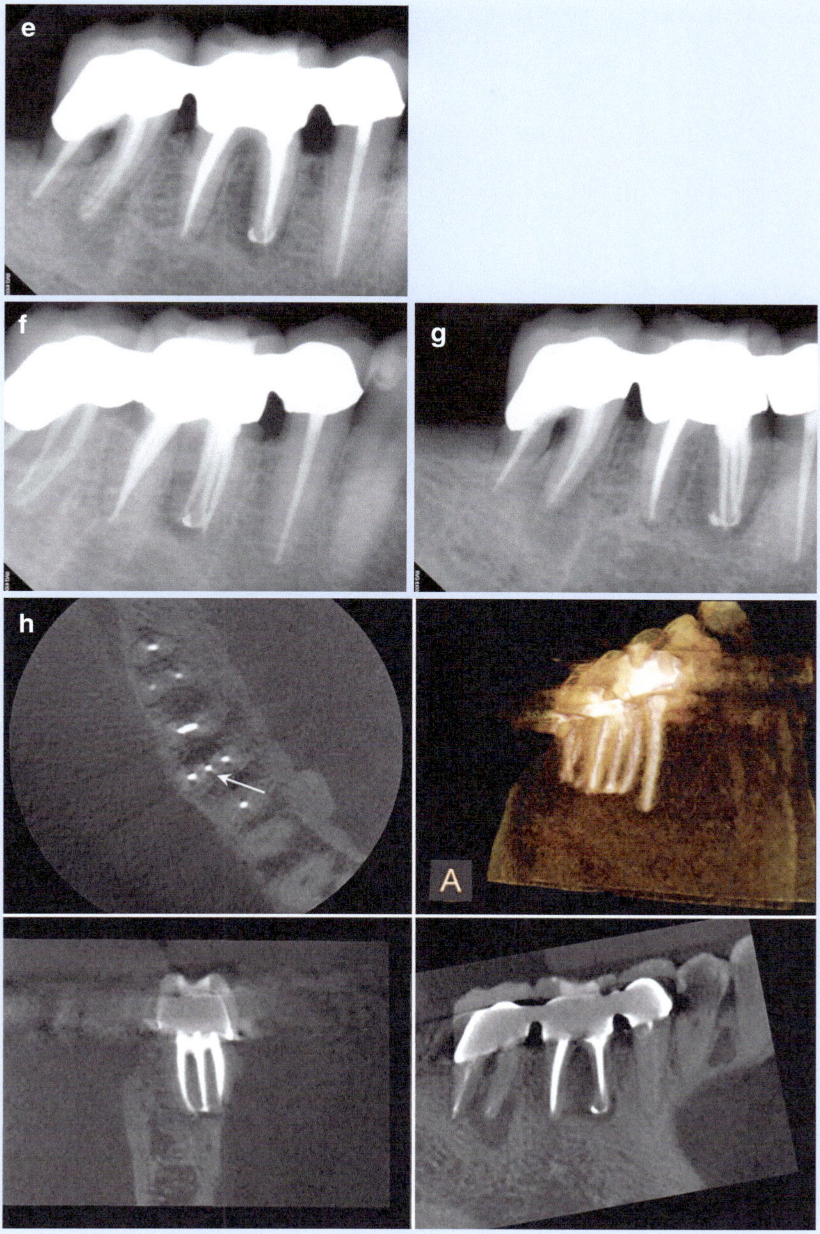
e
f
g
h
A

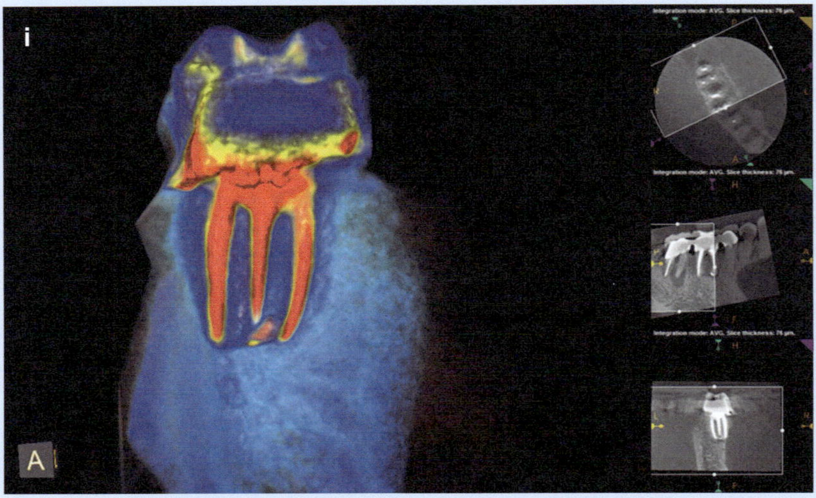

Case 4 Description: The patient was asymptomatic, but presented for evaluation of a "pimple on his gum."

4 a,b: Right-angle and off-angle radiographs reveal PAP on the mesial root of tooth #30. There is also a suggestion of pathology on the mesial root of #31 as well.

4 c: Tracing the sinus tract revealed the source to be the apex of the mesial root of #30. Periodontal probing of the tooth was within normal limits, discounting a vertical root fracture as an etiology.

4 d: The axial and coronal sections of the CBCT scan were suggestive of a middle mesial canal; the distance between the MB and ML canals in the axial section measured 4.3 mm, exceeding the reported minimum span for a third negotiable space. Note also the PAP on the mesial root of #31, with the high probability of the same etiology.

4 e–g: Right-angle and off-angle radiographs reveal 3 separate canals and apical foramen in the completed mesial root. The retreated distal root also had 3 canals, but the final instrumentation created one large, scalloped ribbon canal configuration.

4 h: The axial and coronal sections demonstrate the span of the obturation in the mesial root and the confluence of the canals in the distal.

4 i: The colorized 3-D model highlights the comparative sizes between the retreated MB and ML canals, and the primary instrumentation of the MM canal, terminating in 3 separate apical foramina.

An extremely rare instance of additional mesial canals in mandibular molars is presented in Sect. 6.5, Case #5. The patient had received conservative one-visit endodontic therapy approximately 6 months prior to presentation, with a full coverage crown restoration placed shortly afterward. The patient had been symptomatic since the completion of therapy, and the discomfort was increasing with time. As in the previous case (6.4) conventional 2D radiographs failed to disclose the true nature of the complexity of the root canal system of both the mesial and distal roots. In the axial and coronal sections of the CBCT scan, four canals can be identified in the mesial root. The mesiobuccal and mesiolingual canals had been treated and obturated, but two additional canal spaces are revealed between them; they were designated the buccal middle mesial (BMM) and the lingual middle mesial (LMM). The incidence of four canals in the mandibular first molar mesial root was reported as 3.3% [28], but this was a radiographic study without clinical verification. The only reported clinical treatment of a four-canal mesial root, to date, was published by Reeh in 1998 [29], finding an additional three canals in the distal root of a mandibular first molar.

Case #5: #30 Retreatment: Undiagnosed Buccal MMes/Lingual MMes canals

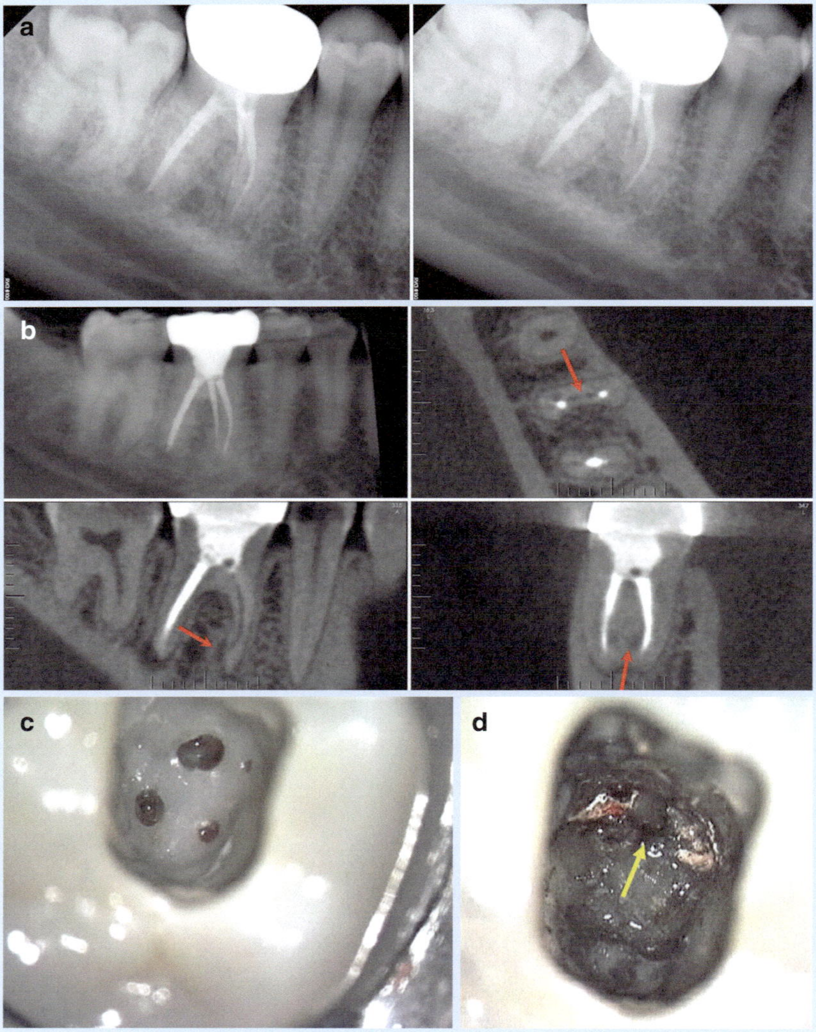

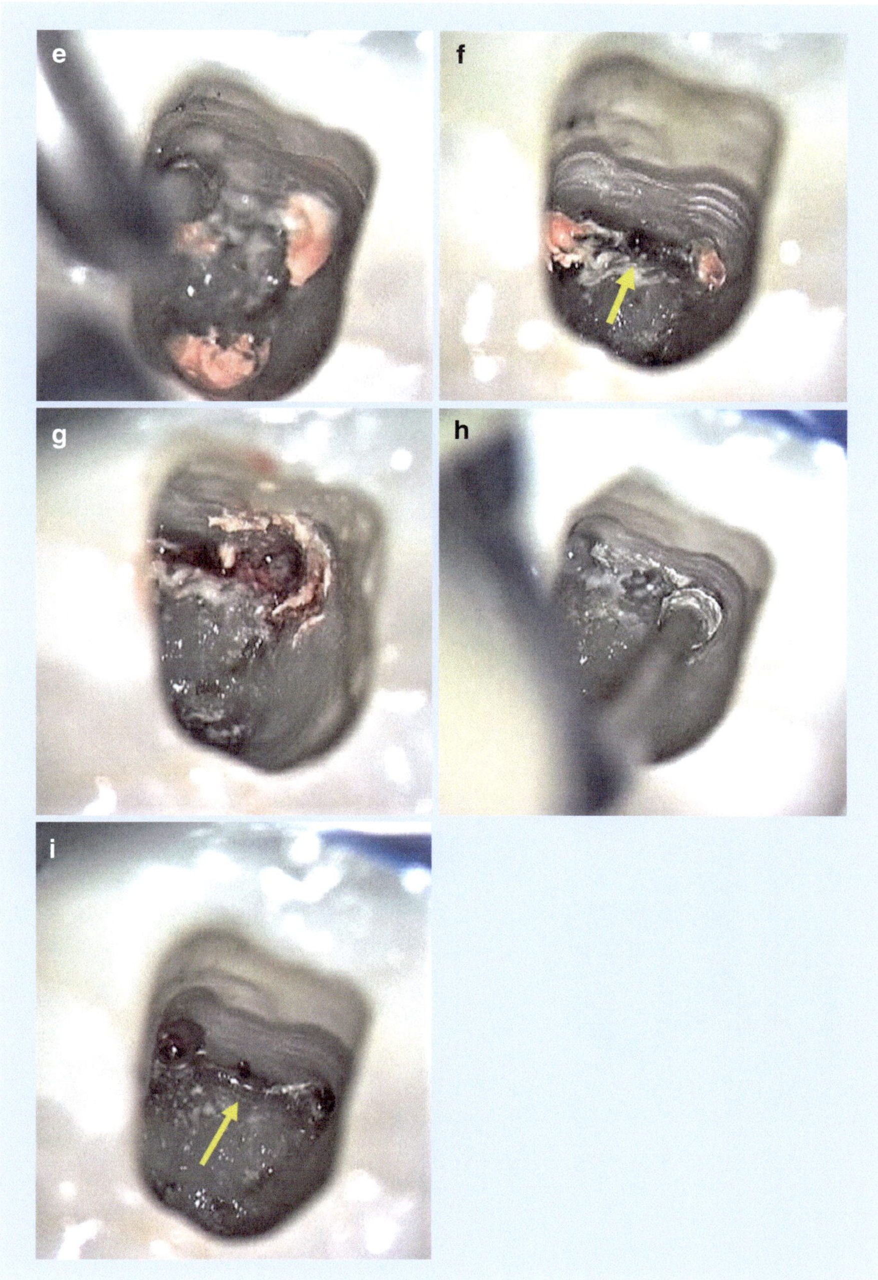
e
f
g
h
i

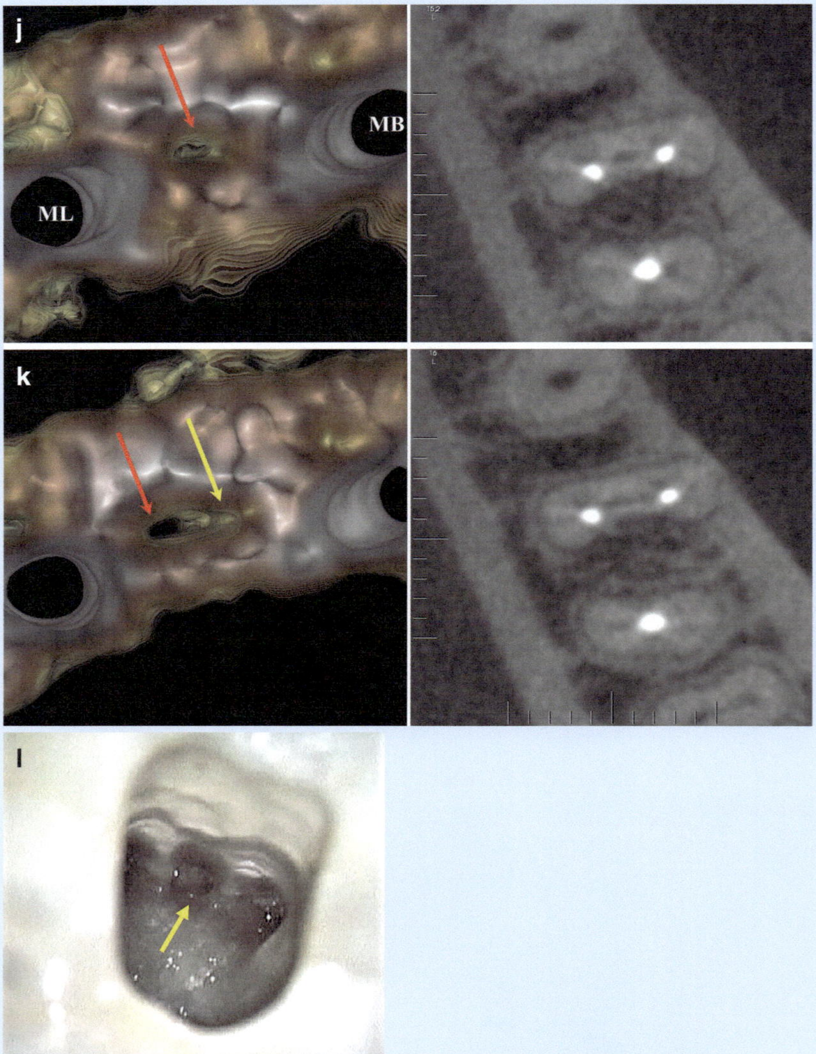
j
MB
ML
k
l

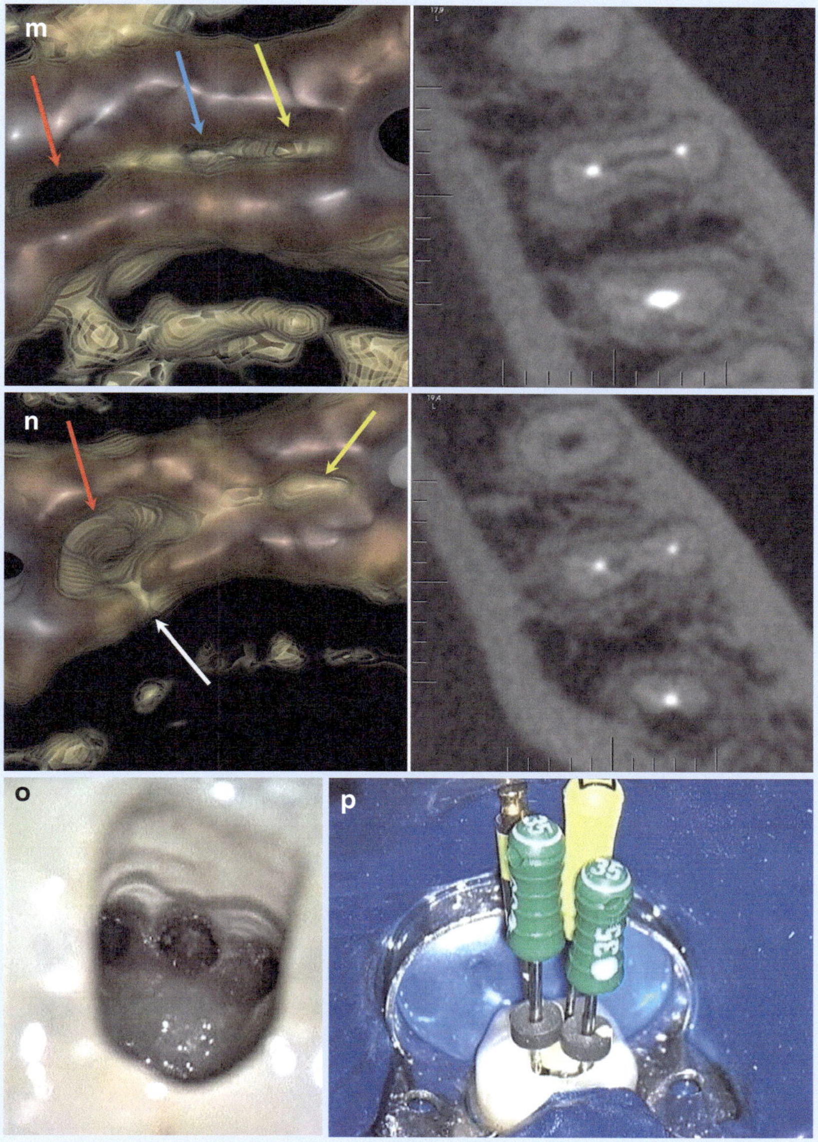
m
n
o
p

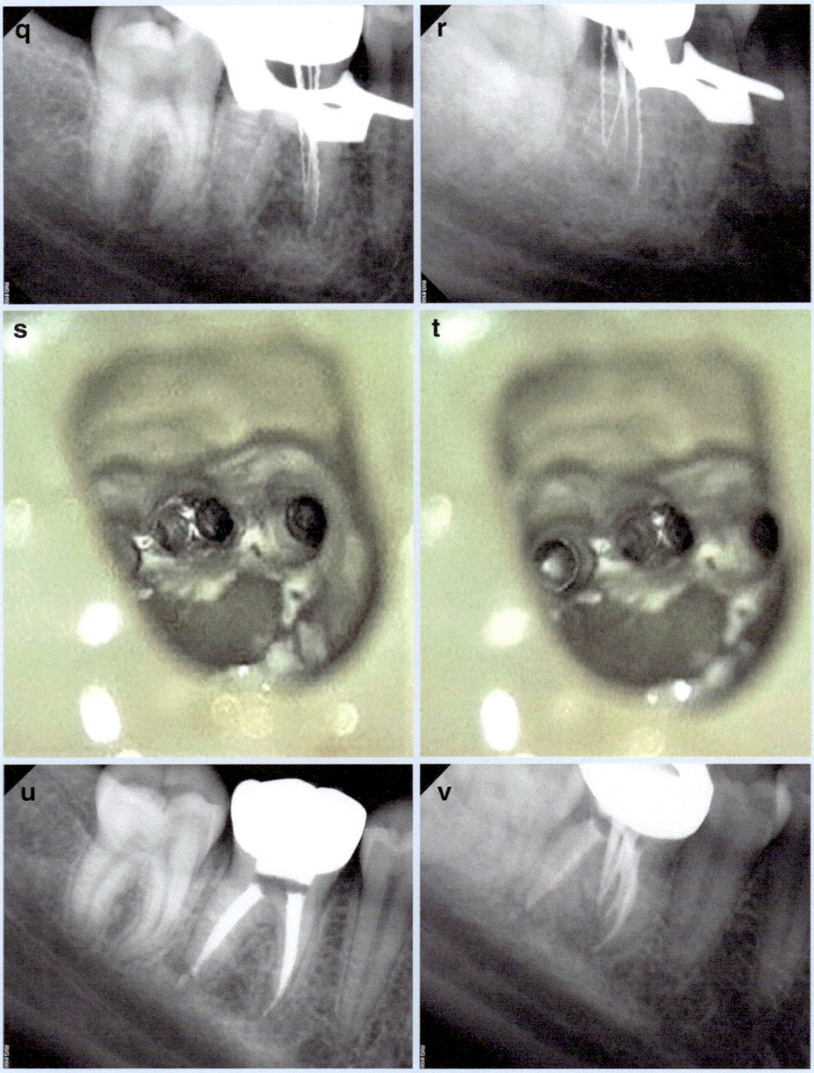
q
r
s
t
u
v

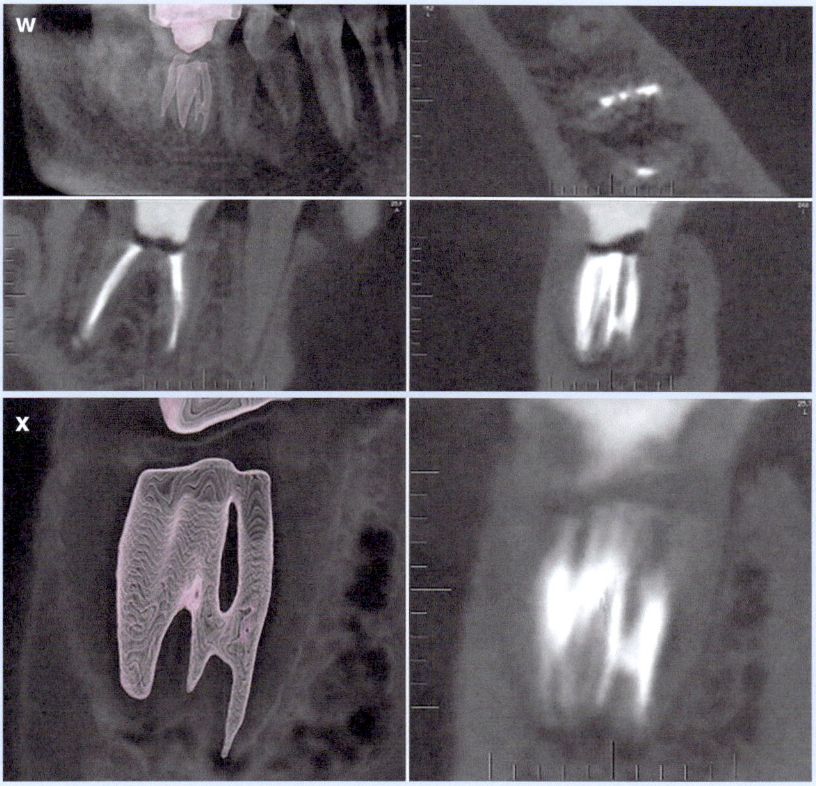
W
X

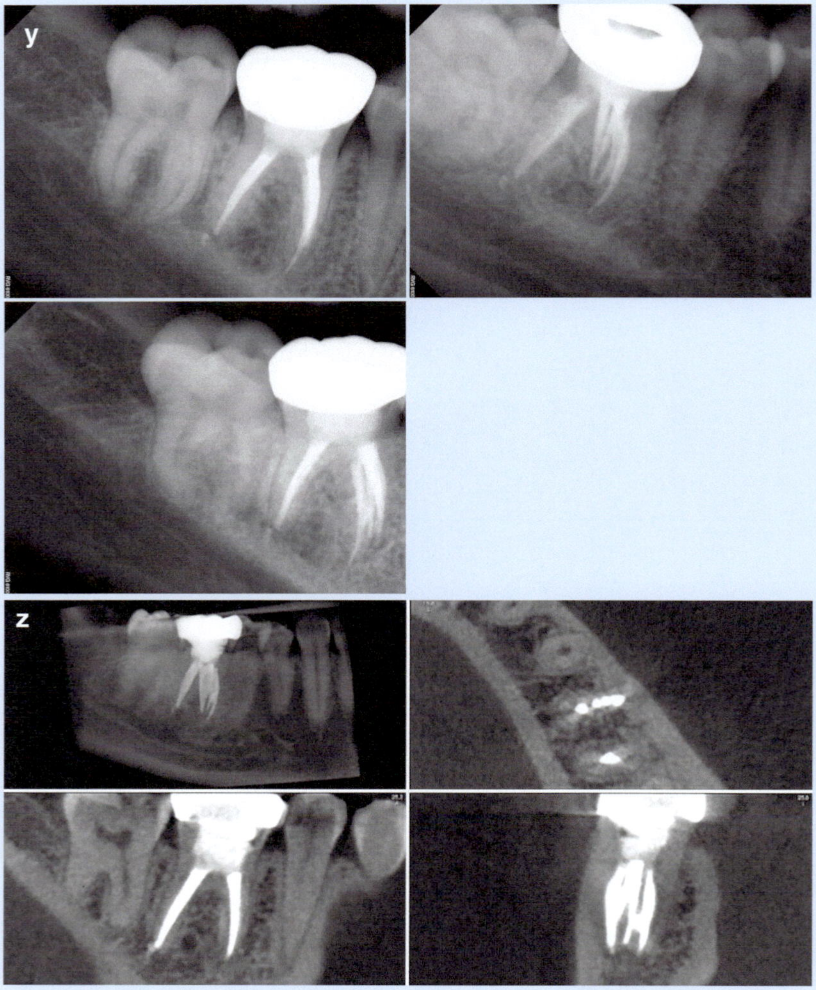

Case 5 Description: The patient presents in persistent pain following NSRCT in tooth #30; diagnosed as an "abscess" associated with tooth #29.

5 a: Radiographs from 2 angles reveal the previous RCT in tooth #30, with a small radiolucency associated with distal root apex. The "abscess" seen at the apical extent of #29 is the Mental Foramen.

5 b: The CBCT scan reveals a patent isthmus in the mesial root of #30 in the axial view (arrow) and areas of lesser density associated with the mesial and distal apices. The sagittal section reveals the apical foramen of an unfilled canal space (arrow).
5 c: Partial removal of the buildup material revealed multiple voids in the core material, with fluid evident on the floor of the chamber.
5 d: Removal of the core reveals the presence of pulp tissue between the mesiobuccal and mesiolingual canal spaces obturated with gutta percha (arrow).
5 e: A football-shaped ultrasonic tip is used to expand the isthmus space.
5 f: A small depression in the isthmus trough (arrow) is revealed after the excavation.
5 g: The gutta percha material in the mesial canals was harvested, precipitating bleeding from the tissue in the isthmus.
5 h: The isthmus space is deepened after complete removal of the obturative material using the same football ultrasonic tip.
5 i: The deeper excavation reveals a bifurcation in the isthmus space (arrow).
5 j: Using the e-VolDX program (CDT Software) with dedicated 3D filters, the axial view level seen in 5f is represented in 2D and 3D. The depression in the isthmus trough is readily seen between the mesiobuccal/mesiolingual spaces (arrow).
5 k: Using the same program the axial view level seen in 5i is represented in 2D and 3D, revealing a bifurcation of the isthmus space. The two additional canals were labeled the buccal middle mesial (BMM) (yellow arrow) and the Lingual middle mesial (LMM) (red arrow).
5 l: Initial exploration with hand files expands the common space into the bifurcation 4 mm apical to the floor of the chamber (arrow).
5 m: Using the e-VolDX program the level 2 mm apical to the isthmus bifurcation revealed the LMM canal (red arrow), BMM canal (yellow arrow), and a cul-de-sac fin extending from the BMM canal towards the LMM canal (blue arrow).
5 n: This level reveals the BMM canal (yellow arrow) and the LMM (red arrow) with its apical foramen exiting the distal aspect of the mesial root (white arrow). The low-density area associated with this canal is also seen in 5b.
5 o: Final instrumentation enables the visualization of the four canal orifices in the mesial root.

5 p: Clinical image showing #35 H files in the MB/ML canals, and #20 K files in the BMM/LMM canals.
5 q, r: Radiographs demonstrating the extent and distribution of the four canal spaces located and negotiated.
5 s,t: Sealer placed in the four canal spaces highlight the bifurcation and location of the four completed canal orifices.
5 u,v: Radiographs demonstrating the extent and distribution of the four obturated canal spaces in the mesial root and large ribbon-shaped distal canal.
5 w: CBCT scan of the completed retreatment, with the coronal axis centered on the mesial root.
5 x: Using the e-VolDX program, the coronal view of the mesial root is rendered in a 3D filter. The 4 canal spaces are clearly defined, as well as the cul-de-sac fin seen in 5m.
5 y: Six-month recall radiographs from several angles demonstrate resolution of the small periapical area seen at the distal root apex.
5 z: Six-month recall CBCT scan demonstrates the resolution of all the low-density areas seen in the preoperative scan.

Mandibular molars with distolingual supernumerary roots present a unique challenge to any practitioner. First coined *radix entomolaris* by Carabelli [30], they demonstrate great variability in anatomical presentations and ethnic predispositions [31–35]. While the presence of the additional root may be vaguely apparent on conventional radiographs, the precise anatomical variant is readily displayed with the aid of the cone beam scan [36]. It proved an indispensable asset in the next case, the retreatment of tooth #30 (Sect. 6.6, Case #6). The existence of the radix is suggested by the radiographs, but the true nature of the roots position is revealed in the axial sections of the scan. The coronal and sagittal views disclose the extent of the periapical involvement preoperatively and the resolution 12 months later.

Case #6: #31 Retreatment: Radix Entomolaris

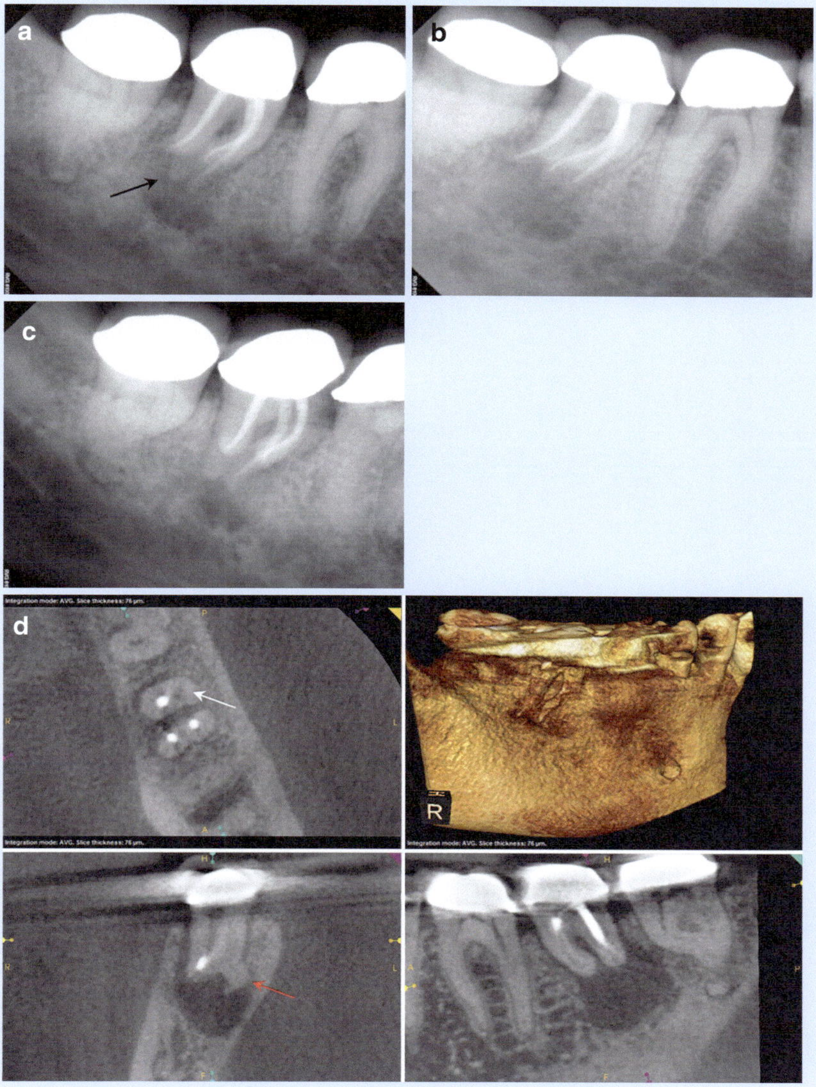

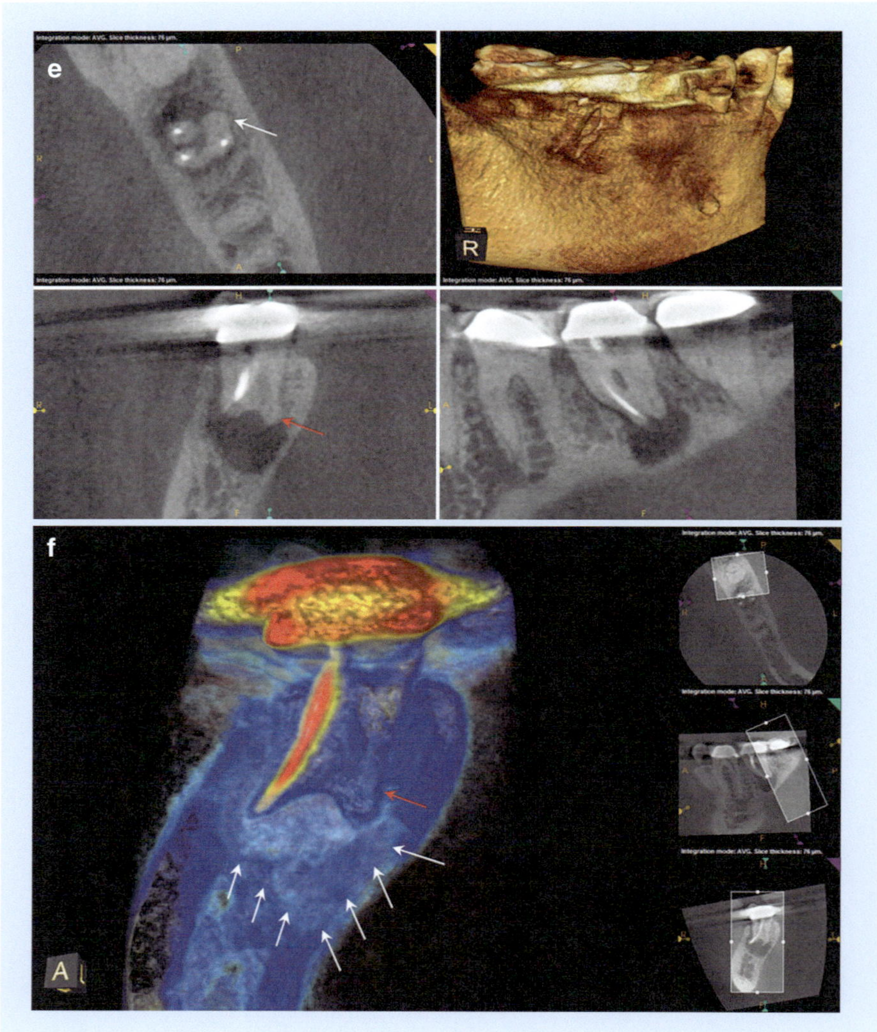
e
R
f
A

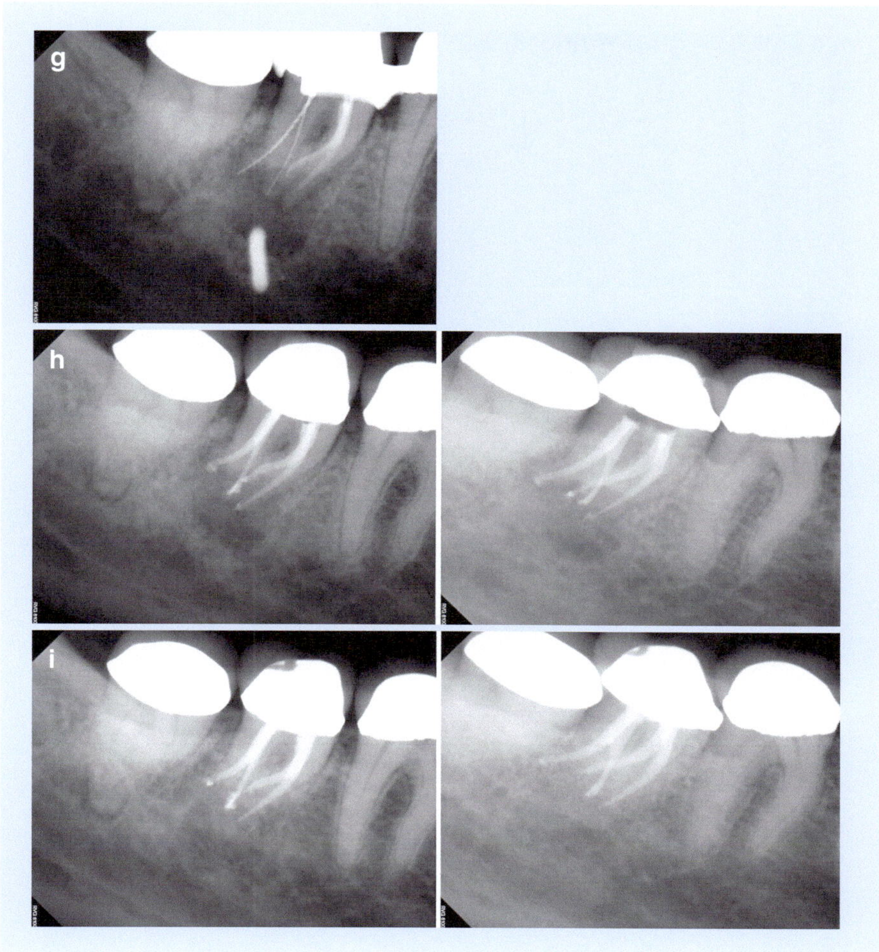
g
h
i

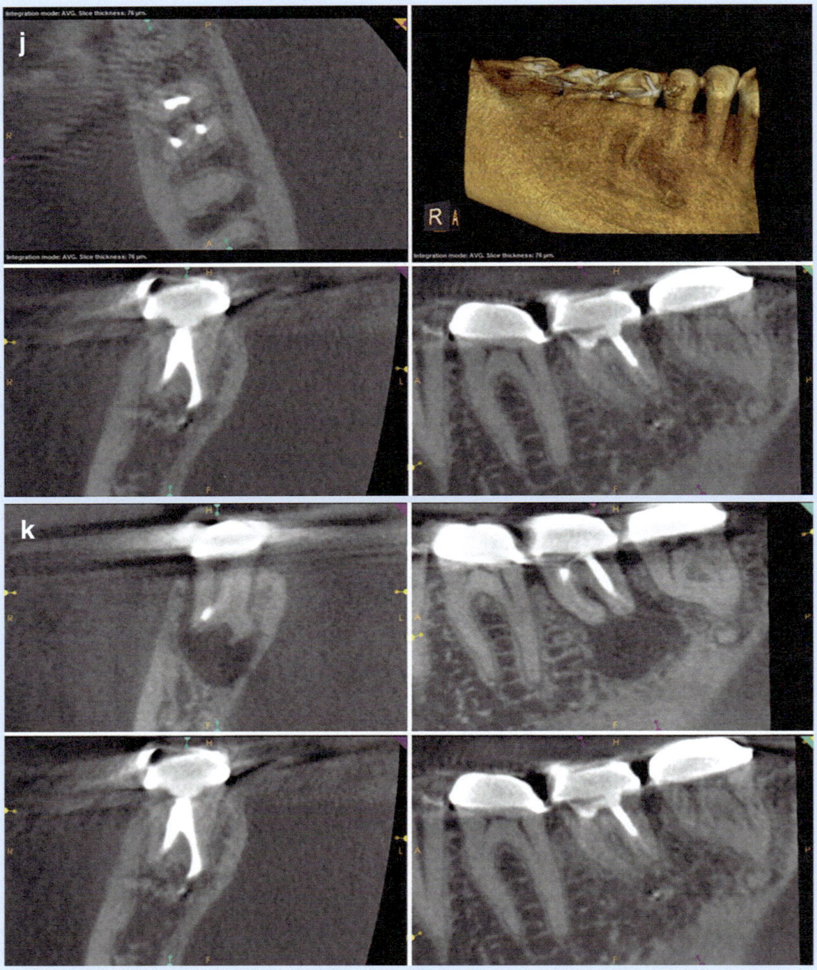

Case 6 Description: the patient presented with a diagnosis of Symptomatic Apical Periodontitis, localized to a tooth that was endodontically treated 3 years previously.

6 a–c: Right-angle and off-angle radiographs reveal a large PAA at the apices of tooth #30. There is a suggestion of an auxiliary root in 5(a) (black arrow), but its origin within the chamber and buccal-lingual position is not disclosed in any of the conventional images.

6 d: The axial view in the scan 2 mm apical to the CEJ confirms the presence of a second canal in the distal root, 2 mm lingual to the DB (white arrow). The coronal section reveals a sharp dilacerations of this root towards the buccal as it nears its terminus (red arrow); this change in direction will be explained in the next figure.
6 e: The axial view 2 mm from the terminus shows the DL root fusing with the ML root (white arrow), but their respective canal spaces do not join. At this level, the canal assumes a more linear path (red arrow).
6 f: The colorized 3-D coronal section highlights the juxtaposition of the DB and DL roots (red arrow) as well as the extent of the PA lesion and the thinning of the lingual cortical plate (white arrows).
6 g: Working length radiograph with files in the DB and DL canals. The gutta percha is yet to be removed from the mesial canals (the radio-opaque pin in the image is a 5 mm reference in the film holder).
6 h: Final radiographs of the completed retreatment. Note the overlapping of the mesial roots and the DL root.
6 i: Twelve-month recall radiographs; the lesion appears to be resolved, but overlying structures can mask underlying spaces.
6 j: Twelve-month CBCT scan demonstrates complete resolution after a thorough review of all the slices in all planes. This slice level corresponds to the location of the largest dimension of the lesion preoperatively.
6 k: A comparison of the preoperative (top) and 12-month postoperative (bottom) coronal and sagittal slices at almost identical levels, exhibiting complete resolution of the lesion.

The variability of canal morphology in maxillary molars is not confined solely to the MB root, as the following case demonstrates (Sect. 6.7, Case #7). The initial radiographic exam was not encouraging, but, despite the evidence to the contrary, the tooth's mobility was between a 1 and 2, with no depression into the socket. The lone region of deep periodontal probing depth was at the mesial aspect of the tooth, coincident with the vertical defect seen in the pretreatment radiographs. However, conservative reflection and examination with the SOM failed to disclose any crown-root fractures. The patient reported being told that the dentist had encountered some difficulties during the procedure, including an unexplained "obstruction" and possibly a separated instrument.

Case #7: #2 Retreatment: Undiagnosed DB canal

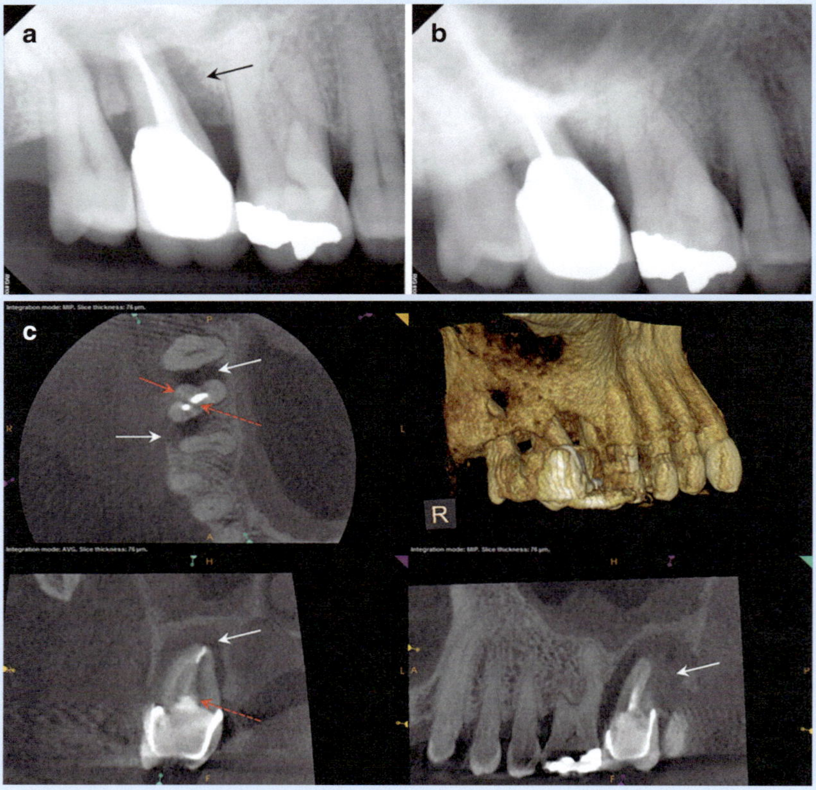

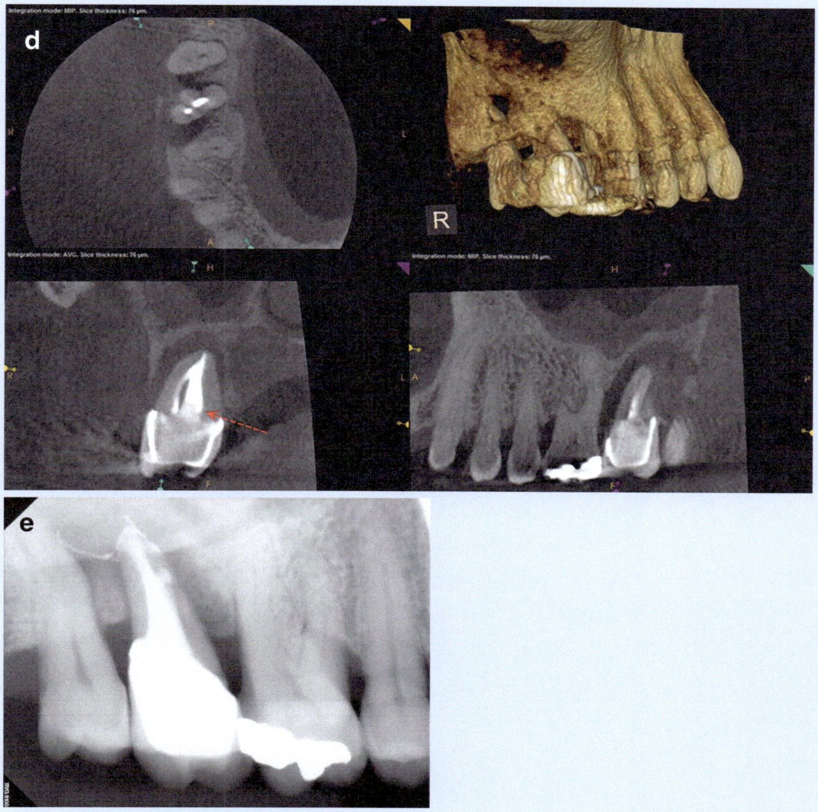
d
R
e

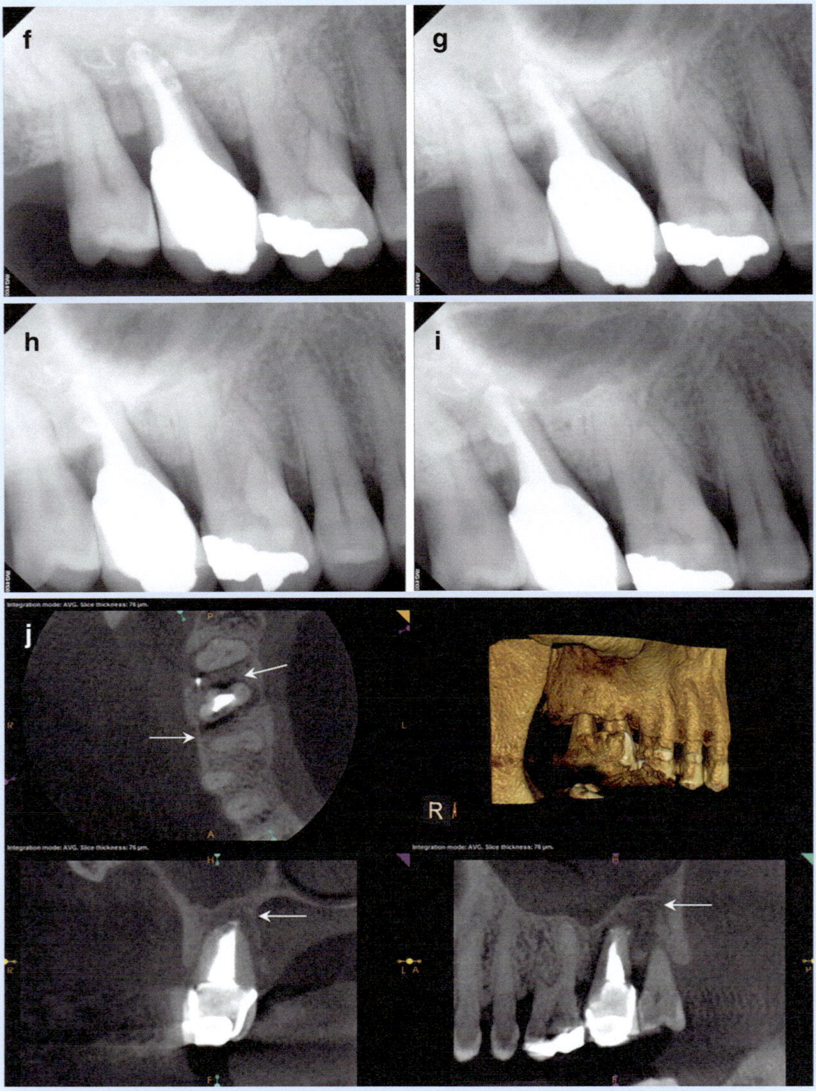

Case 7 Description: The patient presents for evaluation of tooth #2. It has been treated within the previous 9 months, and has developed deep periodontal probing at the mesial aspect of the root. The tooth is mobile but not depressible in the socket. Initial micro-reflection of the area and inspection with the SOM did not disclose any vertical fracture.

7 a,b: Preoperative radiographs demonstrating the extent of the bone loss at the mesial aspect of the root and the appearance of a 3-walled defect (black arrow).
7 c,d: The axial view reveals the extent of the bone loss at the mesial and distal aspects, with only the palatal wall intact (white arrows). The bulbous portion of the root at the distal suggests the location of the DB canal (red arrow). The coronal view shows the approximate location of the suspected perforation (red dashed arrows); the invagination of the root form and the proximity of the obturative material were suggestive of this iatrogenic event. Re-access of the canal spaces confirmed the presence of the DB canal and the perforation in the palatal canal.
7 e: Final post-treatment radiograph; note the multiple apical foramina in the mesial and distal aspects of the apical third of the root, and the dramatic change in the width of the obturation.
7 f, g: Recall radiographs 6 months after initial treatment. The probing depth was reduced dramatically, and the tooth became more stable in the alveolus. Multiple apical foramina can be seen in the mesial and distal aspects of the apical third of the root.
7 h, i: Twelve-month recall radiographs reveal resolution of the mesial defect, although the PDL is widened and indicates possible occlusal trauma. The periodontal probing depths are within normal limits.
7 j: Twelve-month recall CBCT scan demonstrates approximately 80% resolution of the presenting lesion, with a re-establishment of the buccal cortical plates and periapical bone matrix (white arrows).

Initial analysis of the CB scan was even less encouraging; the bone loss appeared to be circumferential around the fused roots, with the only competent attachment at the palatal aspect. However, two observations were made during the slice by slice assessment: an asymmetrical root form at the DB portion of the root (suggestive of a missing canal) and the close proximity of the existing obturation to the mesial aspect of the root in the apical third of the tooth (consistent with a possible root perforation). These findings were presented to the patient, who desired to retain the tooth if at all possible. The retreatment was agreed to, after detailed informed consent and full disclosure of the poor prognosis.

Re-entry into the chamber revealed an atypical C-shaped canal, coursing from the normal DB orifice location toward the palatal aspect of the chamber. Partial removal of the gutta-percha in the palatal canal confirmed that this C-shaped isthmus, containing small fragments of necrotic tissue, indeed joined the body of the palatal canal space. This anomaly is extremely rare in appearance, with a reported incidence in first molars of 0.091% [37]. In second molars, this irregularity has only been associated clinically with the palatal root [38] or in the study of sectioned extracted teeth [39]. It also appears to be genetically determined, which could provide insights into the ethnic origins of those patients with this morphologic variation [40].

Complete removal of all the obturative material in the palatal canal uncovered the suspected perforation of the mesial aspect of the space in the coronal third of the root. Following gentle debridement and disinfection, the perforation was sealed with a bioceramic (ProRoot™ MTA, Dentsply Tulsa Dental) and the patient was appointed for the following day to complete the retreatment of the remaining canal space (MB) and placement of the inter-appointment medicament ($Ca(OH)_2$). The patient's treatment was completed 4 weeks later, and the 12-month recall examination displayed remarkable healing and normal mobility.

Occasionally, the discovery of unusual anatomy is serendipitous, often disclosed by the unintentional tracking of the root canal filling material. Such is the case with the next clinical presentation (Sect. 6.8, Case #8). The patient's chief complaint referenced the MB root of tooth #14, which did demonstrate active disease secondary to a missed MB_2. However, the radiographic exam revealed the existence of a bifurcation in the palatal root. The existence of two canals in this root has multiple permutations: it can present as two orifices with two separate canals [41–43], two roots or orifices with a common apical foramen [44], or the most uncommon of all: one orifice with a common canal that bifurcates or trifurcates [45–47]. As with other clinical situations regarding anatomy deep in the canal spaces, it is of paramount importance to have precise knowledge of how deep the anomaly is in the root and what direction(s) they are tracking toward. The CBCT permitted exact measurements in the palatal root to pinpoint the level of the bifurcation, facilitating exact and intentional instrumentation of both canals, with complete obturation of both prepared spaces in the palatal root.

Case 8: Arsenlis #14 Retreatment: Bifurcated Palatal Root

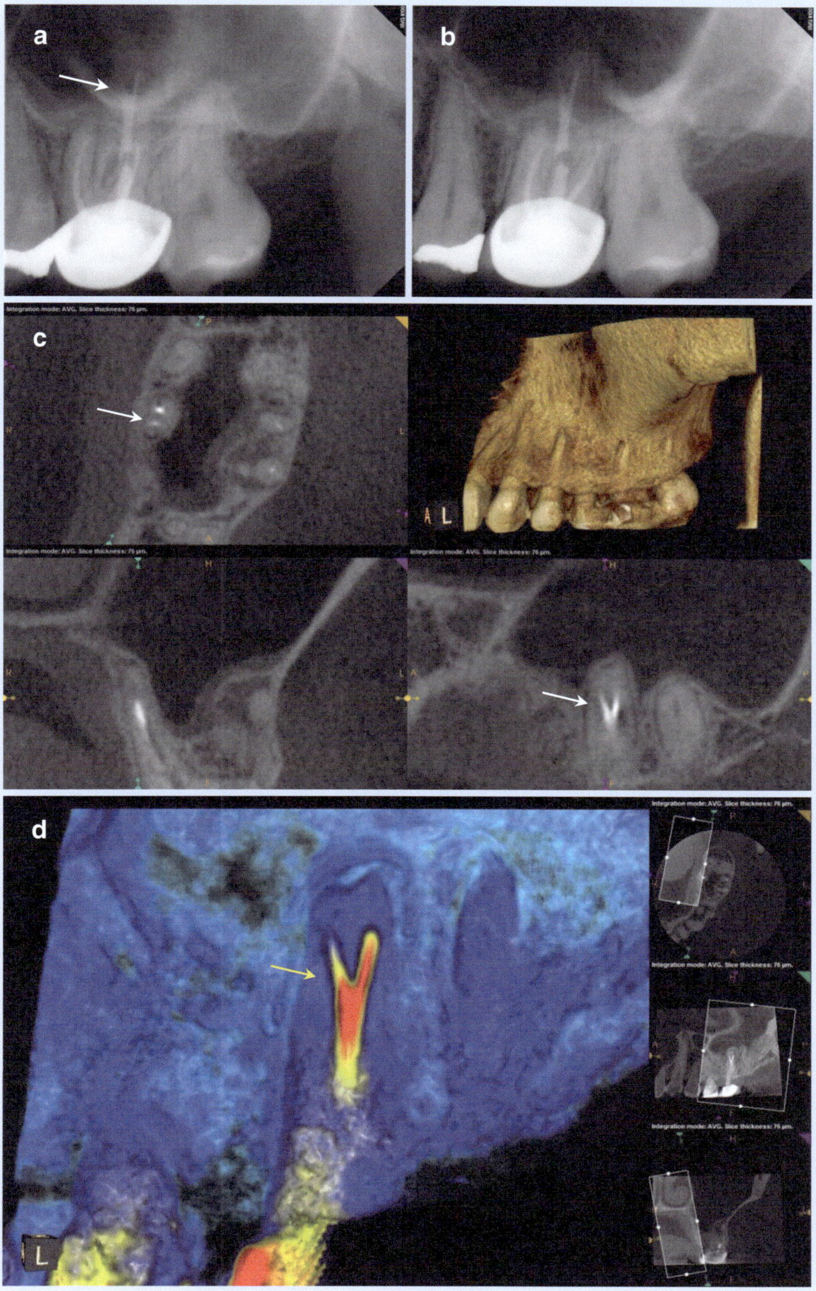

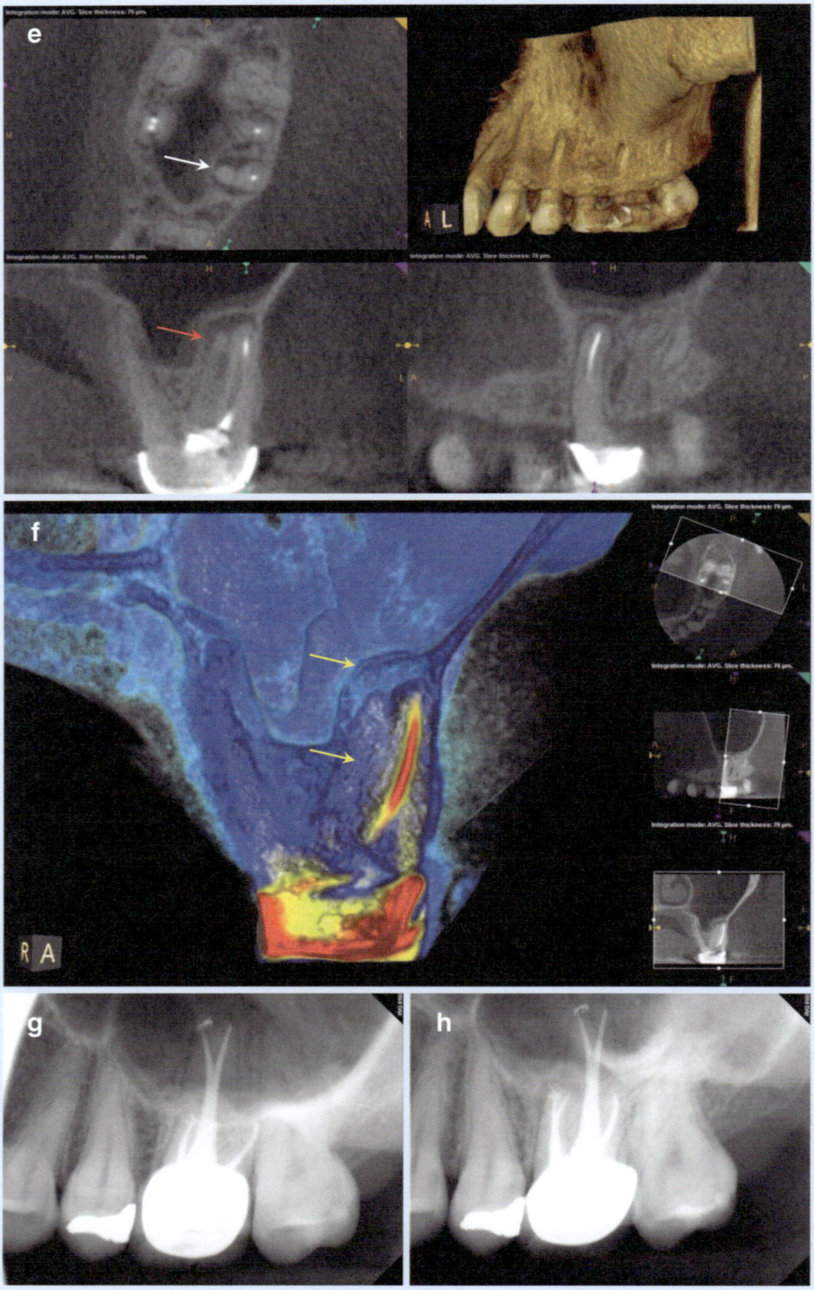
e
A L
f
R A
g
h

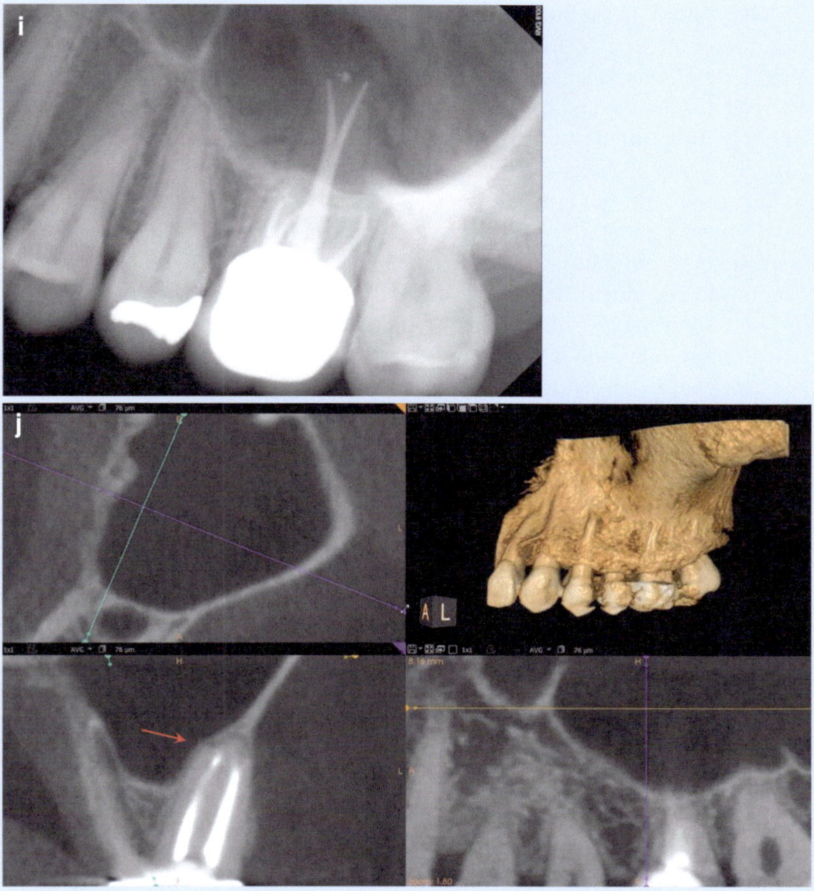

Case 8 Description: The patient presented in pain in a tooth that has been previously treated 1 year ago. Her preliminary diagnosis is Symptomatic Apical Periodontitis.

8 a,b: Preoperative radiographs from different angles reveal PAP on the MB root apex, as well as the suggestion of a bifurcation of the palatal canal. The distal part of the split appears more dense than the mesial, implying that the mesial radiopacity is a sealer tract.

8 c: The CBCT scan shows definitively two separate canals in the palatal root. Accurate measurements place the level of the bifurcation 4.3 mm from the terminus of the distopalatal canal. The higher density spot in the axial and sagittal sections of the palatal root is the gutta percha; the lower density object is the sealer tract (white arrows).

8 d: This colorized sagittal section has been magnified to ascertain the angle of the bifurcation; the deviation is less than 40°, so an appropriately angled instrument should be able to engage the orifice without difficulty (white arrow). When the angle of bifurcation is 60° or more, the dilaceration may be too abrupt to allow easy insertion of the file without additional coronal modification of the common canal space.
8 e: The axial section of the MB root demonstrates the eccentric placement of the MB root canal filling, indicative of the presence of an MB_2 canal (white arrow). The coronal view of the same root suggests that the MB_2 may, in fact, be a separate root fused to the MB_1 (red arrow).
8 f: The colorized coronal section highlights the MB_2 root, and the distension/expansion of the floor of the maxillary sinus from the developing apical lesion (yellow arrows).
8 g,h: Final treatment radiographs presenting the obturation of the separate MB_1/MB_2 canals as well as the Mesiopalatal and Distopalatal canals.
8 i: Twelve-month recall radiograph: the lesion at the MB root appears healed, and the patient is asymptomatic.
8 j: Twelve-month recall CBCT: the lesion at the MB root appears healed, and the patient is asymptomatic. Note the resolution of the sinus floor distension/expansion when compared to the preoperative CBCT in Fig. 8 f (red arrow).

Two canals in one root are also an uncommon occurrence in the tooth considered in the next example (Sect. 6.9, Case #9): the mandibular first premolar. A recent literature review [48] reported that two or more canals were found in 24.2% of the teeth studied, with 21.1% having two or more apical foramina. Higher incidences of teeth with additional canals and roots have been reported in Chinese, Australian, and sub-Saharan Africa populations, with the lowest incidence in Western Eurasian, Japanese, and American Arctic populations. As is the case with mandibular anterior teeth with two canals, the lingual canal of the pair is the most often misdiagnosed and missed. Careful pretreatment assessment using the CBCT assisted in the successful discovery and acquisition of this auxiliary canal.

Case 9: #28 Retreatment: Undiagnosed Lingual canal

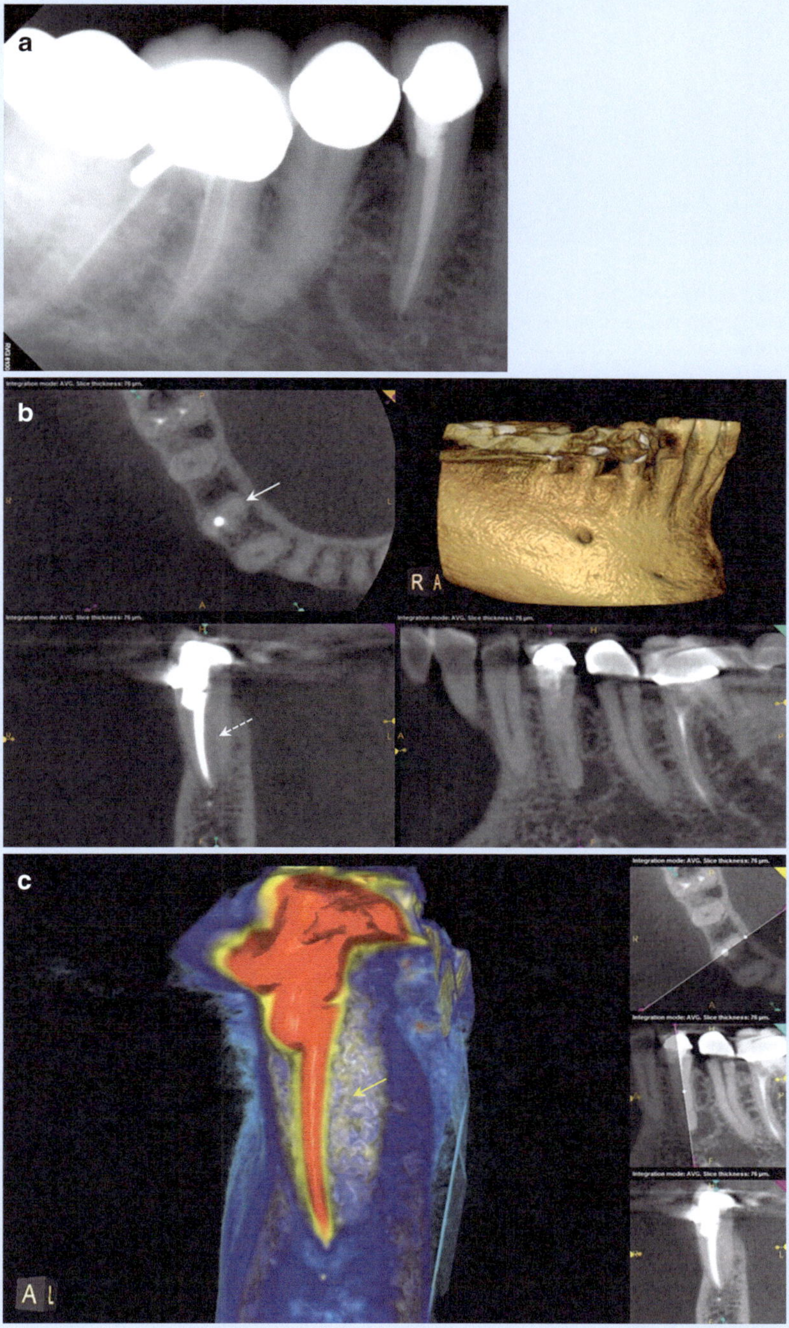

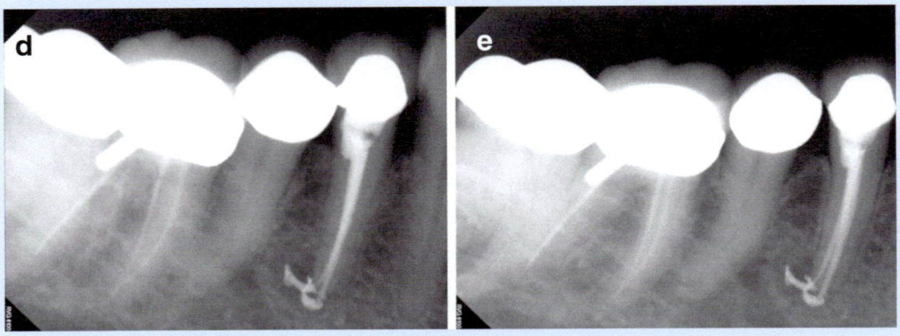

Case 9 Description: The patient presents with the chief complaint of biting sensitivity. The tooth was endodontically treated the previous year, and was referred for evaluation of vertical fracture.

9 a: Preoperative radiograph of tooth #28. The tooth has been restored with a full coverage crown, and there is a periapical area at the apex of the tooth. Periodontal probing is minimal, with no deep probing evident circumferentially. The tooth is, however, sensitive to percussion and biting.

9 b: Survey of the axial sections in the CBCT reveals the asymmetry of the existing root canal filling, highly suggestive of an additional canal space (white arrow). A faint low-density line can be seen in the coronal section (broken white arrow) bifurcating from the buccal canal at the junction of the coronal and middle thirds of the root. This most likely represents the lingual canal space.

9 c: The colorized coronal section demonstrates the buccal displacement of the existing obturation; the yellow arrow points to the area of the suspected canal location.

9 d,e: Post-treatment radiographs from different angles, displaying the deep point of the bifurcation (middle third of the root) and sealer extrusions into the periapical area.

Despite the best efforts at pretreatment planning, the excavation process in teeth with canal systems that have undergone a "calcific" transformation presents a unique challenge. Repeated insults to the pulpal tissues in the form of multiple or deep restorations or occlusal trauma elicit varied responses from those tissues. If the stimulation is overt and overwhelming, the most common response is pulpal necrosis. However, if the stimulation doesn't exceed that threshold, reparative dentin is elaborated by the pulp to insulate itself from the site of injury. Occasionally this response continues, with the coronal pulpal tissues becoming displaced by a haphazard elaboration of dentin, termed dystrophic obliteration or, more commonly, calcification. When this process extends into the canals themselves, discovery and negotiation is often realized several millimeters below the floor of the pulp chamber in the roots themselves. Visualization is limited, even with an operating microscope, and excessive dentin removal and/or perforations are not uncommon. Conventional radiographs, even from several angles, fail to disclose critical dimensions and directions from strategic corresponding clinical and radiographic landmarks. Canal acquisition guided by dynamic navigation is promising, but the technology is expensive and not widespread [49–51]. An alternative is using the CBCT scan as an intraoperative means to observe the excavation that has been performed previously. Adjustments to the depth/direction are planned, and this step can be repeated until the location of the canal(s) is realized. The next case (Sect. 6.10, Case #10) is an example of this technique.

Case 10 #12: Continuation of initiated treatment

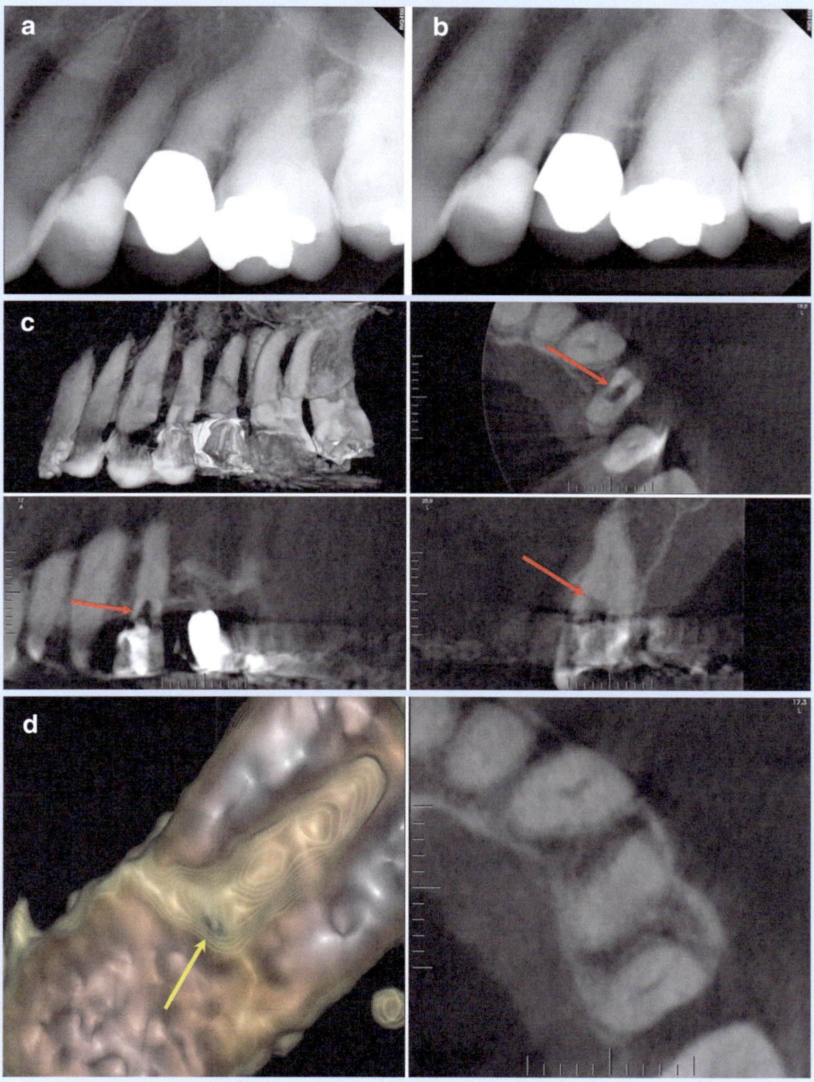

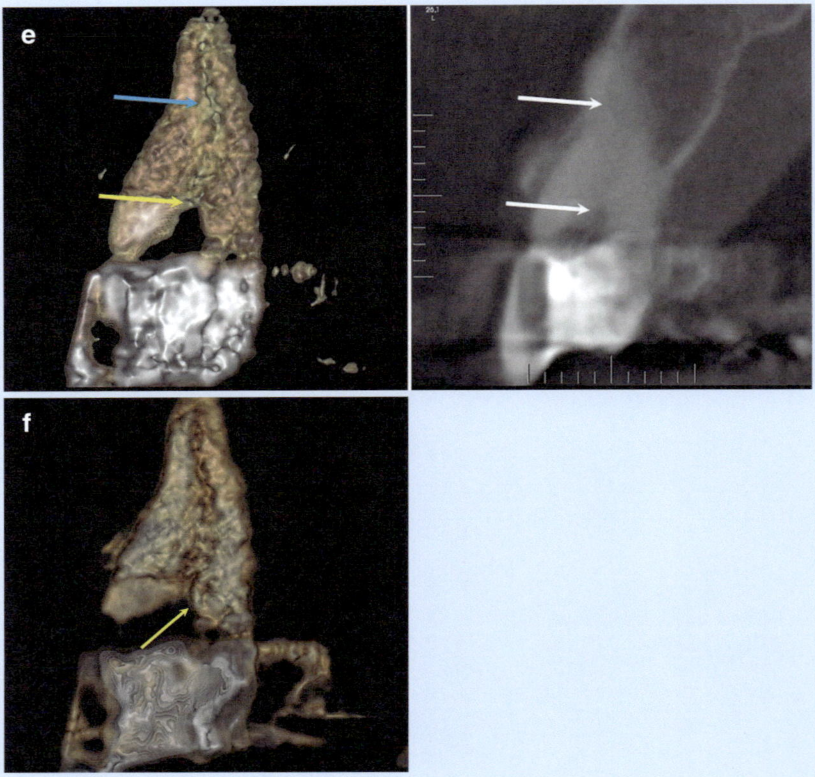

Case 10 Description: The patient presents for continuation of treatment of tooth #12 initiated at the general dentist's office.

10 a: The patient presented with the pretreatment radiograph from the referral dentist showing the dystrophic nature of the canal space(s) and dilacerated root geometry.

10 b: The pretreatment radiograph taken prior to the commencement of therapy demonstrates the excavation into the root approximately 3 mm below the CEJ.

10 c: The CBCT scan revealed the extent and direction of the attempt to locate the canal space(s), with a bias toward the buccal aspect of the root. The red arrows reveal the excavated spaces in the axial, coronal, and sagittal views.

10 d: Employing the e-VolDX program (CDT Software) with dedicated 3D filters, the "calcified" canal space is located at the palatal extent of the excavation in the axial view. The yellow arrow pinpoints the entrance to this space. Note the lack of disclosure of the space in the radiographic axial section.

10 e: Using the same program and 3D filter, compare the presence and course of the dystrophic canal space (yellow arrow) and the patent space in the apical third of the root (blue arrow) with the coronal view from the scan.
10 f: Adjusting the range in the filter demonstrates the canal entrance (yellow arrow), the dystrophic deposition of dentin in the coronal portion of the space, and the patent canal space more apically.

The presentation is similar to Case #1, with an important distinction: there was more than one operator involved. Access had been previously attempted by the referring practitioner, essentially obliterating any anatomical clues to the canal locations normally observed under higher magnification. Although by definition this is not a retreatment because there is no existing root canal filling material, the absence of coronal tooth structure via dentistogenic means warrants this designation. This placed the second practitioner at a distinct disadvantage, not having the subtle shading and color changes in the dentin to aid in the discovery of the canal positions. The extent of this excavation is clearly seen in the preoperative scanned images, with a displacement of the attempted access toward the buccal aspect of the root. What is also evident is the pattern and distribution of the dystrophic dentin, demonstrating the merging of the obliterated buccal canal with the more patent palatal canal space and its course to the apex of the tooth. These insights were crucial to the successful treatment of this tooth.

The final clinical case (Sect. 6.11, Case #11) is testimony to the diversity of endodontic filling materials. Virtually every dental material has been employed for endodontic obturation, from amalgam and silver cones to various paste formulations and polymerized rubber. They all present varying degrees of postoperative complications and retreatment difficulties [52–55] and many have been discontinued. One variant of the paste filling is prevalent in Europe, especially in the Eastern European countries. Its chemical name is resorcinol-formalin paste, but it is commonly known as “Russian red” due to its color and popularity among the former Soviet bloc countries. It has no standardized application or instrumentation protocols and stains the surrounding tooth structures a distinctive rouge color [56, 57]. Its effect on pulpal tissues has been ascribed as “mummifying” or “resinifying” [58, 59] with a complication rate of 95% [60]. This material is notoriously difficult to retrieve and harvest from the canal spaces, owing to its insolubility to various solvents common to other retreatment techniques [61, 62]. Instead, the use of rotary burs and ultrasonic excavation, in conjunction with continual observation through the operating microscope, is advocated for safer negotiation and recovery of this material [62]. In this instance, both teeth #18 an #19 were treated with this material, and the CBCT was indispensable in the assessment and planning of this successful revision.

Case 11: #18,19 Retreatment of paste obturation (Russian Red)

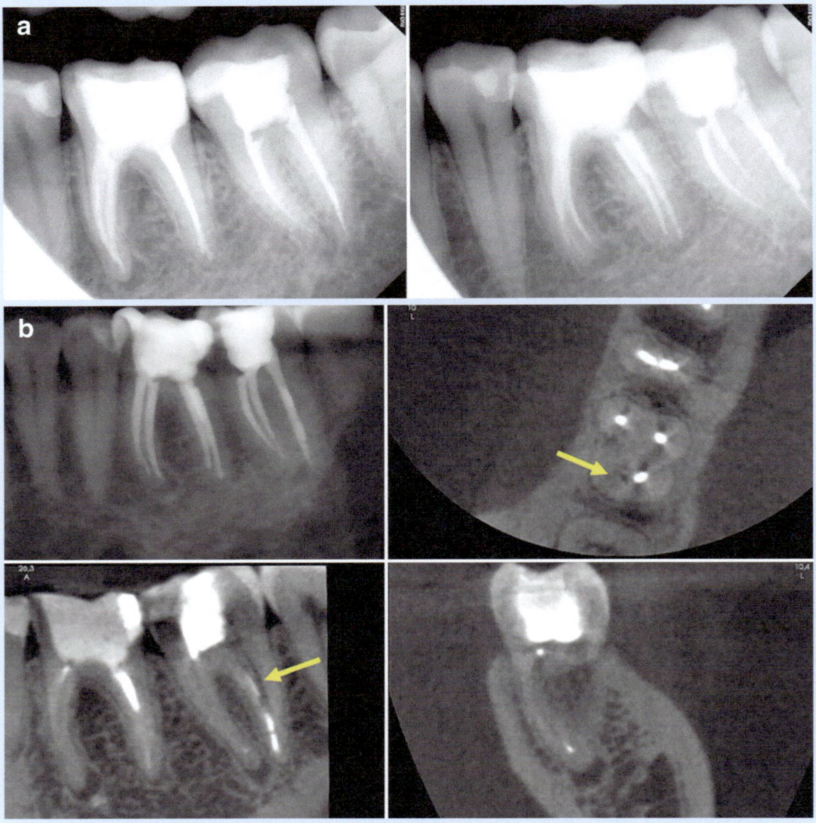

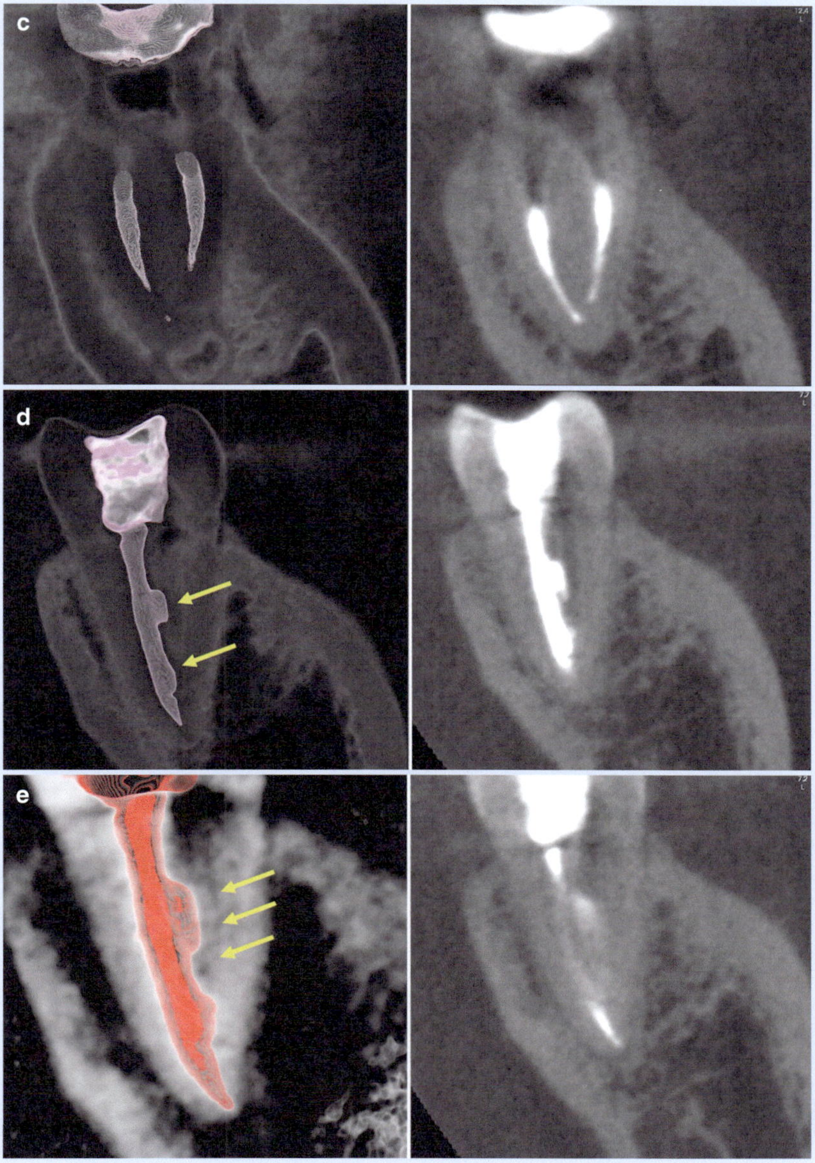
c
d
e

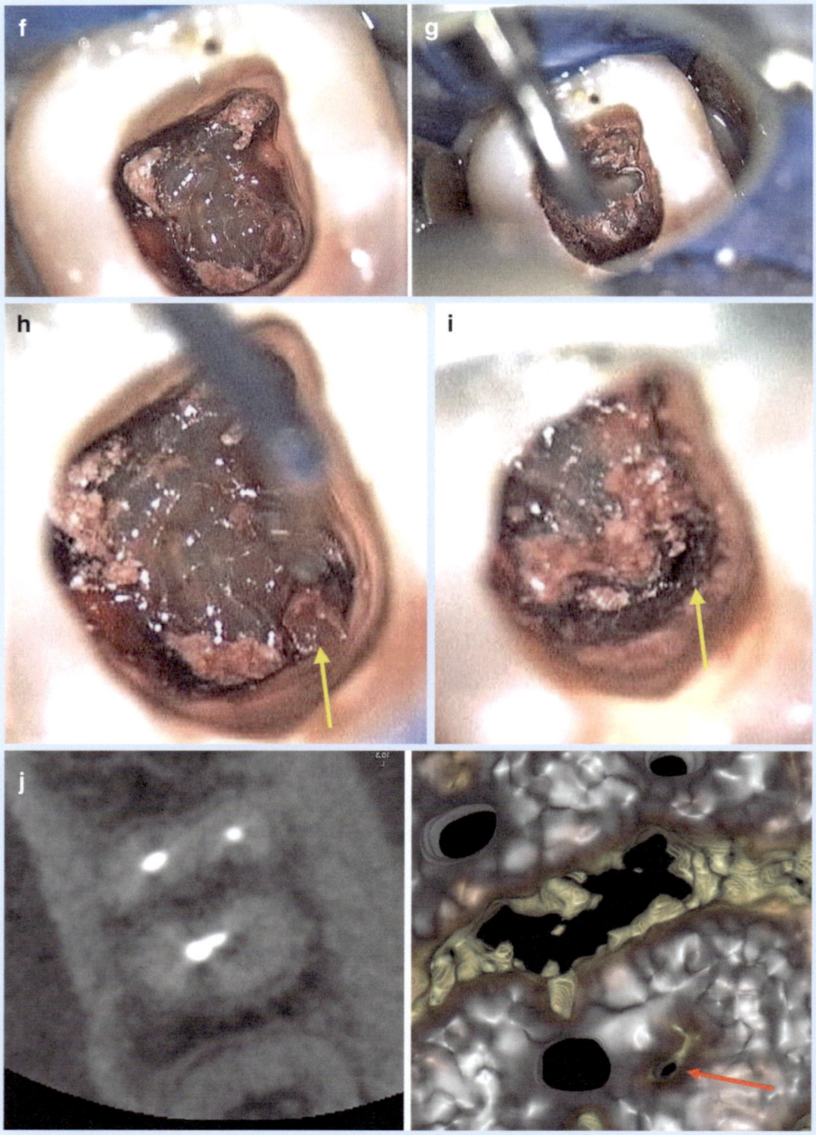
f
g
h
i
j

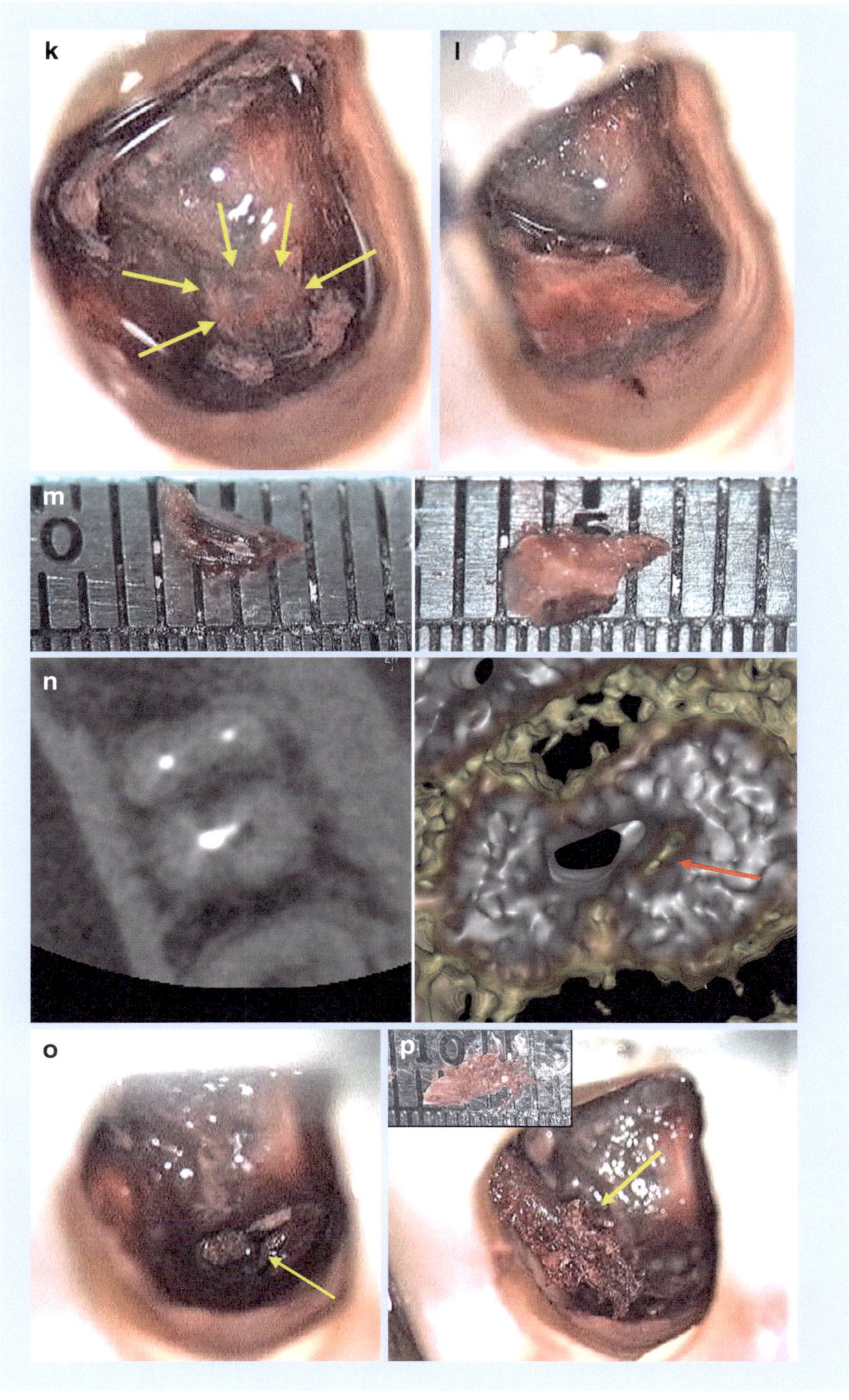
k
l
m
0
5
n
o
p

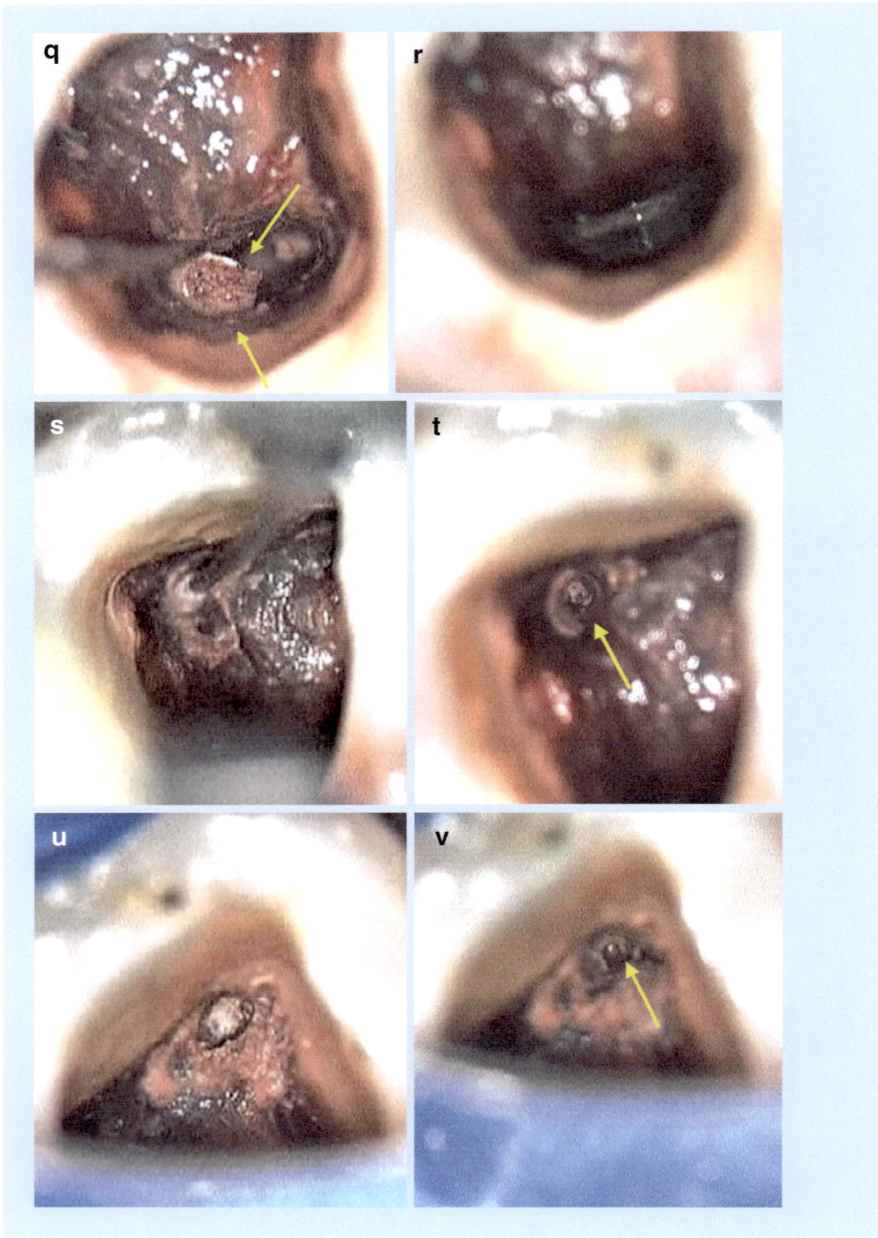
q
r
s
t
u
v

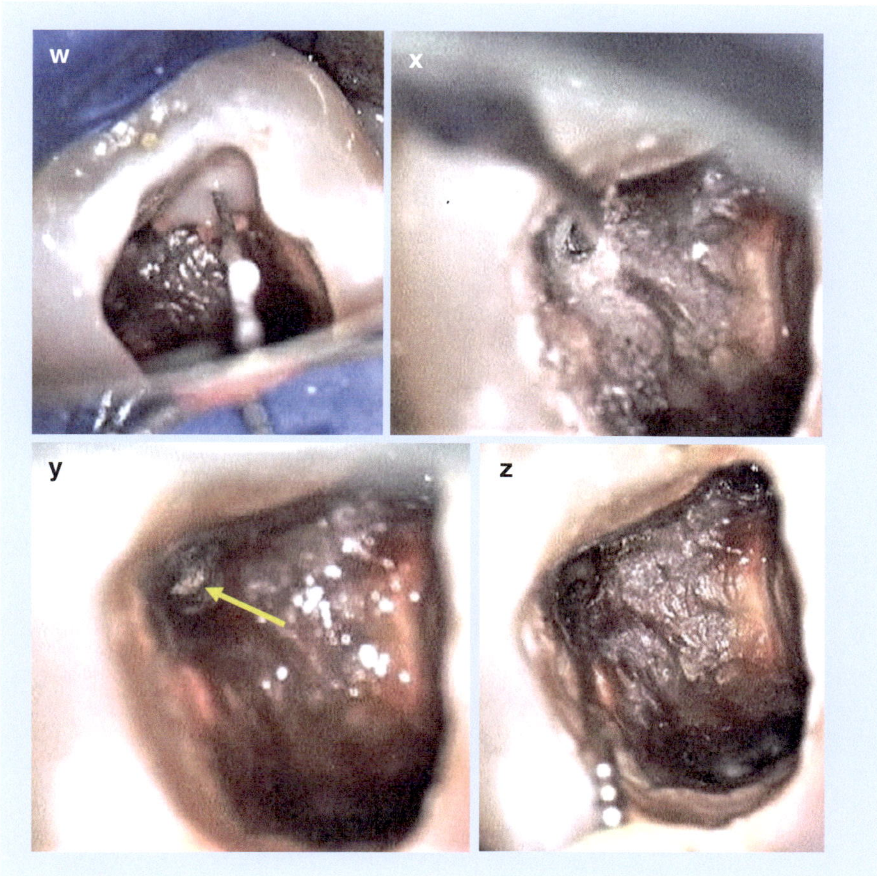
w
x
y
z

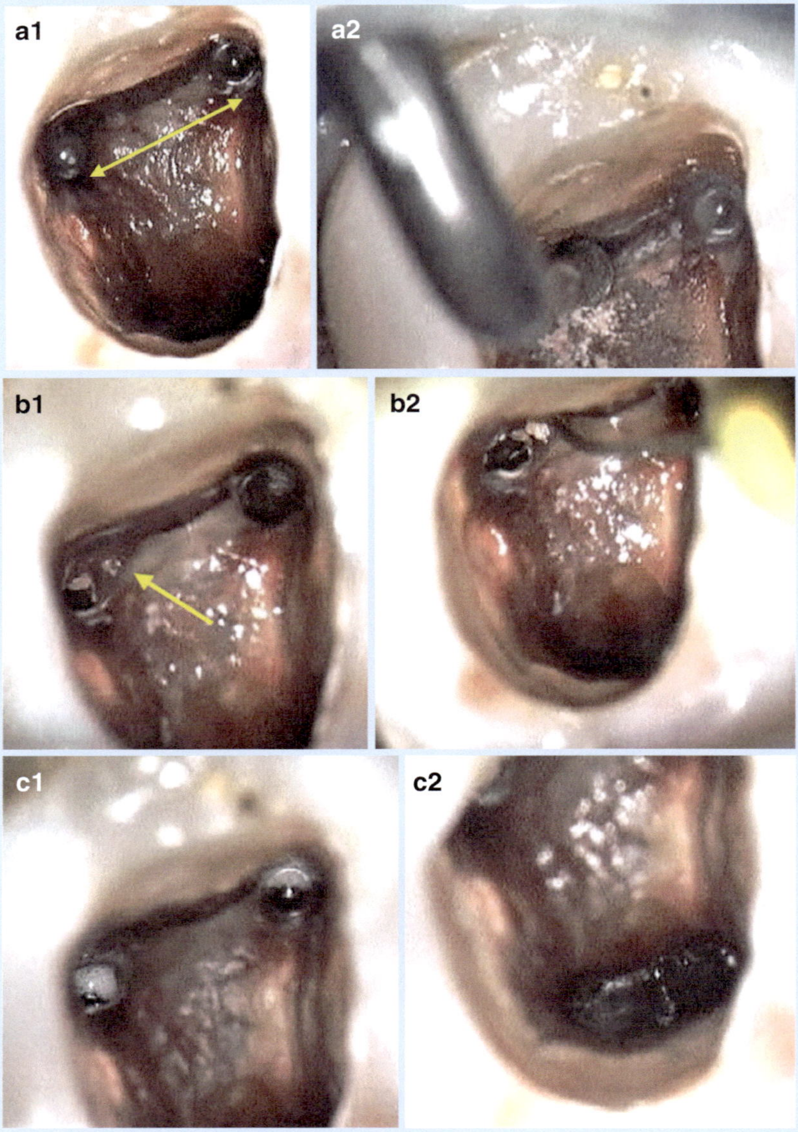
a1
a2
b1
b2
c1
c2

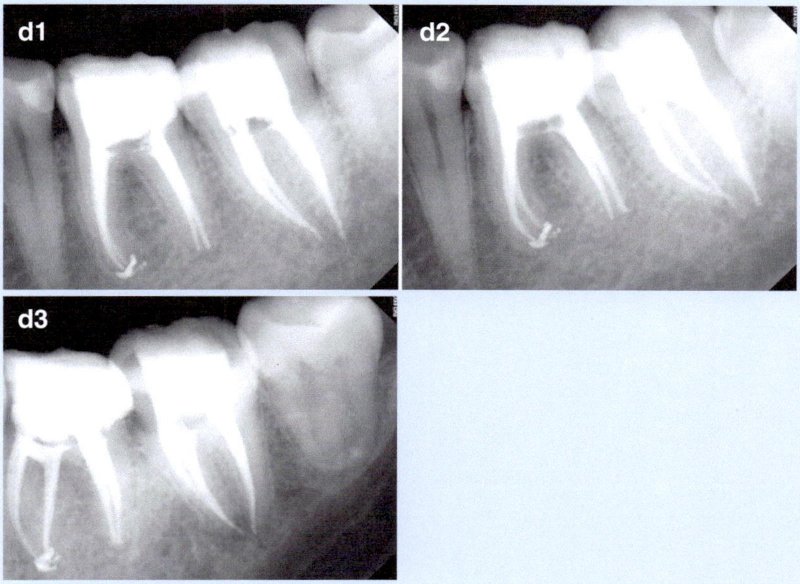
d1
d2
d3

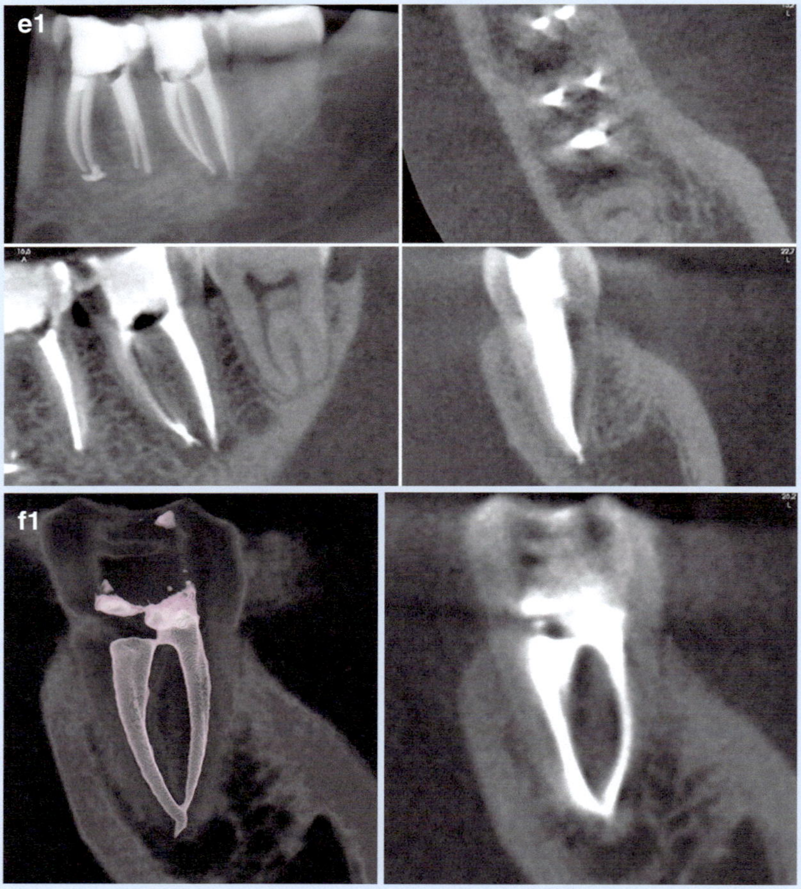
e1
f1

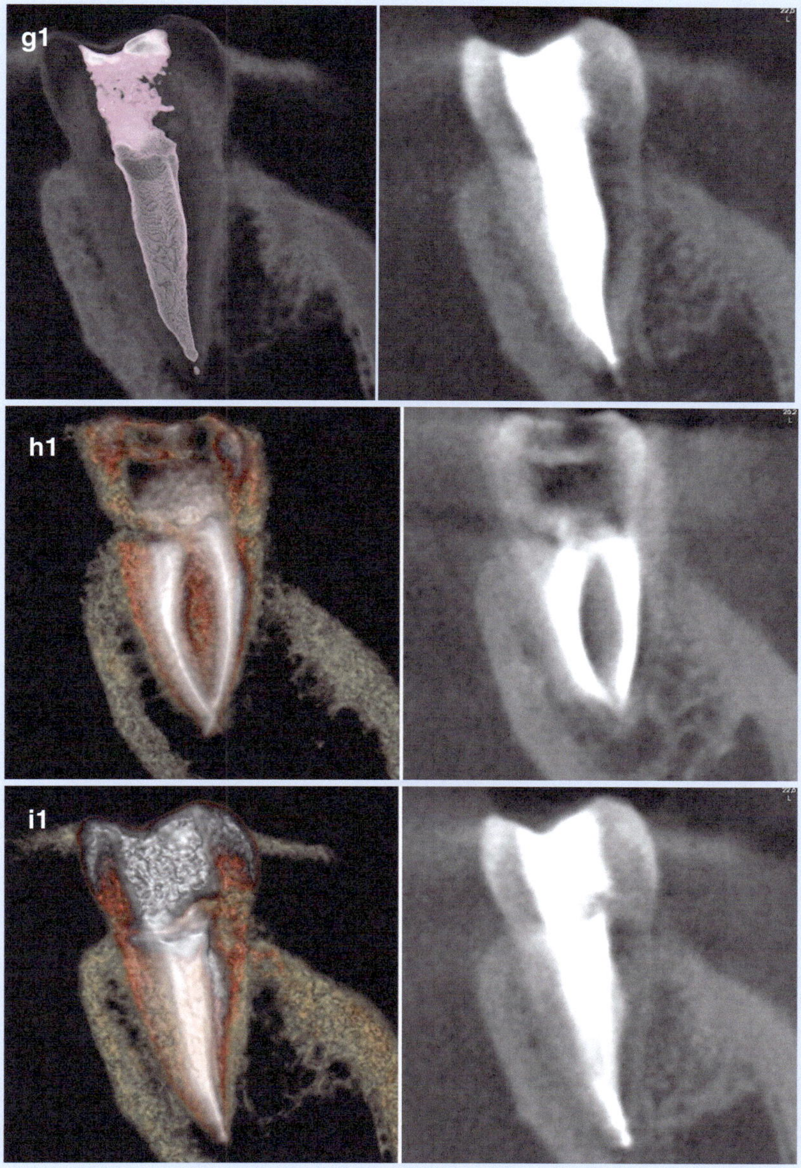
g1
h1
i1

Case 11 Description: The patient presents retreatment of teeth #'s 18/19. Initial treatment rendered in Ukraine 8 years ago. Diagnosis: Previous RCT/ Symptomatic Apical Periodontitis.

11 a: Preoperative radiographs revealing the presence of root canal treatment in teeth #18/19, with periapical lesions on all apices.
11 b: CBCT scan demonstrating low-density areas on the mesial root apices of #18/19, with an undiagnosed distolingual canal space in #18 (yellow arrow).
11 c: CBCT coronal view using the e-VolDX program (CDT Software) demonstrates the incomplete obturation and associated low-density area apically in the mesial root.
11 d: CBCT coronal view using the same software reveals the undiagnosed distolingual canal space and incomplete obturation (yellow arrows).
11 e: Using a different 3D filter, the "resinyfied" pulpal tissues are identified with regard to their extent, density, and location (yellow arrows).
11 f: Upon access to the previous pulp chamber, the obturative material was identified as resorcinol-formalin paste ("Russian Red") due to the rigidity of the material and the characteristic red staining of the surrounding tooth structure.
11 g: A football-shaped ultrasonic tip is used to refine the boundaries of the pulp chamber and remove the stained dentin overhangs and begin to define the canal orifices.
11 h: A small pulp stone is located and removed from the orifice of the distolingual canal space (yellow arrow).
11 i: Upon removal a patent space can be visualized apically in the root (yellow arrow).
11 j: Using the e-VolDX program the space located in 11i is visualized in the 3D filter (red arrow).
11 k: With the aid of irrigation fluid in the chamber, the outline of the "resinyfied" pulp tissue is identified (yellow arrows). This will enable discreet dislodgement using small ultrasonic tips.
11 l: A large fragment of resinyfied pulp tissue is delivered from the distal canal space.
11 m: The delivered fragment resembles petrified wood in appearance and texture, and is stained the characteristic deep ruby color of the paste.
11 n: Using the e-VolDX program the large fragment from 11l/m was virtually dissected from the distal canal space, with insight into its extent and shape. It also disclosed additional fragments more apically in the canal (red arrow).
11 o: An additional resinyfied piece of pulp tissue is dislodged using ultrasonic tips and displaced to the buccal aspect of the canal space (yellow arrow).

11 p: The fragment is delivered and is similar to the previous fragment in appearance and texture (yellow arrow).
11 q: A small piece of the hardened paste was dislodged in toto and delivered from the canal for identification and inspection (yellow arrows). Note the color and granular appearance. When fully set, it has the color and hardness of die stone used to pour dies in a dental laboratory.
11 r: Visualization of the evacuated distal canal space into the apical third of the root.
11 s: Using a pear-shaped ultrasonic tip (E6D, Helse Endodontics, Ocoee, FL) the paste in the coronal aspect of the mesiobuccal canal is removed. The thin profile of the tip allows for visualization of the excavation in real time without the microscope vision obstructed by a conventional handpiece. The depth and direction has been determined preoperatively using the CBCT scan and the 3D filters.
11 t: After approximately 3 mm, the excavation in the MB is halted for inspection. There is still a considerable thickness of paste, but a different pattern of ultrasonic tip will be employed for further excavation.
11 u: The mesiolingual canal was excavated to approximately the same level as the MB, but a void in the paste can be visualized.
11 v: Using a D-11T spreader, the void is penetrated (yellow arrow) to allow the insertion of an endodontic file (yellow arrow).
11 w: A hand file is inserted into the space and patency is confirmed.
11 x: Using an arrow-shaped ultrasonic tip termed the Flatsonic (R2, Helse Endodontics, Ocoee, FL) the paste in the middle third of the MB canal is removed. The thinner profile of this tip allows for improved visibility without undue excavation.
11 y: After an additional 1.5 mm of paste removal, inspection of the space reveals a void in the paste similar to 11u (yellow arrow). This is expanded in the same manner using the D-11T.
11 z: The void is penetrated into the canal space and patency is achieved.
11 a1: Both the MB and ML canal spaces have been negotiated and cleaned. There is greater than a 3 mm space between the canal orifices, and a middle mesial canal is suspected (yellow arrow).
11 a2: A football-shaped ultrasonic is used to deepen the trough between the two canal orifices.
11 b1: A small orifice is observed and penetrated with the D-11T spreader.
11 b2: The orifice is engaged with a hand file and threaded into the space; it merged with the MB canal space in the middle third of the root.
11 c1/2: Final appearance of the fully instrumented canal spaces and pulp chamber. Note the difference in color from the original presentation in the access. Tooth #19 was retreated in exactly the same manner with regard to technique and materials because of the presence of this paste in that tooth as well.

11 d1,2,3: Postoperative radiographs from different angles showing the extent and distribution of the retreated canal spaces.
11 e1: Postoperative CBCT specifically of tooth #18.
11 f1: Postoperative CBCT coronal slice of the mesial root of tooth #18; note the distribution of the filling as compared to the preoperative, and the small dilaceration of the canal space in the apical 1.5 mm.
11 g1: Postoperative CBCT coronal slice of the distal root of tooth #18; note the distribution of the filling as compared to the preoperative scan and the wide ribbon-shaped configuration.
11 h1/i1: Postoperative CBCT coronal slice of the mesial and distal roots of tooth #18 using a different 3D filter to detect any voids or inconsistencies in the obturation. (None were found.)

Non-surgical retreatment has been, and will continue to be, a challenging, rewarding, and frustrating aspect of specialty practice. But with the evolving techniques and imaging technologies, the practitioner can take consolation in the fact that they can provide the most effective and appropriate service for their patients via the least invasive means possible.

References

1. Grossman LIOS, Del Rio CE. Endodontic Practice. Eleventh ed. Philadelphia, PA: Lea & Febiger; 1988. p. 182–90.
2. Weine F. Endodontic therapy. Saint Louis, MO: The C.V. Mosby Company; 1972.
3. Krasner P, Rankow HJ. Anatomy of the pulp-chamber floor. J Endod. 2004 Jan;30(1):5–16.
4. Schwarze T, Baethge C, Stecher T, Geurtsen W. Identification of second canals in the mesiobuccal root of maxillary first and second molars using magnifying loupes or an operating microscope. Aust Endod J. 2002 Aug;28(2):57–60.
5. Kulild JC, Peters DD. Incidence and configuration of canal systems in the mesiobuccal root of maxillary first and second molars. J Endod. 1990 Jul;16(7):311–7.
6. Stropko JJ. Canal morphology of maxillary molars: clinical observations of canal configurations. J Endod. 1999 Jun;25(6):446–50.
7. Suter B, Lussi A, Sequeira P. Probability of removing fractured instruments from root canals. Int Endod J. 2005 Feb;38(2):112–23.
8. Roda RS. Root perforation repair: surgical and nonsurgical management. Pract Proced Aesthet Dent: PPAD. 2001;13(6):467–72. quiz 74
9. Koch K. The microscope. Its effect on your practice. Dent Clin N Am. 1997 Jul;41(3):619–26.
10. Hess W. The anatomy of the root canals of the teeth of the permanent dentition. London: John Bale, Sons & Danielsson Ltd; 1925.
11. FJ V. Root canal anatomy of the mandibular anterior teeth. JADA. 1974;89(2):369–71.
12. Neaverth EJ, Kotler LM, Kaltenbach RF. Clinical investigation (in vivo) of endodontically treated maxillary first molars. J Endod. 1987 Oct;13(10):506–12.
13. Bellizzi R, Hartwell G. Radiographic evaluation of root canal anatomy of in vivo endodontically treated maxillary premolars. J Endod. 1985 Jan;11(1):37–9.

14. Fogel HM, Peikoff MD, Christie WH. Canal configuration in the mesiobuccal root of the maxillary first molar: a clinical study. J Endod. 1994 Mar;20(3):135–7.
15. Niemczyk S. CBCT: The Virtual Surgery© in Endodontic Diagnosis. Dental economics–oral hygiene. 2012 (February):80–1.
16. Michetti J, Maret D, Mallet JP, Diemer F. Validation of cone beam computed tomography as a tool to explore root canal anatomy. J Endod. 2010 Jul;36(7):1187–90.
17. Baratto Filho F, Zaitter S, Haragushiku GA, de Campos EA, Abuabara A, Correr GM. Analysis of the internal anatomy of maxillary first molars by using different methods. J Endod. 2009 Mar;35(3):337–42.
18. Matherne RP, Angelopoulos C, Kulild JC, Tira D. Use of cone-beam computed tomography to identify root canal systems in vitro. J Endod. 2008 Jan;34(1):87–9.
19. Badole GP, Warhadpande MM, Shenoi PR, Lachure C, Badole SG. A rare root canal configuration of bilateral maxillary first molar with 7 root canals diagnosed using cone-beam computed tomographic scanning: a case report. J Endod. 2014 Feb;40(2):296–301.
20. Llena C, Fernandez J, Ortolani PS, Forner L. Cone-beam computed tomography analysis of root and canal morphology of mandibular premolars in a Spanish population. Imaging Sci Dent. 2014 Sep;44(3):221–7.
21. Silva EJ, Nejaim Y, Silva AI, Haiter-Neto F, Zaia AA, Cohenca N. Evaluation of root canal configuration of maxillary molars in a Brazilian population using cone-beam computed tomographic imaging: an in vivo study. J Endod. 2014 Feb;40(2):173–6.
22. Torres A, Jacobs R, Lambrechts P, Brizuela C, Cabrera C, Concha G, et al. Characterization of mandibular molar root and canal morphology using cone beam computed tomography and its variability in Belgian and Chilean population samples. Imaging Sci Dent. 2015 Jun;45(2):95–101.
23. Mahendra M, Verma A, Tyagi S, Singh S, Malviya K, Chaddha R. Management of complex root canal curvature of bilateral radix entomolaris: three-dimensional analysis with cone beam computed tomography. Case reports in dentistry. 2013;2013:697323.
24. Low KM, Dula K, Burgin W, von Arx T. Comparison of periapical radiography and limited cone-beam tomography in posterior maxillary teeth referred for apical surgery. J Endod. 2008 May;34(5):557–62.
25. Bornstein MM, Lauber R, Sendi P, von Arx T. Comparison of periapical radiography and limited cone-beam computed tomography in mandibular molars for analysis of anatomical landmarks before apical surgery. J Endod. 2011 Feb;37(2):151–7.
26. Witherspoon DE, Small JC, Regan JD. Missed canal systems are the most likely basis for endodontic retreatment of molars. Tex Dent J. 2013 Feb;130(2):127–39.
27. Karapinar-Kazandag M, Basrani BR, Friedman S. The operating microscope enhances detection and negotiation of accessory mesial canals in mandibular molars. J Endod. 2010 Aug;36(8):1289–94.
28. Goel NK, Gill KS, Taneja JR. Study of root canals configuration in mandibular first permanent molar. J Indian Soc Pedod Prev Dent. 1991 Mar;8(1):12–4.
29. Reeh ES. Seven canals in a lower first molar. J Endod. 1998 Jul;24(7):497–9.
30. Carabelli G. Systematiches Handbuch Der Zahnheikunde. 2nd ed. Vienna: Braumuller and Seidel; 1844.
31. Steelman R. Incidence of an accessory distal root on mandibular first permanent molars in Hispanic children. ASDC J Dent Child. 1986 Mar-Apr;53(2):122–3.
32. de Souza-Freitas JA, Lopes ES, Casati-Alvares L. Anatomic variations of lower first permanent molar roots in two ethnic groups. Oral Surg Oral Med Oral Pathol. 1971 Feb;31(2):274–8.
33. Garg AK, Tewari RK, Kumar A, Hashmi SH, Agrawal N, Mishra SK. Prevalence of three-rooted mandibular permanent first molars among the Indian population. J Endod. 2010 Aug;36(8):1302–6.
34. Schafer E, Breuer D, Janzen S. The prevalence of three-rooted mandibular permanent first molars in a German population. J Endod. 2009 Feb;35(2):202–5.
35. De Moor RJ, Deroose CA, Calberson FL. The radix entomolaris in mandibular first molars: an endodontic challenge. Int Endod J. 2004 Nov;37(11):789–99.

36. Hannah R, Kandaswamy D, Jayaprakash N. Endodontic management of a mandibular second molar with radix entomolaris: a case report. Restor Dent Endod. 2014 May;39(2):132–6.
37. De Moor RJ. C-shaped root canal configuration in maxillary first molars. Int Endod J. 2002 Feb;35(2):200–8.
38. Singla M, Aggarwal V. C-shaped palatal canal in maxillary second molar mimicking two palatal canals diagnosed with the aid of spiral computerized tomography. Oral Surg Oral Med Oral Pathol Oral Radiol Endod. 2010 Jun;109(6):e92–5.
39. Carlsen O, Alexandersen V, Heitmann T, Jakobsen P. Root canals in one-rooted maxillary second molars. Scand J Dent Res. 1992 Oct;100(5):249–56.
40. Alavi AM, Opasanon A, Ng YL, Gulabivala K. Root and canal morphology of Thai maxillary molars. Int Endod J. 2002 May;35(5):478–85.
41. Harris WE. Unusual root canal anatomy in a maxillary molar. J Endod. 1980 May;6(5):573–5.
42. Benenati FW. Maxillary second molar with two palatal canals and a palatogingival groove. J Endod. 1985 Jul;11(7):308–10.
43. Bond JL, Hartwell G, Portell FR. Maxillary first molar with six canals. J Endod. 1988 May;14(5):258–60.
44. Thews ME, Kemp WB, Jones CR. Aberrations in palatal root and root canal morphology of two maxillary first molars. J Endod. 1979 Mar;5(3):94–6.
45. Stone LH, Stroner WF. Maxillary molars demonstrating more than one palatal root canal. Oral Surg Oral Med Oral Pathol. 1981 Jun;51(6):649–52.
46. Cecic P, Hartwell G, Bellizzi R. The multiple root canal system in the maxillary first molar: a case report. J Endod. 1982 Mar;8(3):113–5.
47. Wong M. Maxillary first molar with three palatal canals. J Endod. 1991 Jun;17(6):298–9.
48. Cleghorn BM, Christie WH, Dong CC. The root and root canal morphology of the human mandibular first premolar: a literature review. J Endod. 2007 May;33(5):509–16.
49. Jain SD, Carrico CK, Bermanis I. 3-dimensional accuracy of dynamic navigation Technology in Locating Calcified Canals. J Endod. 2020 Jun;46(6):839–45.
50. Dianat O, Nosrat A, Tordik PA, Aldahmash SA, Romberg E, Price JB, et al. Accuracy and efficiency of a dynamic navigation system for locating calcified canals. J Endod. 2020 Nov;46(11):1719–25.
51. Jain SD, Saunders MW, Carrico CK, Jadhav A, Deeb JG, Myers GL. Dynamically navigated versus freehand access cavity preparation: a comparative study on substance loss using simulated calcified canals. J Endod. 2020 Nov;46(11):1745–51.
52. Rising DW, Goldman M, Brayton SM. Histologic appraisal of 3 experimental root canal filling materials. J Endod. 1975 May;1(5):172–7.
53. Spradling PM, Senia ES. The relative sealing ability of paste-type filling materials. J Endod. 1982 Dec;8(12):543–9.
54. Tanzilli JP, Nevins AJ, Borden BG. A histologic study comparing Hydron and gutta-percha as root canal filling materials in monkeys. J Endod. 1981 Sep;7(9):396–401.
55. van der Burgt TP, Plasschaert AJ. Bleaching of tooth discoloration caused by endodontic sealers. J Endod. 1986 Jun;12(6):231–4.
56. Schwandt NW, Gound TG. Resorcinol-formaldehyde resin "Russian red" endodontic therapy. J Endod. 2003 Jul;29(7):435–7.
57. Wu MKWM. Pink teeth resulting from Russian endodontic therapy. J Am Dent Assoc. 2000;131:1598–9.
58. Sikri VKSP, Singh J, Manjri M, Khanna S. Clinical and experimental observations on resinifying therapy. Oral Surg Oral Med Oral Pathol Oral Radiol. 1986;62:441–8.
59. Sikri VK, Sikri P, Singh J, Manjri M, Khanna S. Resinifying therapy in endodontics. II--Histological and bacteriological evaluation. Ind J Dent Res. 1996 Apr-Jun;7(2):51–3.
60. Kaminska-Litwin KWD. Clinicoradiographic evaluation of dental treatment using the extirpation method. Czas Stomatol. 1983;36:721–4.
61. Vranas RN, Hartwell GR, Moon PC. The effect of endodontic solutions on resorcinol-formalin paste. J Endod. 2003 Jan;29(1):69–72.
62. Gambrel MG, Hartwell GR, Moon PC, Cardon JW. The effect of endodontic solutions on resorcinol-formalin paste in teeth. J Endod. 2005 Jan;31(1):25–9.

Surgical Treatment Utilizing Cone Beam Computed Tomography

7

Mohamed I. Fayad and Bradford R. Johnson

Abstract

Cone beam computed tomography (CBCT) is a diagnostic imaging modality that provides a high-quality, dimensionally accurate three-dimensional (3D) representation of the osseous elements of the maxillofacial skeleton. CBCT has the potential to transform the practice of endodontic microsurgery, much in the same way that other new technologies introduced over the past two decades—such as microscopes, ultrasonic devices, and new root-end filling materials—have led to enhanced safety and treatment outcomes. The different applications of CBCT in diagnosis, treatment planning, and long-term outcome evaluation of periapical surgery will be reviewed. In this chapter, cases will be presented to demonstrate the value of CBCT imaging in presurgical assessment, case selection, and treatment planning in endodontic microsurgery. The use of CBCT to identify and manage cases involving close proximity to important anatomical structures (e.g., maxillary sinus, the inferior alveolar, mental, and nasopalatine neurovascular bundles) and to evaluate the outcome of periapical microsurgery will be presented and discussed.

7.1 Potential Applications of CBCT in Treatment Planning of Endodontic Microsurgery

Cone beam computed tomography (CBCT) is a radiographic method which allows the clinician to visualize an individual tooth or teeth in relation to the surrounding structures and to create a three-dimensional (3D) image of the area. Traditional

M. I. Fayad (✉) · B. R. Johnson
Department of Endodontics, University of Illinois Chicago, Chicago, IL, USA
e-mail: mfayad1@uic.edu; bjohnson@uic.edu

M. I. Fayad, B. R. Johnson (eds.), *3D Imaging in Endodontics*,
https://doi.org/10.1007/978-3-031-32755-1_7

radiographic examinations are usually limited to two-dimensional views captured using radiographic film or digital sensors. Two-dimensional methods reproduce the three-dimensional anatomy as a 2D image. Essential information of the three-dimensional anatomy of the tooth/teeth and adjacent structures may be obscured, and, even with paralleling techniques, distortion and superimposition of dental structures in periapical images is unavoidable.

The role of CBCT in planning for periapical microsurgery has been well documented [1–4]. A major advantage of CBCT is the three-dimensional geometric accuracy compared with conventional radiographs. Comparing CBCT with periapical films, the CBCT has been reported to be a more sensitive means to detect changes in density of the bony structures [5] and the presence of periapical rarefaction. Three-dimensional visualization of the location of lesions and increased accuracy in the diagnosis of the true periapical status have been reported [6, 7]. The different spatial views of CBCT images eliminate the superimposition of anatomical structures. Periapical microsurgery involving maxillary and mandibular molars is often challenging. Difficulties include the close proximity of the apices or periapical lesions to vital structures. In the posterior maxillary region, the roots of maxillary teeth overlap with anatomic structures such as the maxillary sinus and the zygomatic process. The roots of maxillary posterior teeth and their periapical tissues can be visualized separately and in all three orthogonal planes without superimposition of the overlying zygomatic process, alveolar bone, and adjacent roots. In the posterior mandibular region, the roots of the mandibular premolars and molars are associated with close proximity of the apices or periapical pathology to the mental foramen and mandibular canal.

Both medical CT and CBCT have been used for planning endodontic microsurgery [8, 9]. Three-dimensional imaging allows for a more precise preoperative analysis of the anatomical relationship of the root apices to important neighboring structures such as the mandibular canal, mental foramen, and maxillary sinus. Velvart et al. [8] found that the relationship of the mandibular canal to the root apices could be determined in every case when using medical CT but in less than 40% of cases when using conventional radiography. It is likely that similar results could be achieved with CBCT using considerably less radiation. Rigolone et al. [9] concluded that CBCT may play an important role in periapical microsurgery of palatal roots of maxillary first molars. The distance between the cortical plate and the palatal root apex can be measured, and the presence or absence of the maxillary sinus between the roots could be assessed. In addition, the thickness of the cortical plate, the cancellous bone pattern, fenestrations, the shape of the maxilla and mandible, as well as the inclination of the roots of teeth planned for periapical surgery can be determined before starting surgery. Root morphology can be visualized in three dimensions, as can the number of root canals and whether they converge or diverge from each other. Missed (and untreated) root canals in root-filled teeth may be identified using axial slices, allowing for a level of diagnostic precision that is usually not possible, even with several angled 2D radiographs. The true size, location, and extent of periapical disease can be appreciated using CBCT, and the actual root, or roots, associated with a periapical lesion can be identified with confidence.

In two recent studies, the thickness and the anatomic characteristics of the Schneiderian membrane and cortical bone were evaluated using CBCT in patients planned for periapical surgery in the maxillary molar region [10, 11]. The Schneiderian membrane in the vicinity of roots with apical lesions tends to be significantly thicker when compared to the roots of teeth without apical pathosis [10].

Close proximity and even contact of the root apices of mandibular posterior teeth and the mandibular canal are not rare and must be taken into consideration when planning apical microsurgery to decrease the risk of iatrogenic nerve damage [12]. The mean distance between the mandibular canal and the apices of the adjacent teeth was evaluated in a recent study [13]. A total of 821 second mandibular premolars and 597 first, 508 second, and 48 third mandibular molars were included in this study. The mean distances were 4.2, 4.9, 3.1, and 2.6 mm, respectively. The occurrence of a direct relationship between the root tips and the mandibular canal was noted in 3.2%, 2.9%, 15.2%, and 31.3% of the teeth. Women were almost twice as often affected as men. No significant differences were found concerning the location (right/left) of the teeth ($P > 0.05$). Significantly shorter distances from the mandibular canal to the root apices were found in patients younger than 35 years old compared with older patients.

CBCT enables periapical disease at the root apex to be detected earlier than on conventional radiographs [14]. CBCT scans resulted in 62% more periapical radiolucent areas being detected on individual roots of posterior mandibular and maxillary teeth when compared with two angled periapical radiographs. In situations where patients have poorly localized symptoms associated with an untreated or previously root-filled tooth and clinical and periapical radiographic examination shows no evidence of disease, CBCT may be indicated to detect the presence of previously undiagnosed periapical disease. Simon et al. [15] compared the ability of CBCT and biopsy with histological examination to differentiate between periapical cysts and granulomas in teeth with large periapical lesions. It was found that gray scale value measurements of periapical lesions on CBCT images were able to differentiate solid (granulomas) from cystic- or cavity (cyst)-type lesions. If confirmed, these findings could influence the decision-making process when considering a nonsurgical or surgical approach to endodontic retreatment.

A recent study evaluated the concordance of two- and three-dimensional radiography with histopathology in the diagnosis of periapical lesions [16]. The final histological diagnosis of the periapical lesions included 55 granulomas (94.8%) and 3 cysts (5.2%). Radiographic assessment overestimated cysts by 28.4% (CBCT imaging) and 20.7% (periapical radiography), respectively. In contrast to Simon et al. [15], it was concluded that in order to establish a definitive diagnosis of an apical lesion, the tissue specimen should be evaluated histologically. Analysis of two-dimensional and three-dimensional radiographic images results only in a tentative diagnosis that should be confirmed with biopsy.

One of the more interesting areas in which CBCT may be applied in endodontics is evaluating the outcome of treatment [17, 18]. CBCT scans should result in a more objective and therefore more accurate determination of the outcome of endodontic treatment. CBCT images are geometrically accurate, and there is no distortion of the teeth being assessed or superimposition of overlying anatomy as often seen with conventional film and digitally captured periapical radiographs. Recently, clinical studies have compared the diagnostic value of 2D and 3D radiography for the post-surgical assessment of periapical healing following periapical microsurgery [19–21]. There was higher agreement when evaluating healing using CBCT compared to the 2D imaging. The results of these studies demonstrated that the percentage of repair was different for both methods. More remaining osseous defects were detected after periapical microsurgery on CBCT images than on periapical radiographs. The lower rate of healing observed on CBCT could be attributed to the type of the bony defect that might require regenerative procedures, or longer observation periods for healing assessment may be necessary. There is a need to define the criteria for radiographic healing when using CBCT for microsurgical outcome assessment.

Future research may show that root-filled teeth that appear to have "healed" using conventional radiographs may still have signs of periapical disease (e.g., widened periodontal ligament space, periapical radiolucency) when imaged using CBCT. This in turn may have implications for restorative treatment planning, in situations where evidence of healing using 2D radiographs is one of the criteria to move forward with a new restoration.

Figures 7.1, 7.2, 7.3, 7.4, 7.5, 7.6, 7.7, 7.8, 7.9, 7.10, 7.11, 7.12, 7.13, 7.14, 7.15, 7.16, 7.17, 7.18, 7.19, 7.20, 7.21, 7.22 and 7.23 demonstrate a series of surgical cases where CBCT was a valuable aid in accurate diagnosis and treatment planning prior to surgical treatment.

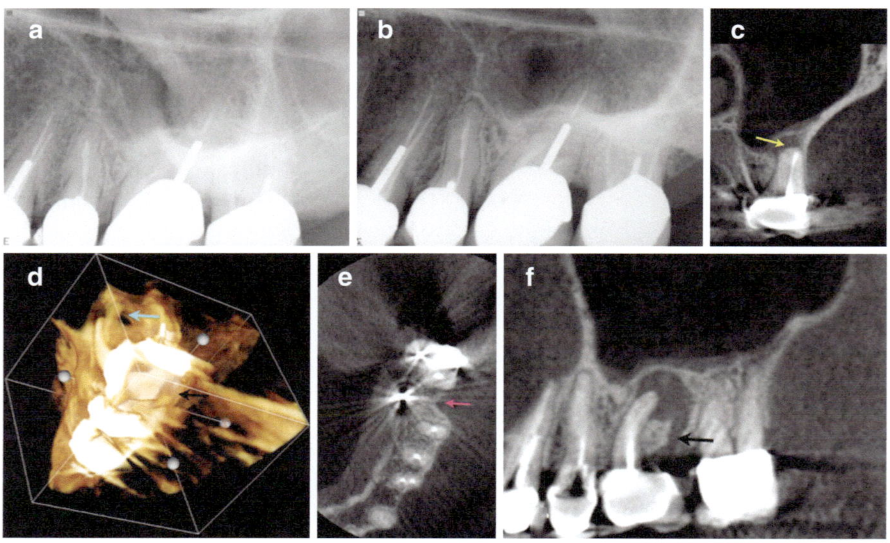

Fig. 7.1 Periapical radiographs of tooth #14, mesial and distal angles, respectively (**a** and **b**). Coronal view of the mesiobuccal root showing a missed mesiobuccal canal and periapical pathology not detected on the 2D radiograph (yellow arrow) (**c**). 3D reconstruction showing a crestal bony defect (blue arrow) (**d**). Axial view showing a previous distobuccal root amputation site (pink arrow) that was not detected on the periapical radiographs (**e**). (**f**) Sagittal view showing the crestal defect (black arrow) communicating with the periapical lesion and elevating the floor of the maxillary sinus, with no evidence of sinus perforation (**f**)

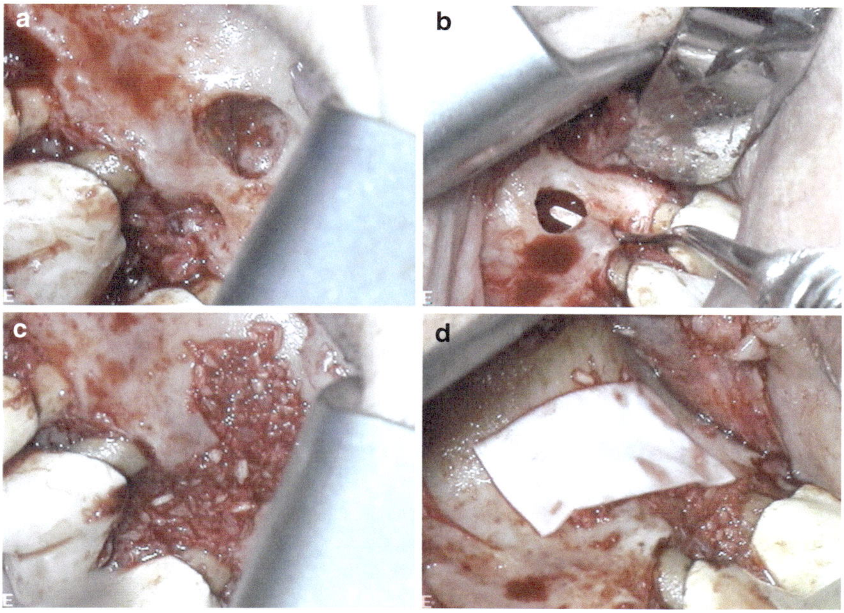

Fig. 7.2 Continuation of case presented in Fig. 6.1: Clinical picture after flap reflection showing both crestal and periapical lesions (**a**). Communication between both defects (**b**). Both defects grafted with enCore™ combination allograft (Osteogenics Biomedical, Lubbock, TX) (c). CopiOs™ pericardium membrane (Zimmer, Warsaw, IN) (**d**)

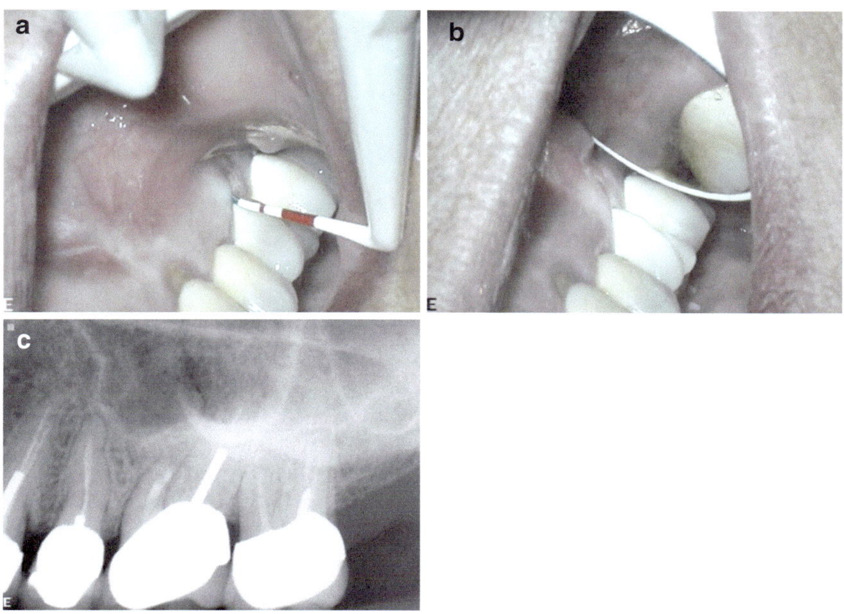

Fig. 7.3 Continuation of case presented in Figs. 6.1 and 6.2: Clinical soft tissue healing one year postoperative (**a** and **b**). One-year postoperative recall radiograph (**c**)

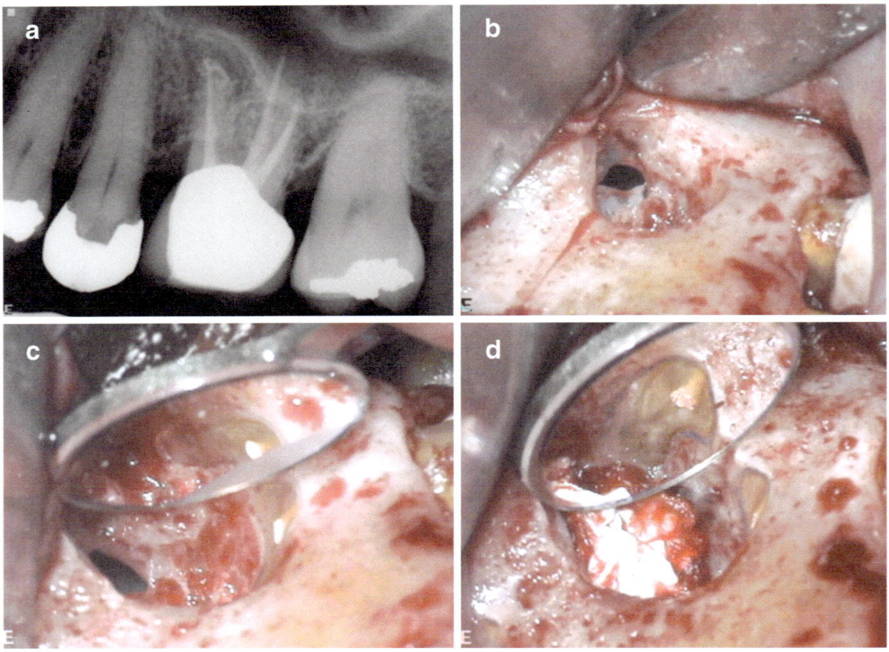

Fig. 7.4 Periapical radiograph of tooth #14 referred for periapical surgery (**a**). Clinical picture demonstrating sinus communication after degranulation of the defect (**b** and **c**). Clinical picture demonstrating the protection of the sinus communication with Collacote™ and methylene blue staining of the MB root resection to confirm complete resection and locate the untreated mesio-palatal canal prior to ultrasonic root-end preparation (**d**)

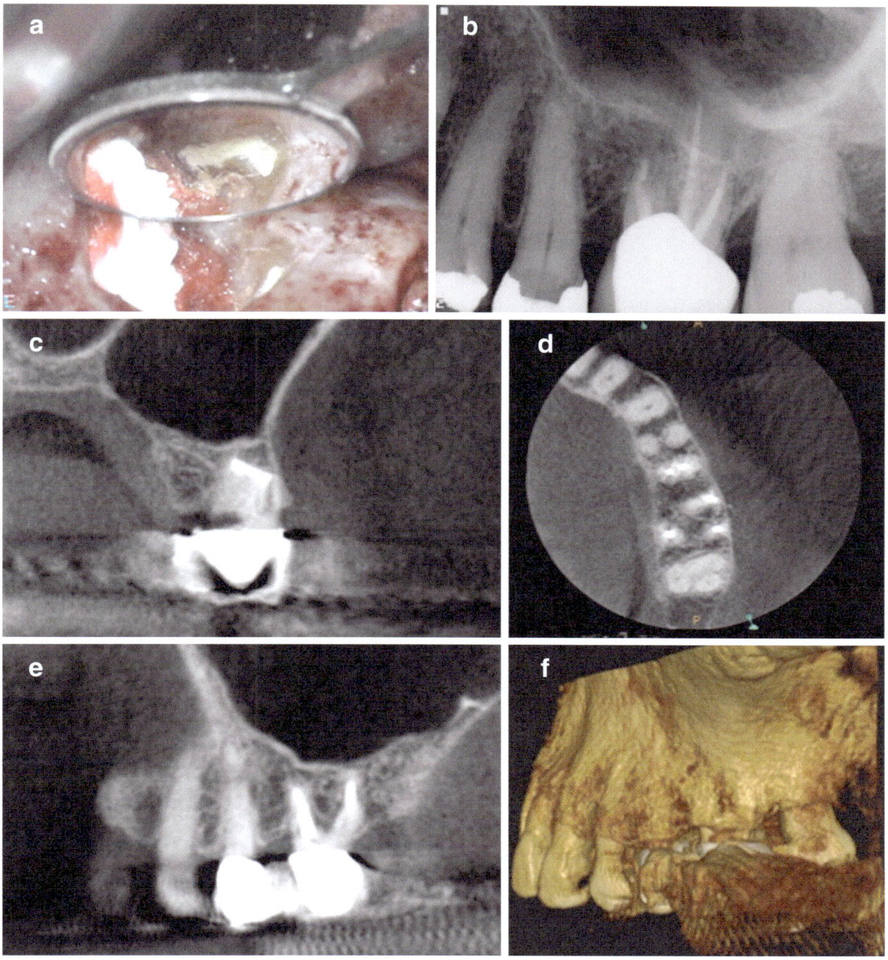

Fig. 7.5 Continuation of case presented in Fig. 6.4: Root-end filling with MTA (**a**). Postoperative radiograph (**b**). Eight-year recall CBCT demonstrating the coronal (**c**), sagittal (**e**), axial (**d**), and 3D rendering (**f**). Complete bone regeneration of the buccal plate as well as the floor of the sinus can be visualized

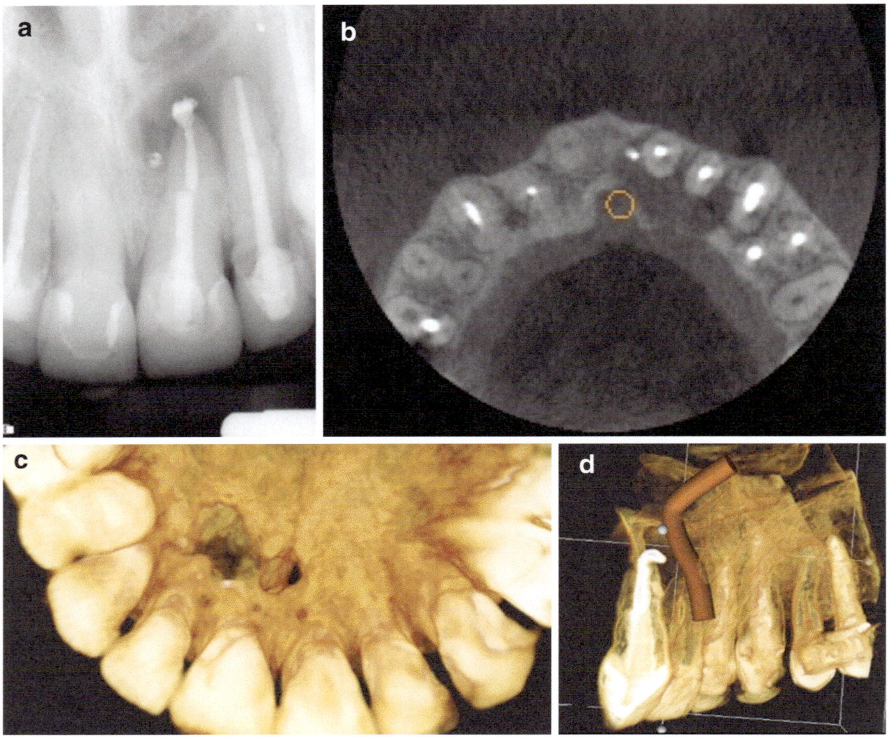

Fig. 7.6 Periapical radiograph of the maxillary anterior region showing a periapical lesion associated with tooth #9 (**a**). (B) Axial view showing the extent of the lesion, palatal plate perforation, and relationship of the nasopalatine neurovascular bundle to the periapical lesion (**b**). Palatal view of the 3D reconstruction showing perforation of the palatal plate (**c**). 3D reconstruction showing the nasopalatine bundle (**d**)

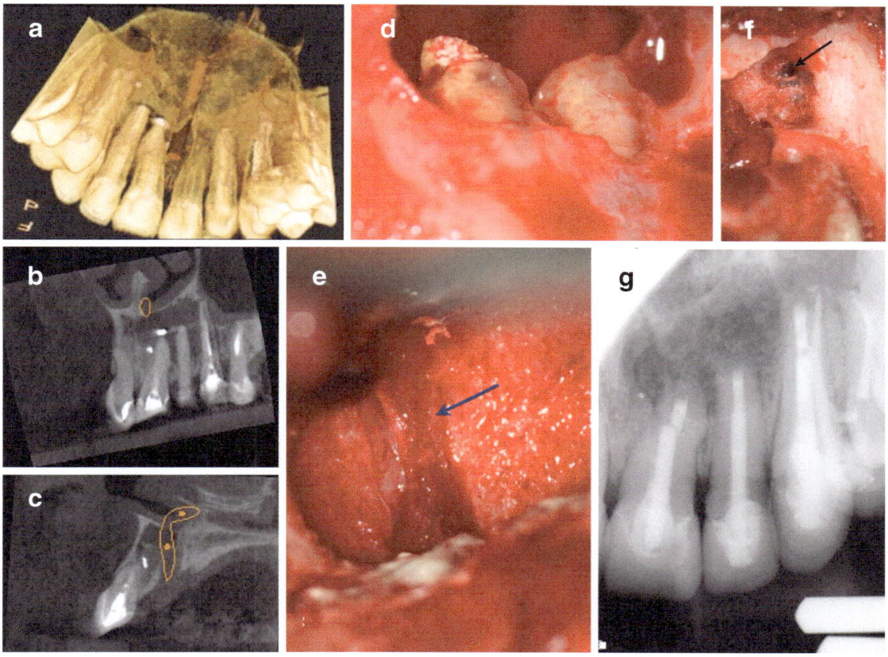

Fig. 7.7 Continuation of case presented in Fig. 6.6: Palatal view CBCT reconstruction showing the exit of the nasopalatine bundle from the incisive canal (**a**). Coronal view showing periapical radiolucency involving teeth #9, 10, and 11 (**b**). Sagittal view of the exit of the nasopalatine bundle from the incisive canal (**c**). Periapical defect after degranulation showing the apices of teeth #9 and 10 before resection (**d**). (E) A clinical picture of the intact nasopalatine neurovascular bundle (blue arrow) after degranulation (**e**). Lateral wall of the maxillary sinus distal to tooth #11 (black arrow) (**f**). An immediate postoperative radiograph (**g**) after grafting the through-and-through defect with Puros allograft™ (Zimmer Dental, Warsaw, IN) material and, CopiOs™ membrane

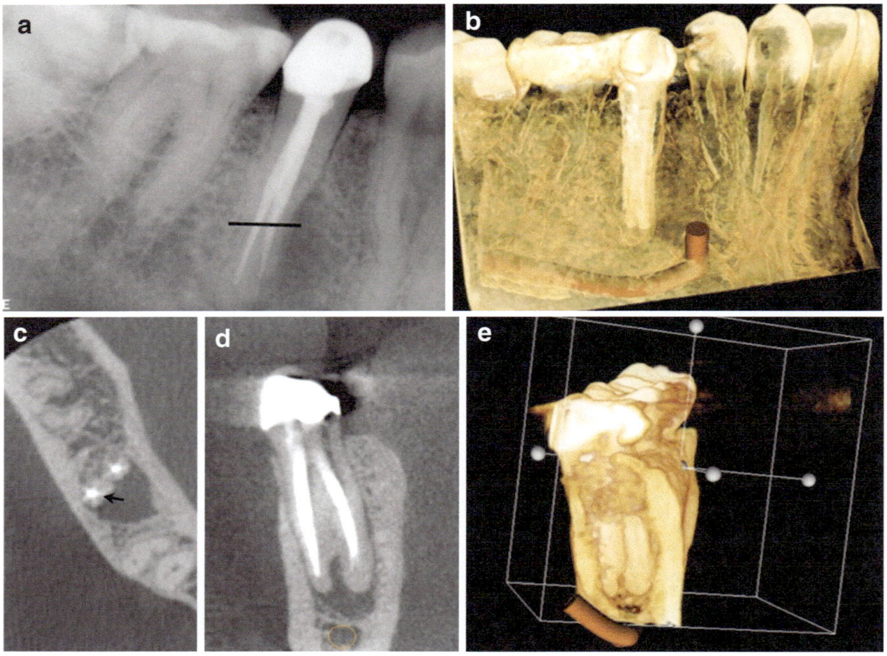

Fig. 7.8 Periapical radiograph of tooth #29 that was referred for apical microsurgery (**a**). The line corresponds to the level of the axial view in (**c**). Note the C-type-shaped canal (black arrow). 3D rendering demonstrating the relationship and proximity of the inferior alveolar nerve (IAN) and mental foramen to the apex of tooth #29 (**b**). Axial view of the apical one-third demonstrating the extent of the periapical defect (**c**). Coronal view demonstrating the relationship and the proximity of the IAN canal (**d**). 3D rendering demonstrating the relationship and the proximity of the IAN to the periapical defect as well the apex of tooth #29 (**e**)

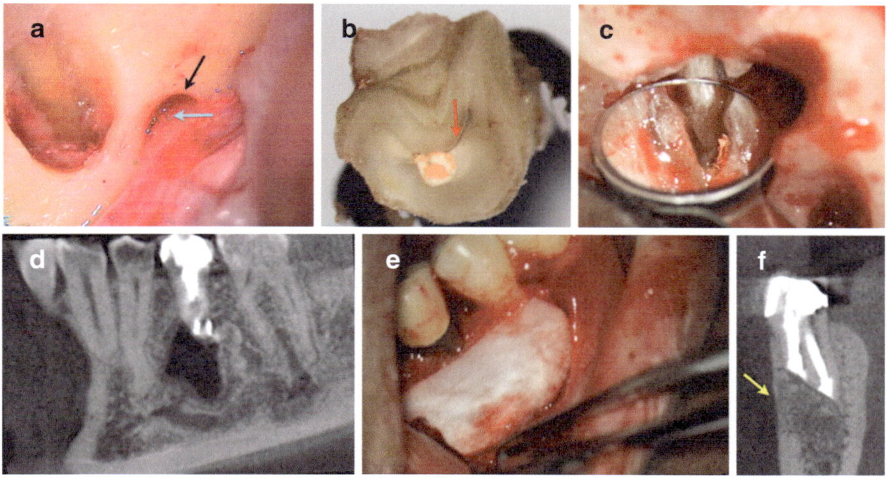

Fig. 7.9 Continuation of case presented in Fig. 6.8: Clinical picture of the mental foramen (black arrow) and the neurovascular bundle (blue arrow) being identified (**a**). Clinical picture of the resected apex of tooth #29 after extraction and root-end resection, in preparation for root-end preparation, filling, and intentional replantation (**b**). Note the C-shaped anatomy which is similar to the axial view (**c**). Replanted tooth after ultrasonic apical preparation of the C-shaped canal and MTA root-end filling of the apical preparation (**d**). Bony defect grafted with Puros™ allograft (Zimmer Dental, Warsaw, IN) and, CopiOs™ membrane (**e**). One-year coronal view CBCT recall demonstrating complete remodeling of the defect including the buccal cortical plate (**f**)

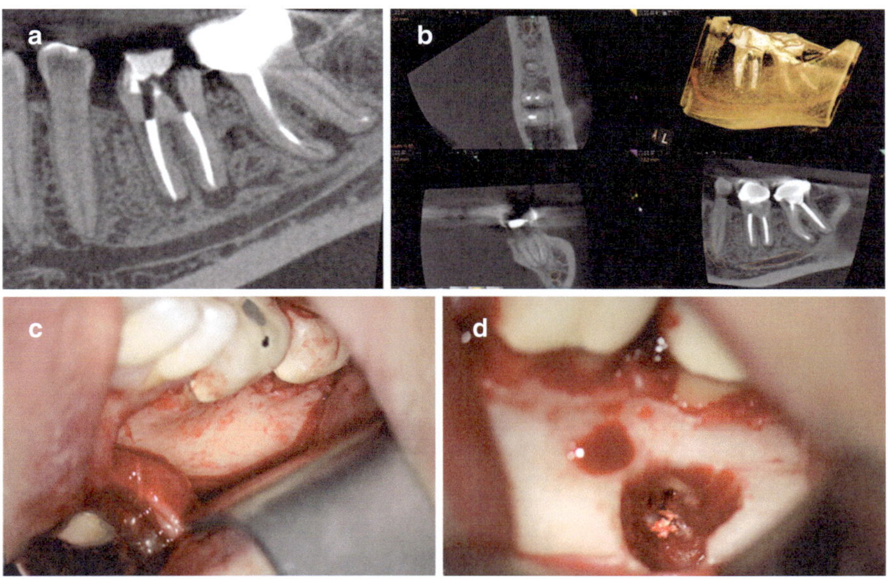

Fig. 7.10 CBCT sagittal view of tooth #18 that was referred for periapical microsurgery (**a**). CBCT of the axial, coronal, sagittal views and 3D rendering demonstrating the proximity of the IAN to the mesial root of tooth #18 (**b**). Clinical picture after surgical flap reflection showing the buccal cortical plate (**c**). Osteotomy and resection of the mesial root (**d**)

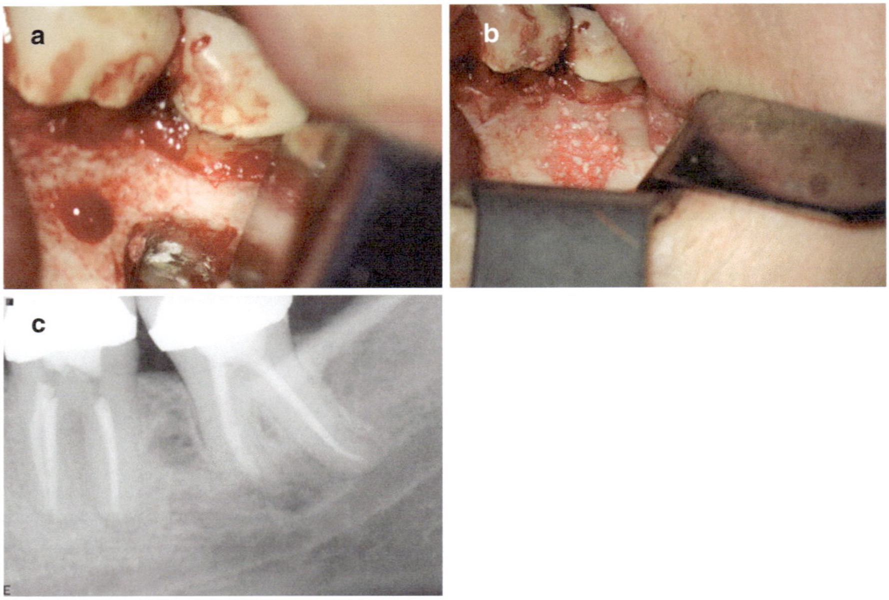

Fig. 7.11 Continuation of case presented in Fig. 6.10: Clinical picture demonstrating the MTA root-end filling (**a**). Periapical defect grafted with Puros™ allograft (Zimmer Dental, Warsaw, IN) material and, and before placing CopiOs™ membrane (**b**). Immediate postsurgical radiograph (**c**)

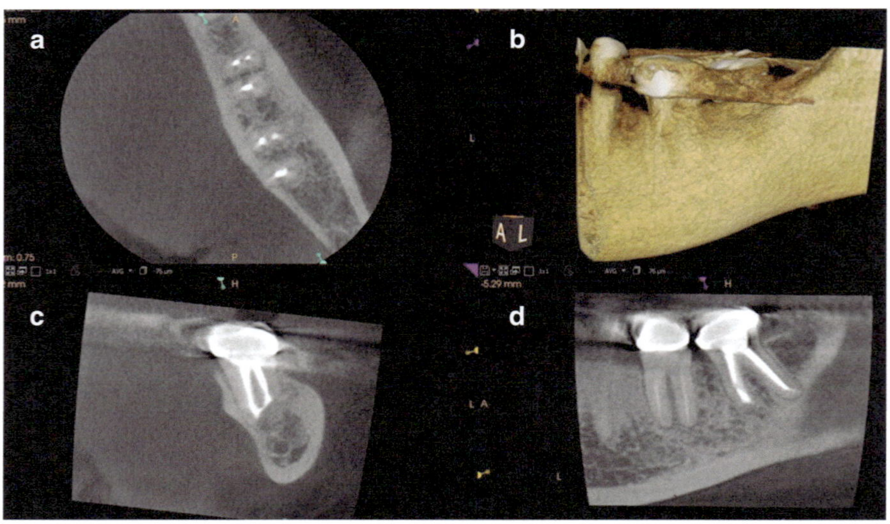

18 months recall

Fig. 7.12 Continuation of case presented in Figs. 6.10 and 6.11: 18-month postoperative CBCT scan demonstrating complete remodeling of the defect and the buccal plates (**a**, **b**, **c**, and **d**)

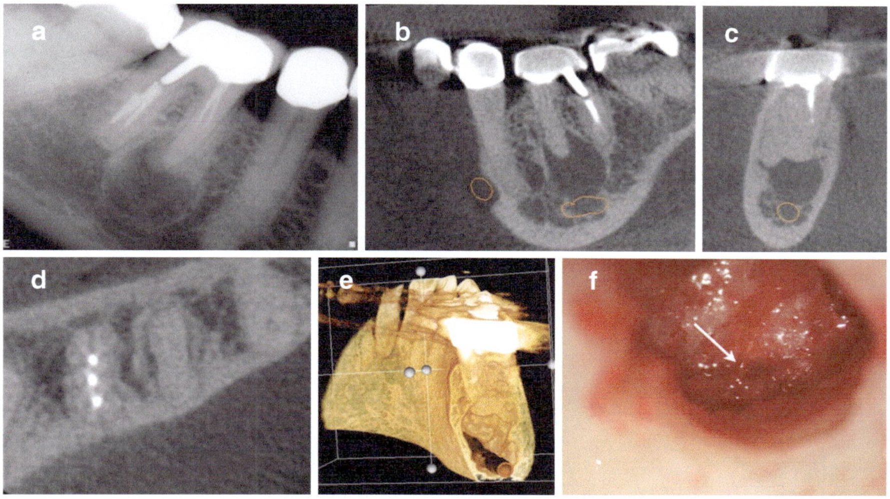

Fig. 7.13 Periapical radiograph of tooth #30 that was referred for periapical surgery (**a**). CBCT of the sagittal, coronal, and axial views, and 3D rendering demonstrating the proximity and communication of the defect and IAN to the mesial root of tooth #18 (**b**, **c**, **d**, and **e**). Clinical picture after surgical flap reflection, mesial root resection, and degranulation of the defect (**f**). The IAN was detected (white arrow) at the base of the defect

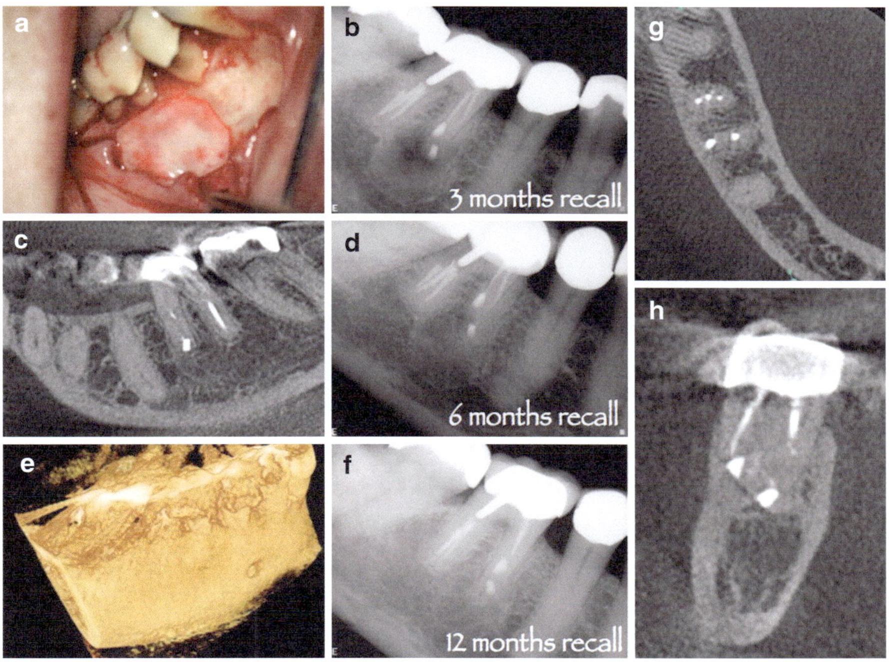

Fig. 7.14 Continuation of case presented in Fig. 6.13: Clinical picture of CopiOs™ membrane without graft material (**a**). Periapical radiograph of 3-month recall (**b**). CBCT sagittal view, periapical radiograph, and 3D rendering at 6-month recall (**c**, **d**, and **e**). Periapical radiograph, axial and coronal views of tooth #30 at 12-month recall demonstrating complete remodeling of the defect including the buccal cortical plate (**f**, **g**, and **h**)

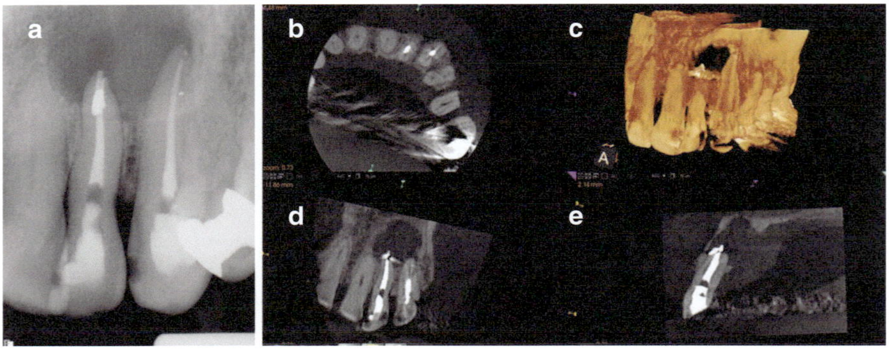

Fig. 7.15 Periapical radiograph of teeth # 10 and 11 (**a**). The 2D radiograph does not allow for appreciation of the true size and extent of the defect. CBCT scan demonstrating the actual size of the defect (**b**, **c**, **d**, and **e**). Perforation and loss of palatal bone can be clearly seen in the sagittal view (**e**)

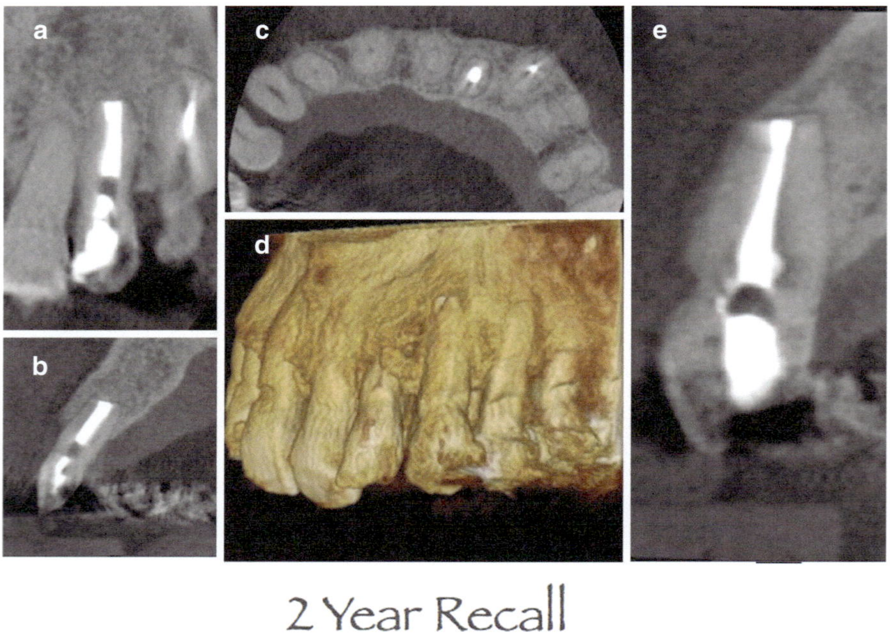

Fig. 7.16 Continuation of case presented in Fig. 6.15: 2-year recall CBCT scan of teeth #10 and 11 demonstrating complete remodeling of the defect including the buccal and palatal cortical plates (**a**, **b**, **c**, d, and e)

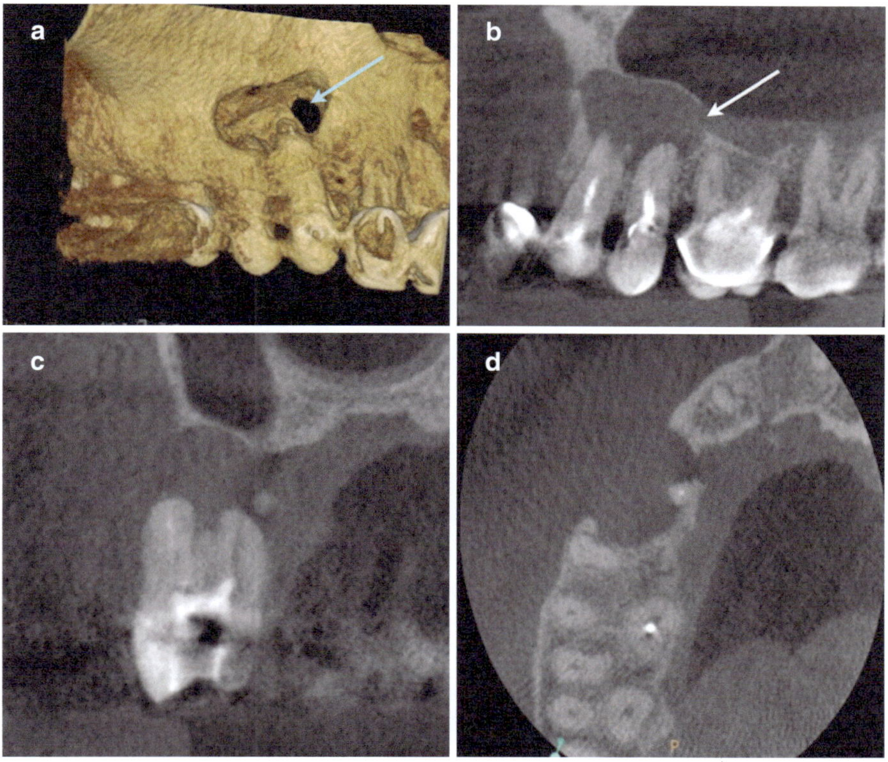

Fig. 7.17 CBCT 3D rendering of teeth #12 and 13 referred for periapical surgery (**a**). Perforation of the maxillary sinus can be visualized (blue arrow). Sagittal view of teeth #12 and 13 (**b**). Perforation of the maxillary sinus noted (white arrow). Coronal view of tooth #12 demonstrating the through-and-through nature of the periapical defect (**c**). Axial view demonstrating the mesio-distal extent of the periapical defect (**d**)

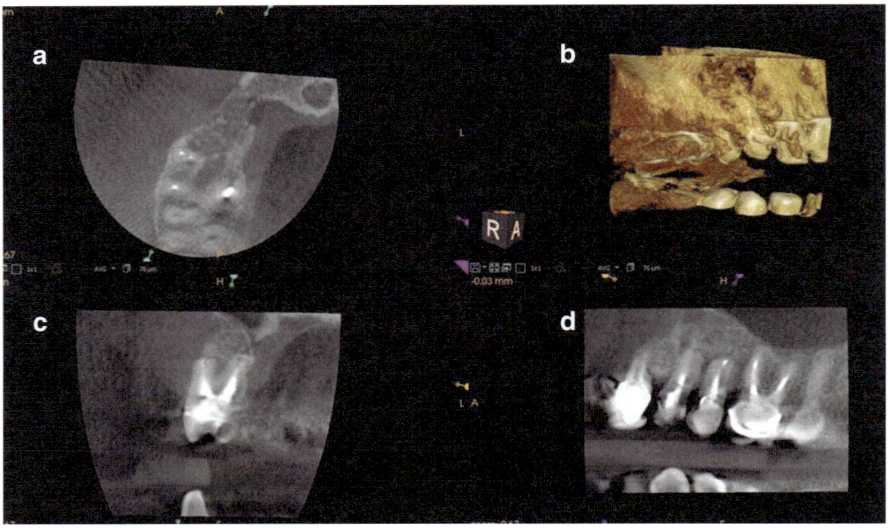

Fig. 7.18 Continuation of case presented in Fig. 6.17: 12-month postoperative CBCT scan of teeth #12 and 13 demonstrating bone remodeling observed in axial (**a**), 3D rendering (**b**), coronal (**c**), and sagittal (**d**)

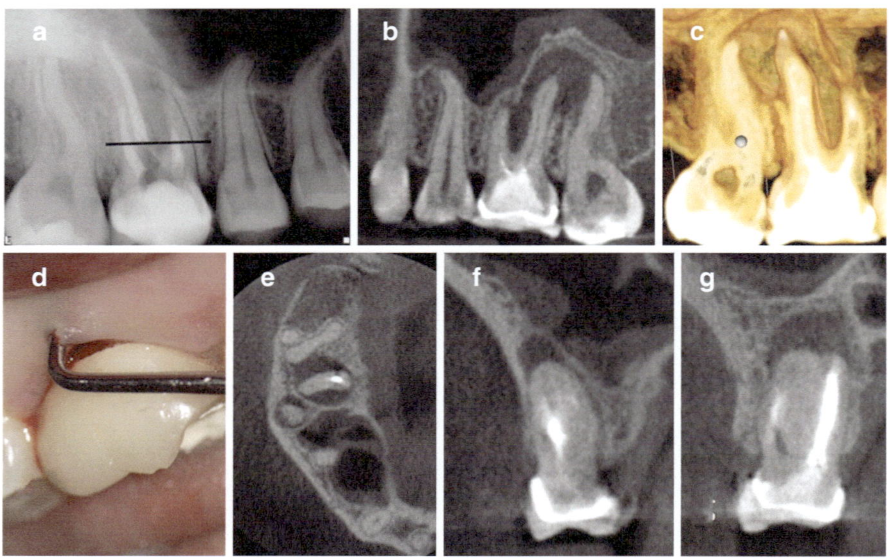

Fig. 7.19 Periapical radiograph of tooth #3 that was referred for periapical surgery (**a**). A nonsurgical retreatment attempt was performed prior to periapical microsurgery. The mesiobuccal canal was blocked. The black line in (**a**) corresponds to the level of the axial view in (**e**). Sagittal view demonstrating the extent of the periapical defect (**b**). 3D rendering of the periapical defect (**c**). Clinical picture demonstrating the endodontic/periodontal communication (**d**). Axial view of the mesiobuccal, distobuccal, and palatal roots (e). Note the fused distal and palatal roots. Coronal view of the mesiobuccal root and the fused distal-palatal roots (**f** and **g**)

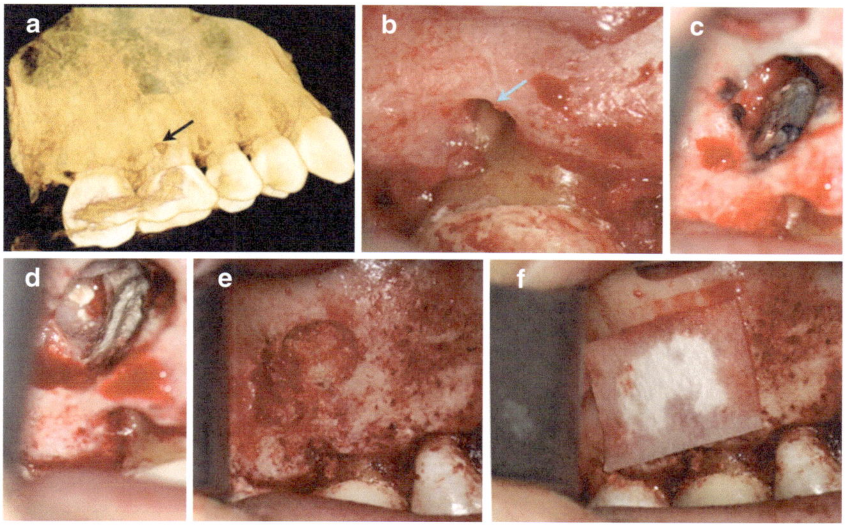

Fig. 7.20 Continuation of case presented in Fig. 6.19: 3D rendering demonstrating the periodontal defect (black arrow) (**a**). After full-thickness flap reflection, the periodontal defect was determined to communicate with the periapical defect (blue arrow) (**b**). Root resection of the fused distal and palatal roots prior to ultrasonic preparation (**c**). (D) MTA root-end filling of the ultrasonically prepared distal and palatal preparation (**d**). Periodontal and periapical defects grafted with Puros™ allograft (Zimmer Dental, Warsaw, IN) material (**e**). Grafted defect covered with CopiOs™ membrane (Zimmer Dental, Warsaw, IN) (f)

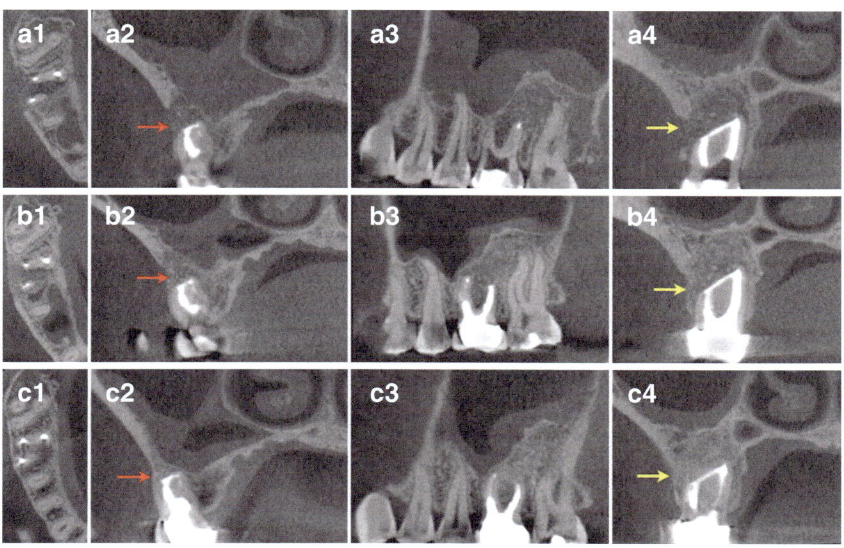

Fig. 7.21 Continuation of case presented in Figs. 6.19 and 6.20: Immediate postsurgical CBCT scan (a.1, a.2, a.3, and a.4). Note buccal defect (red and yellow arrows) (B1, 2, 3, and 4). 6-month recall CBCT scan (b.1, b.2, b.3, and b.4). Note the initial regeneration of the defect including the buccal cortical plate. 1-year recall CBCT scan demonstrating complete remodeling of the defect and the buccal plate (red and yellow arrows) (c.2, c.2, c.3, and c.4)

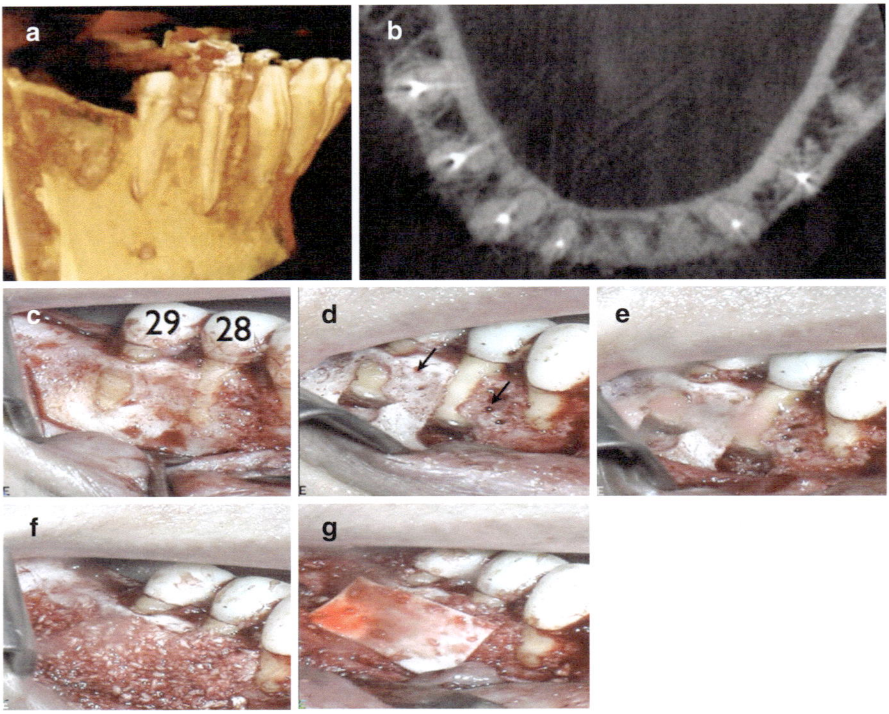

Fig. 7.22 3D CBCT rendering and axial view of teeth #28 and 29 that were referred for apical surgery (**a** and **b**). Complete dehiscence of the root of tooth #28 and fenestration of tooth #29 was observed. Clinical picture after surgical flap reflection confirming the CBCT findings (**c**). Root-end resection, conditioning, and root-end filling with MTA. Size #2 round bur cortical holes were placed (black arrow) for the rapid acceleration phenomenon (R.A.P.) to ensure blood supply to the bone graft (**d** and **e**). Periodontal and periapical defect grafted with enCore™ combination (70% cortical and 30% cancellous) from Osteogenics Biomedical Lubbock, TX. CopiOs™ membrane (Zimmer Dental, Warsaw, IN) was placed over the grafting material (**f** and **g**)

The integration of CBCT and other technologies, such as e-Vol DX software, piezosurgery, static surgical guides, and dynamic navigation systems have revolutionized surgical endodontics.

Recently, a sophisticated post-processing software, e-Vol DXS (CDT Software, São José dos Campos, SP, Brazil), with multiple task-specific-rendering features, has been introduced to enhance the data of CBCT scans [22].

The need for high-quality images to visualize complex anatomical structures, precise identification of lesions, and reduced artifacts has led to the development of the e-Vol DX software.

Figures 7.24, 7.25, 7.26, 7.27, 7.28, 7.29, 7.30 and 7.31 demonstrate a series of surgical cases where CBCT DICOM images were imported into e-Vol DX software and utilized for the visualization of dental anatomy, maxillary sinus structure, and vascular bundles using task-specific-rendering filters.

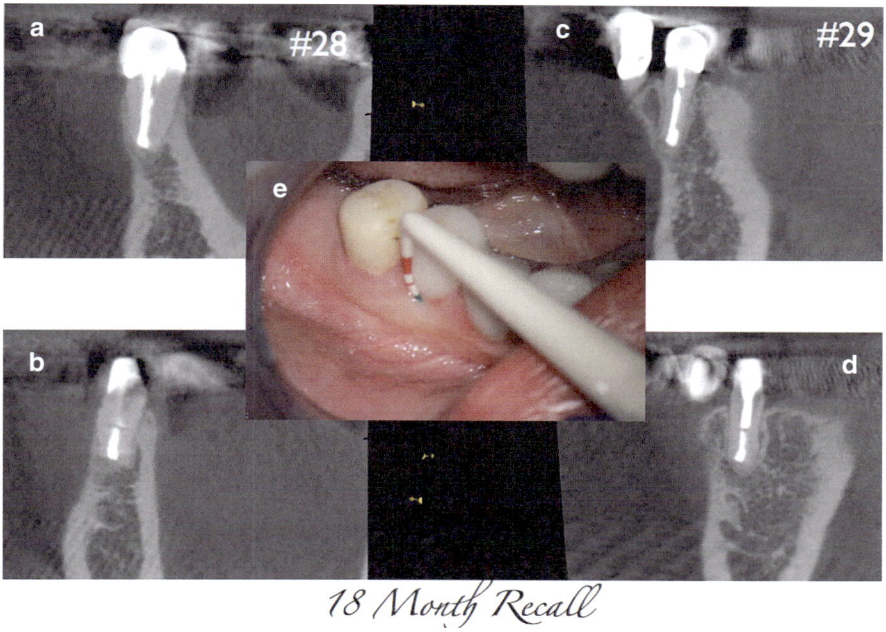

Fig. 7.23 Continuation of case presented in Fig. 6.22: 18-month CBCT coronal and sagittal views demonstrating complete remodeling of the defect and the buccal plates (**a**, **b**, **c**, and **d**). Clinical picture of 18-month recall demonstrating normal color, texture, and periodontal attachment (**e**)

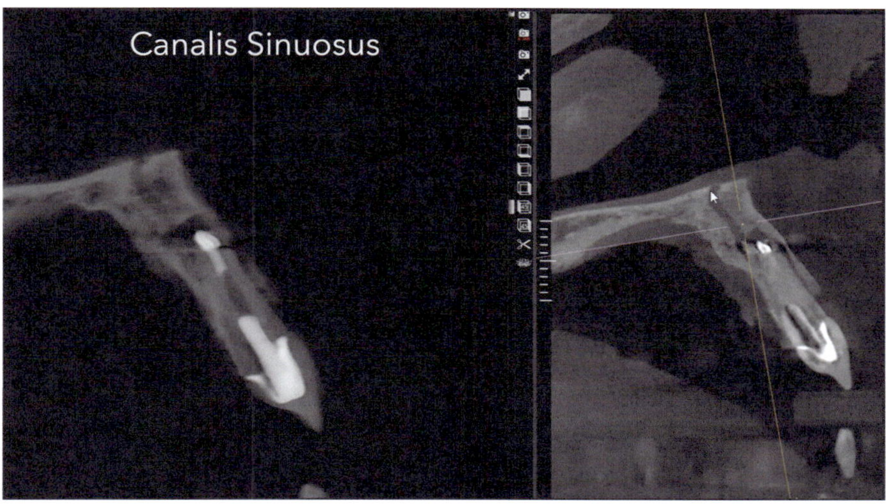

Fig. 7.24 CBCT Dicom images imported into e-VOLDX software. Tooth # 8 was evaluated for apicoectomy. Canalis sinuosus path can be visualized (white arrow) and communicating with the low-density area at the apex of tooth #8. Canalis sinuosus is a neurovascular canal, a branch of the infraorbital canal, through which the anterior superior alveolar nerve passes and travels medially in course between the nasal cavity and the maxillary sinus, reaching the premaxilla in the canine and incisor region. Visualization of Canalis sinuosus is crucial in preoperative microsurgical treatment planning as manipulation or damage to the neurovascular bundle can cause paresthesia of the upper lip

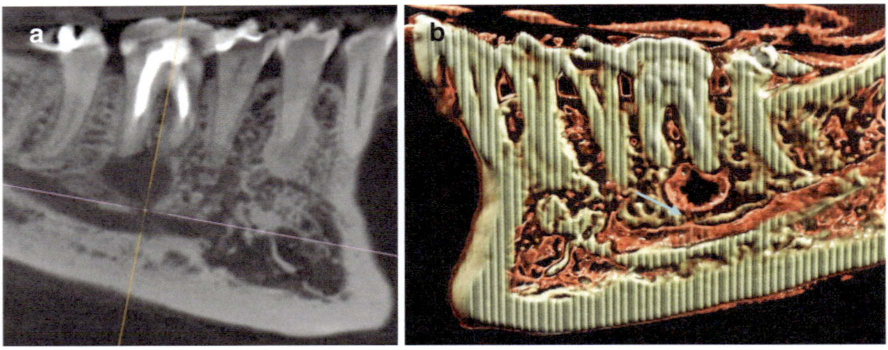

Fig. 7.25 CBCT coronal view of tooth #30 (**a**). The base of the low-density area communicating with the inferior alveolar nerve canal (IANC) was detected (the intersection of the purple lines in figure a and the blue arrow in figure b). CBCT dicom images imported into e-VOLDx software and utilizing the lesion task-specific realistic rendering filter. The lesion as well as the IAN bundle can be visualized

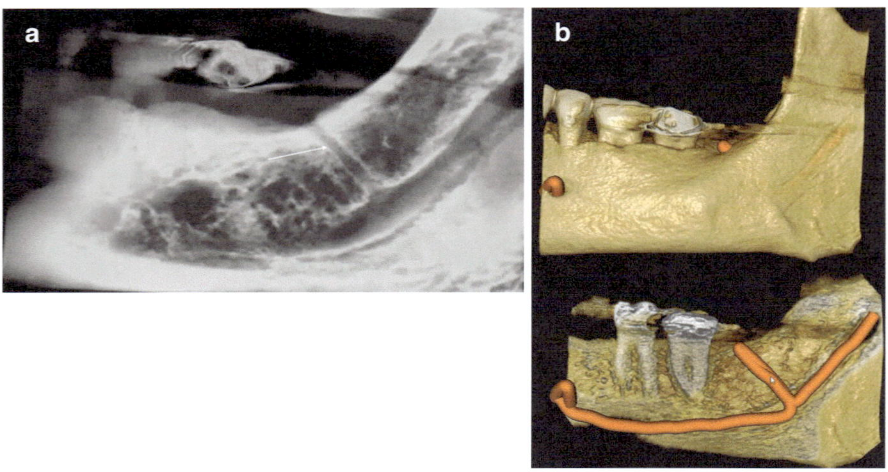

Fig. 7.26 e-VOLDX coronal view of tooth #18. Tooth #18 presented with marginal ridge crack that extended halfway into the distal root and was planned for surgical extraction (**a**). The retromolar canal (RMC) which is an anatomical variant of the mandibular canal was detected (white arrow). Apart from blood vessels it also contains accessory nerve fibers and is clinically important, because its presence can account for failures of mandibular block anesthesia and in rare cases, injuries of its neurovascular bundle can lead to complications such as hemorrhages and dysesthesias. CBCT 3D rendering demonstrating the bifid anatomy of the RMC (**b**)

Recently, the effect of the piezoelectric device on intraoperative hemorrhage control during surgery and the quality of life of patients after endodontic microsurgery was evaluated [23]. Piezoelectric surgery resulted in improved quality of life of patients in the first week post-surgery with lower levels of pain and swelling as well as the number of analgesics taken and better hemorrhage control during surgery.

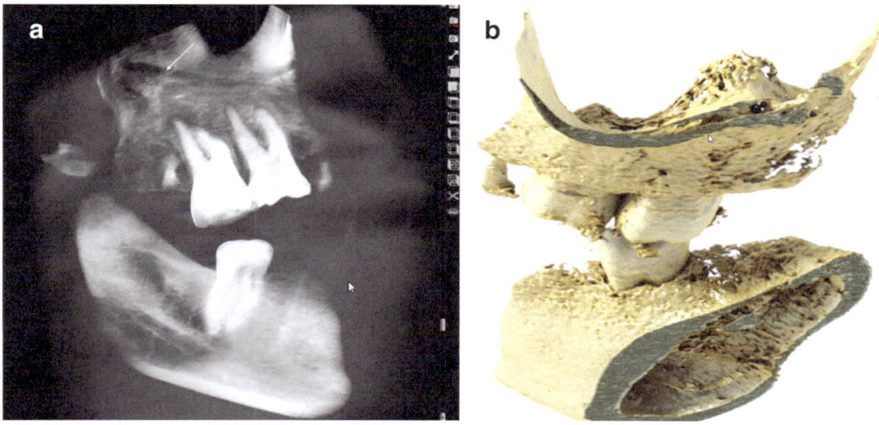

Fig. 7.27 e-VOLDx coronal view utilizing the sinus filter to visualize the posterior superior alveolar (PSA) bundle (white arrow) (**a**). A task-specific realistic rendering visualizing the channel for the PSA bundle (**b**)

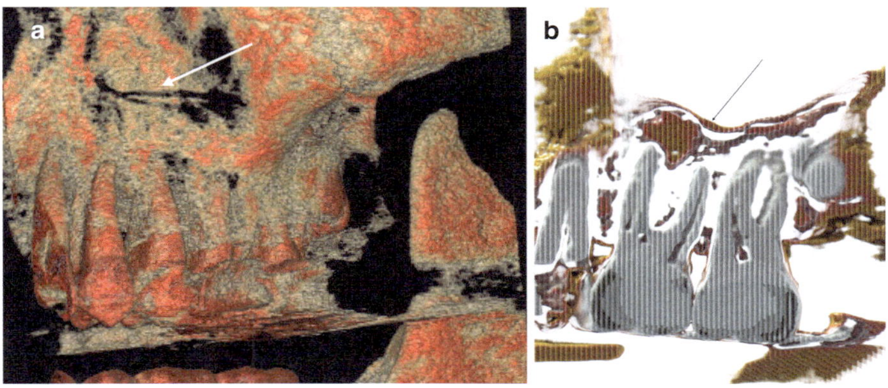

Fig. 7.28 e-VOLDx image for the posterior upper left quadrant. Tooth #14 presented with a previous root canal therapy and a low-density area. The PSA bundle can be detected as identified by the arrows in (**a** and **b**). The lesion task-specific rendering filter was utilized. The lesion as well as the sinus membrane elevated as a response to the odontogenic infection

Piezosurgery inserts are utilized for different purposes and techniques. Among these techniques is the bony lid technique. The bony lid technique is utilized when the surgical site involves thick cortical plate and/or vital structures as the maxillary sinus or mandibular nerve bundle. The bony lid technique can be performed utilizing a static navigation or dynamic navigation techniques. The static navigation technique uses digital workflow to virtually plan the surgical procedure, integrating Standard Tessellation Language and Digital Imaging and Communications in Medicine files to create three-dimensional guides with exacting resection locations, levels, and angles [24, 25].

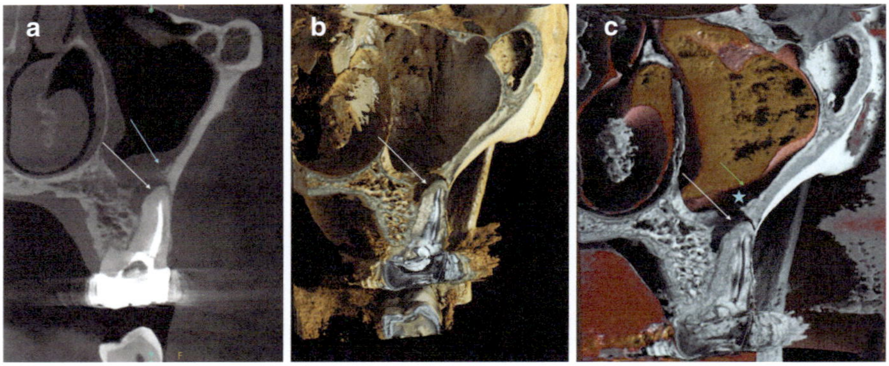

Fig. 7.29 Coronal view of the mesiobuccal root of tooth #14 that was evaluated for apicoectomy. Low density area perforating the maxillary floor was noted (white arrow in (**a**), (**b**), and (**c**))". Maxillary sinus mucositis (blue arrow) (**a**) and blue star (**c**) in response to the odontogenic infection elevating the sinus membrane (green arrow) (**c**)

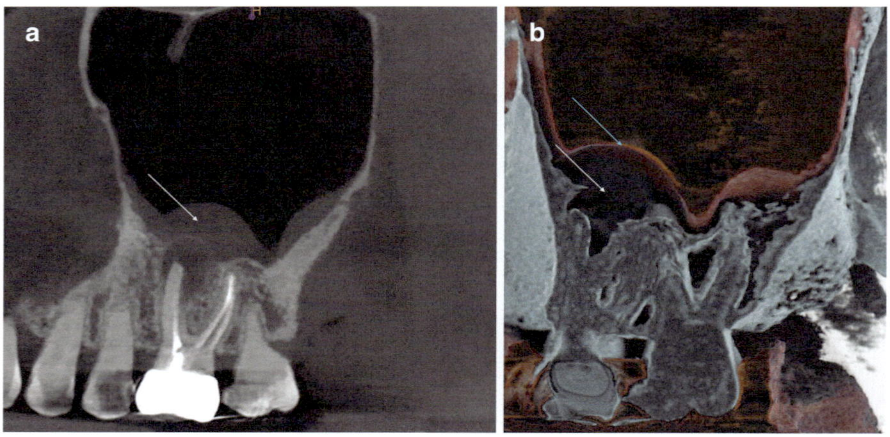

Fig. 7.30 Continuation of case presented in Fig. 7.29. Preoperative CBCT Sagittal view of tooth #14 demonstrating the low-density area related to the MB root as well as the maxillary sinus mucositis (white arrow). e-VOLDX sagittal view utilizing the sinus membrane task-specific realistic rendering (**b**). The periapical defect perforating the sinus floor can be detected and the maxillary mucositis granulation tissue "(white arrowa, (**a**) and (**b**))."elevating the intact sinus membrane (blue arrow)

Niemczyk et al. [24, 25] described the three evolutions of the bony lid technique. The first two evolutions used a surgeon-defined method for site location. The third and final evolution used a digital workflow to virtually plan the surgical procedure, integrating Standard Tessellation Language and Digital Imaging and Communications in Medicine files to create three-dimensional guides with exacting resection locations, levels, and angles. Export of the virtually planned guide in postproduction generates the precision endodontic surgical stent to accurately define the site location and parameters of the procedure.

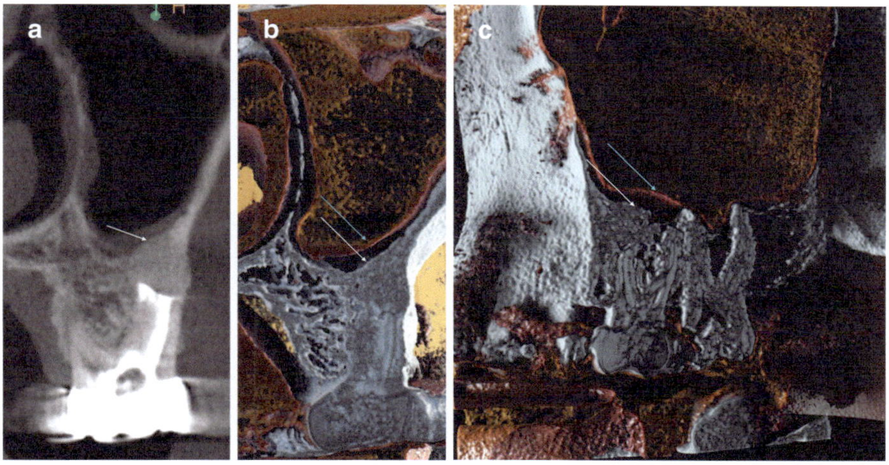

Fig. 7.31 Continuation of case presented in Fig. 7.30: CBCT coronal view of 12 months recall demonstrating bone remodeling as well as the sinus floor (**a**). The resolution of the maxillary sinusitis and remodeling of the sinus floor (white arrow) were noted. e-VOLDx coronal view (**b**) and sagittal view (**c**) demonstrating the remodeling of bone, sinus floor, and the sinus membrane dropping close to its normal original position (blue arrow)

The bony lid technique can be performed utilizing the dynamic navigation. Dynamic navigation integrates surgical instrumentation and radiologic images using an optical positioning device controlled by a dedicated computerized interface. A clinical real-time interface displays and guides users to drill into the targeted position through the prefixed trace according to the output of the preoperative planning software. The guided endodontic concept has been utilized in both nonsurgical and surgical endodontics; however, they have all relied on some form of static guide. The dynamic navigation system offers many advantages versus static guides in nonsurgical and surgical endodontic treatments. Since the clinician visualizes the dental procedure on a monitor in real time, any error in positioning can be immediately detected and corrected in real time. Such a possibility is very helpful in nonsurgical and surgical endodontics because the different steps usually need different orientation of the instruments, which cannot be provided by a single static guide [26, 27].

The utilization of static guides and dynamic navigation has helped clinicians in treatment plan and in performing challenging surgical procedures with more precision and predictability.

Figures 7.32, 7.33, 7.34, 7.35, 7.36, 7.37, 7.38, 7.39, 7.40 and 7.41 demonstrate an example of the utilization of CBCT, Piezosurgery, and dynamic navigation in microsurgical procedures.

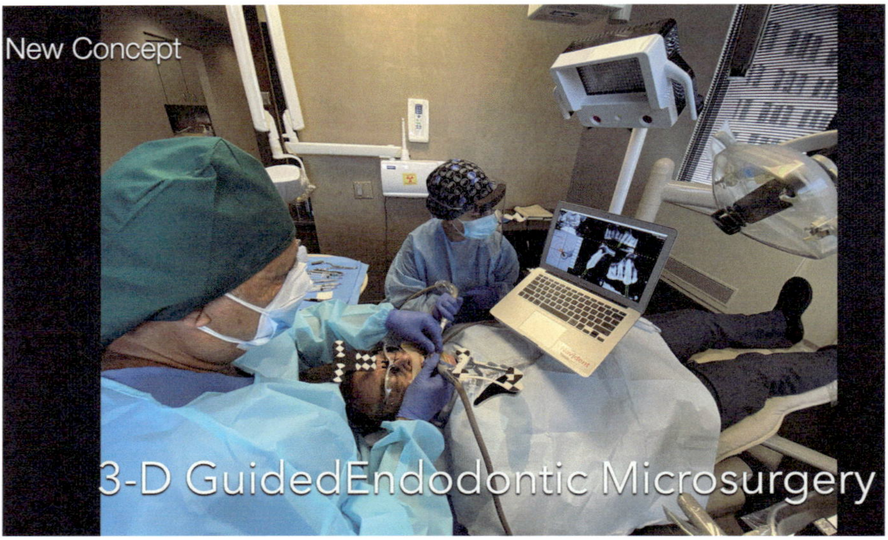

Fig. 7.32 Navident 3 set up demonstrating the patient, doctor, and unit positioning

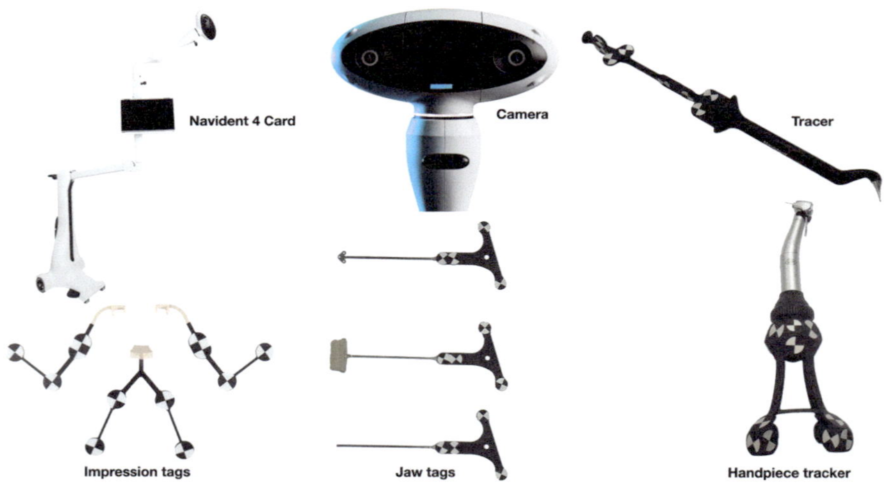

Fig. 7.33 Navident 4 unit and registration parts. The MT4 camera is a high-resolution stereoscopic camera that allows for the small, minimally intrusive tags attached to the instruments and patient be tracked precisely and accurately. With 175 degrees of horizontal and 90 degrees of vertical motion, the robotic camera automatically adjusts to the surgical circumstances ensuring the instruments and the patient are always front and centered

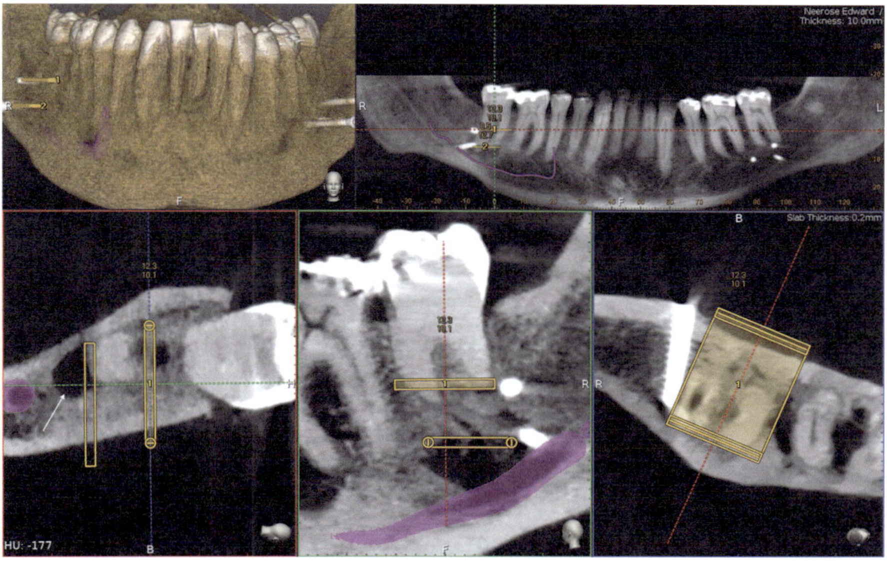

Fig. 7.34 Patient presenting with a low-density area related to the mesial and distal roots of tooth #31. Apicoectomy for tooth #31 was planned due to complete calcified canals, and patient limited mouth opening due to previous jaw surgery. The images are the computer screen of Navident during treatment planning the buccal lid technique. The piezosurgical saw cuts (yellow lines) are planned prior to the surgical procedure to avoid the surgical pins placed from a previous jaw surgery

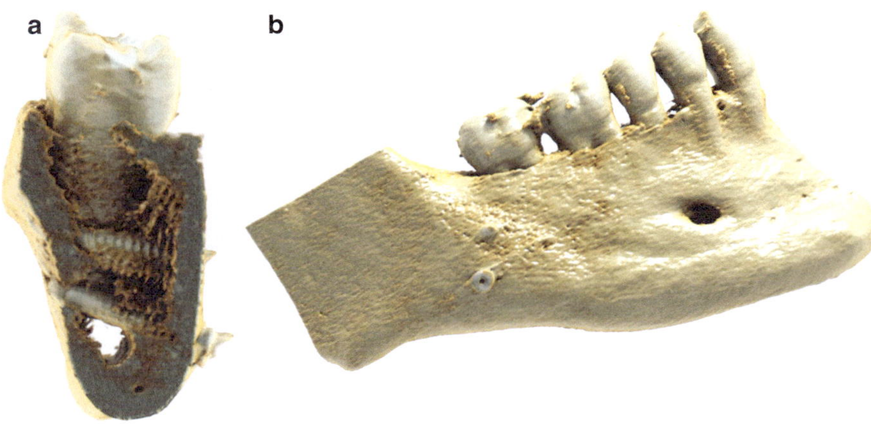

Fig. 7.35 Continuation of case presented in Fig. 7.34: Coronal (**a**) and sagittal e-VOLDx task-specific realistic rendering utilizing the bone filter and demonstrating the close proximity of the dental screws to the distal root (**b**, lower right image)

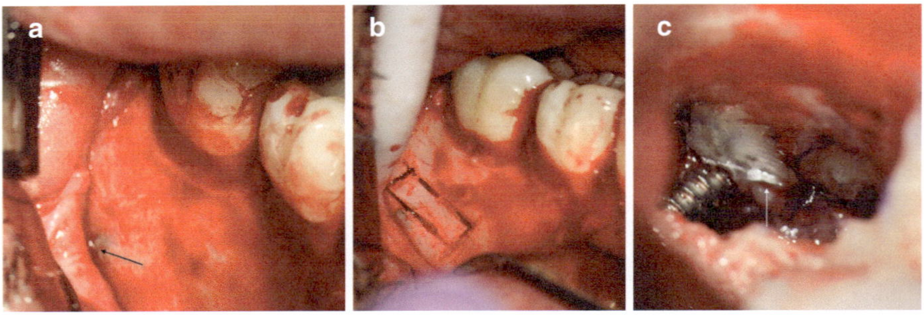

Fig. 7.36 Continuation of case presented in Fig. 7.35: Surgical images after a sulcular buccal flap was reflected. The dental screw can be visualized in (**a**) (black arrow). The buccal lid technique was performed utilizing guided dynamic Piezosurgery (**b**). Root-end resection utilizing dynamic navigation and Piezosurgery. The dental screws were avoided with guided dynamic navigation as planned (**c**)

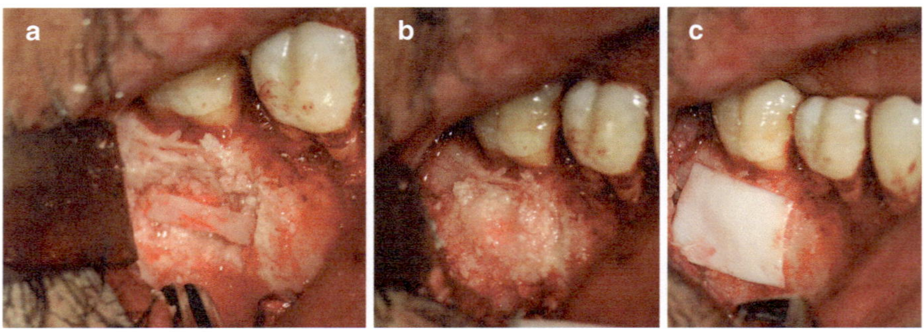

Fig. 7.37 Continuation of case presented in Fig. 7.36: Clinical images after placing the bony lid (**a**), bone graft (**b**), and collagen membrane (**c**)

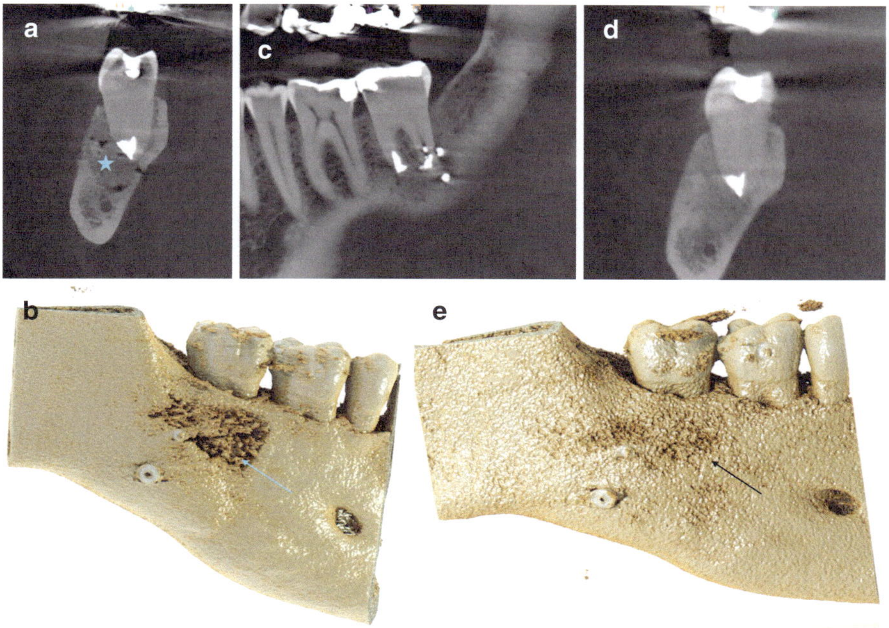

Fig. 7.38 Continuation of case presented in Fig. 7.37: Immediate postsurgical CBCT coronal view demonstrating the bone graft material (blue star) (**a**). e-VOLDx task-specific realistic rendering demonstrating the grafting material as well as the intact surgical dental screws (**b**). Sagittal postsurgical CBCT view demonstrating the root-end filling, grafting material, and the surgical dental screws (**c**). Coronal CBCT view demonstrating complete apical and buccal plate lid remodeling (**d**). e-VOLDx task-specific realistic rendering utilizing the bone filter. Complete buccal bone remodeling around the surgical dental screws can be noted (**e**)

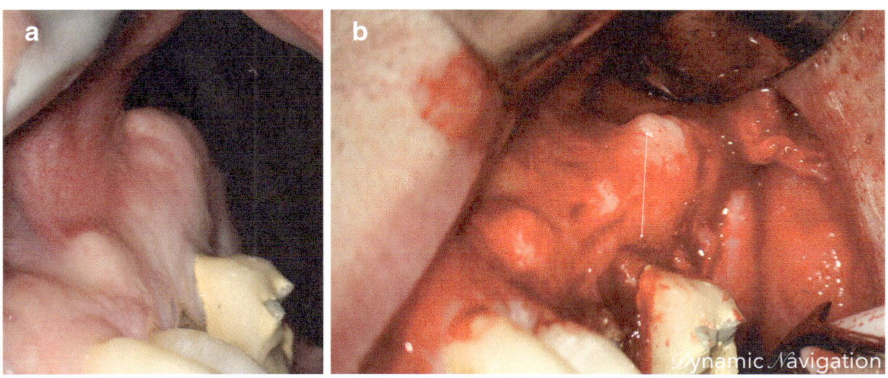

Fig. 7.39 Clinical image of tooth #14. Patient presented for apicoectomy for tooth #14 (**a**). The buccal palate presented with a 15-mm thickness of bony exostosis (white arrow) (**b**)

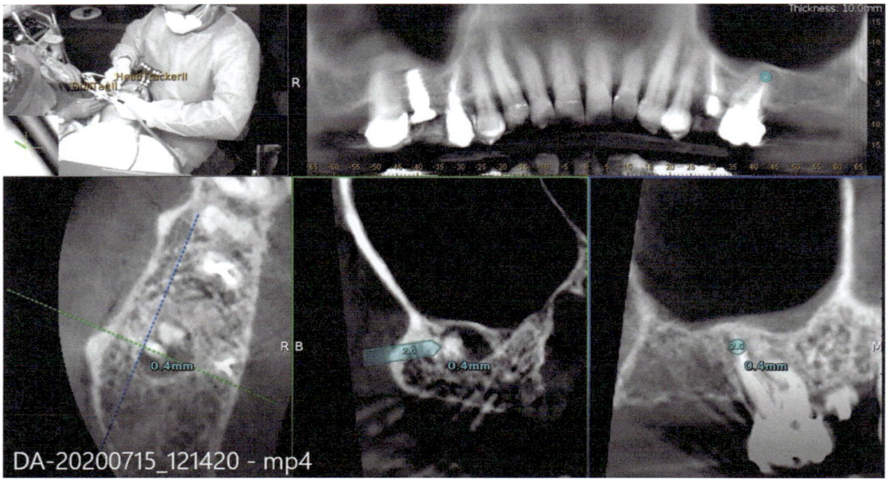

Fig. 7.40 Continuation of case presented in Fig. 7.39: Navident screen image during the real-time dynamic navigation osteotomy towards the target (distobuccal root)

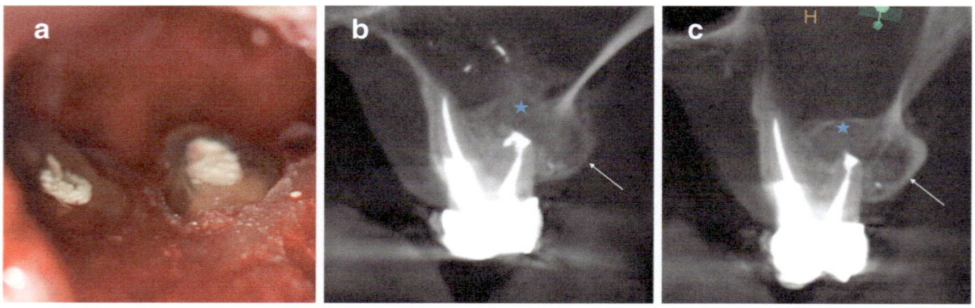

Fig. 7.41 Continuation of case presented in Fig. 7.40: Root-end resection and filling of the mesiobuccal (MB) and distobuccal (DB) roots of tooth #14 (**a**). Coronal CBCT view of the MB (**b**) and DB (**c**) roots demonstrating apical (blue star) and buccal cortical plate remodeling (white arrow)

References

1. Cheung G, Wei WLL, McGrath C. Agreement between periapical radiographs and cone-beam computed tomography for assessment of periapical status of root filled molar teeth. Int Endod J. 2013;46:889–95.
2. Esposito S, Huybrechts B, Slagmolen P, Cotti E, Coucke W, Pauwels R, Lambrechts P, Jacobs R. A novel method to estimate the volume of bone defects using cone-beam computed tomography: an in vitro study. J Endod. 2013;39(9):1111–5.
3. Bornstein MM, Lauber R, Sendi P, von Arx T. Comparison of periapical radiography and limited cone-beam computed tomography in mandibular molars for analysis of anatomical landmarks before apical surgery. J Endod. 2011 Feb;37(2):151–7.

4. Low MTL, Dula KD, Bürgin W, von Arx T. Comparison of periapical radiography and limited cone-beam tomography in posterior maxillary teeth referred for apical surgery. J Endod. 2008;34:557–62.
5. Tsai P, Torabinejad M, Rice D, Azevedo B. Accuracy of cone-beam computed tomography and periapical radiography in detecting small periapical lesions. J Endod. 2012;38:965–70.
6. Tyndall DA, Rathore S. Cone-beam diagnostic applications: caries, periodontal bone assessment, and endodontic applications. Dent Clin N Am. 2008;52:825–41.
7. Cotton TP, Geisler TM, Holden DT, Schwartz SA, Schindler WG. Endodontic applications of cone-beam volumetric tomography. J Endod. 2007;33:1121–32.
8. Velvart P, Hecker H, Tillinger G. Detection of the apical lesion and the mandibular canal in conventional radiography and computed tomography. Oral Surg Oral Med Oral Pathol Oral Radiol Endod. 2001 Dec;92(6):682–8.
9. Rigolone M, Pasqualini D, Bianchi L, Berutti E, Bianchi SD. Vestibular surgical access to the palatine root of the superior first molar: "low-dose cone-beam" CT analysis of the pathway and its anatomic variations. J Endod. 2003;29:773–5.
10. Maillet M, Bowles WR, McClanahan SL, John MT, Ahmad M. Cone-beam computed tomography evaluation of maxillary sinusitis. J Endod. 2011;37(6):753–7.
11. Bornstein MM, Wasmer J, Sendi P, Janner SF, Buser D, von Arx T. Characteristics and dimensions of the Schneiderian membrane and apical bone in maxillary molars referred for apical surgery: a comparative radiographic analysis using limited cone beam computed tomography. J Endod. 2012 Jan;38(1):51–7.
12. Kovisto T, Mansur Ahmad M, Bowles W. Proximity of the mandibular canal to the tooth apex. J Endod. 2011;37(3):311–5.
13. Bürklein S, Carolin Grund C, Schäfer E. Relationship between root apices and the Mandibular Canal: a cone-beam computed tomographic analysis in a German population. J Endod. 2015 Oct;41(10):1696–700.
14. Lofthag-Hansen S, Huumonen S, Grondahl K, Grondahl H-G. Limited cone-beam CT and intraoral radiography for the diagnosis of periapical pathology. Oral Surg Oral Med Oral Pathol Oral Radiol Endodontol. 2007;103:114–9.
15. Simon JHS, Enciso R, Malfaz J-M, Roges R, Bailey-Perry M, Patel A. Differential diagnosis of large periapical lesions using cone-beam computed tomography measurements and biopsy. J Endod. 2006 September;32(9):833–7.
16. Bornstein MM, Bingisser AC, Reichart PA, Sendi P, Bosshardt DD, von Arx T. Comparison between radiographic (2-dimensional and 3-dimensional) and histologic findings of periapical lesions treated with apical surgery. J Endod. 2015 Jun;41(6):804–11.
17. De Paula-Silva FW, Junior MS, Leonardo MR, Consolaro A, daSilva LA. Cone-beam computerized tomographic, radiographic, and histologic evaluation of periapical repair in dogs' post-endodontic treatment. Oral Surg Oral Med Oral Pathol Oral Radiol Endodontol. 2009b;5:796–805.
18. Kourkouta S, Bailey G. Periradicular regenerative surgery in a maxillary central incisor: 7-year results including cone-beam computed tomography. J Endod. 2014;40(7):1013–9.
19. Christiansen R, Kirkevang LL, Gotfredsen E, Wenzel A. Periapical radiography and cone beam computed tomography for assessment of the periapical bone defect 1 week and 12 months after root-end resection. Dentomaxillofac Radiol. 2009 Dec;38(8):531–6.
20. Von Arx T, Janner SF, Hänni S, Bornstein MM. Agreement between 2D and 3D radiographic outcome assessment one year after periapical surgery. Int Endod J. 2015;1-11:915.
21. Tanomaru-Filho M, Jorge EG, Guerreiro-Tanomaru JM, Reis JM, Spin-Neto R, Goncalves M. Two- and tridimensional analysis of periapical repair after endodontic surgery. Clin Oral Investig. 2015;19:17–25.
22. Bueno MR, Estrela C, Azevedo BC, Diogenes A. Development of a new cone-beam computed tomography software for endodontic diagnosis. Braz Dent J. 2018;29:517–29.
23. Bharathi J, Mittal S, Tewari S, Tewari S, Duhan J, Sangwan P, Kumar V. Effect of the piezoelectric device on intraoperative hemorrhage control and quality of life after endodontic microsurgery: a randomized clinical study. J Endod. 2021;47(7):1052–60.

24. Niemczyk SP, Barnett F, Johnson JD, Ordinola-Zapata R, Glinianska A, Bair J, Jang J-H, Sungmin A. PRESS and Piezo Microsurgery (Bony Lid): A 7-year evolution in a residency program part 1: surgeon-defined Site Location. J Endod. 2022;48(6):787–796.e2.
25. Niemczyk SP, Barnett F, Johnson JD, Ordinola-Zapata R, Glinianska A, Bair J, Jang J-H, Sungmin A, Andrew V. PRESS and Piezo Microsurgery (Bony Lid): a 7-year evolution in a residency program—Part 2: PRESS-defined site location. J Endod. 2022;48(6):797–806.e2.
26. Vasudevan A. Dynamic navigation in guided endodontics–a systematic review. European Endodontic J. 2022;7(2):81–91.
27. Aldahmash Sara A, Price Jeffery B, Mostoufi B, Griffin Ina L, Dianat O, Tordik Patricia A, Martinho FC. Real-time 3-dimensional dynamic navigation system in endodontic microsurgery: a cadaver study. J Endod. 2022;48(7):922–9.

The Use of Cone Beam Computed Tomography in Piezosurgery and Static Navigation (PRESS)

8

Stephen P. Niemczyk

Abstract

Treatment of a failing endodontic procedure via microsurgical revision presents better outcomes due, in part, to the integration of the surgical operating microscope (SOM) and CBCT into clinical practice. But challenges still remain with respect to the operational locations and the techniques required to address them. Posterior sites, with substantial cortical plate thicknesses and sensitive anatomy, present the dichotomy of visualization versus post-surgical regeneration of bone. The bony lid technique bridges the gap between these two concepts, and the application of Piezosurgery renders a precise and biocompatible osseous incision.

The primary evolution of the bony lid technique relied on the transfer of measurements from defined landmarks in the CBCT volume to the cortical plate of the surgical site. The secondary evolution utilized a vacuformed stent fabricated with pertinent fiducial markers in gutta-percha defining the surgical site parameters, and a scan exposed with the stent in place. The third and final evolution utilized the digital workflow to virtually plan the surgical procedure, integrating STL and DICOM files to create 3-dimensional guides with exacting resection locations, levels, and angles. Export of the virtually planned guide in post-production generates the precision endodontic surgical stent (PRESS).

The progression from crude on-site measurements to elegant and precise surgical guides enabled the access and manipulations of difficult surgical sites without compromising visibility, post-operative osseous regeneration or patient comfort.

S. P. Niemczyk (✉)
Albert Einstein Medical Center, Dental Department in Philadelphia, Philadelphia, PA, USA

Walter Reed National Medical Center in Bethesda, Bethesda, MD, USA

U. S. Army Endodontic Residency Program in Fort Gordon, Fort Gordon, GA, USA

M. I. Fayad, B. R. Johnson (eds.), *3D Imaging in Endodontics*,
https://doi.org/10.1007/978-3-031-32755-1_8

Apical surgery has long been considered the treatment of choice for failing or refractory non-surgical endodontic therapy, but it was not until the early 1990s, and the introduction of the surgical operating microscope (SOM), that this revision procedure began to realize its potential for success. The coincident increase in illumination and magnification allowed discriminate identification of anatomical structures, precise resection of infected root apices, critical assessment of resected root surfaces, accurate manipulation of ultrasonic root-end instrumentation/preparations, and discreet placement of root-end filling materials. The widespread implementation of the SOM has resulted in a success rate that rivals that of non-surgical endodontic procedures [1–3].

The introduction of maxillofacial cone beam computed tomography (CBCT) in 1996 provided the specialty with the first practical application of volumetric assessment in a clinical setting [4]. While the technology revolutionized the delivery of non-surgical treatment [5–9], the insights gained through the evaluation of a three-dimensional volume were especially enlightening in the surgical environment. Critical dimensions for approach and access to the root apices could be evaluated and measured [10–13]. The location and extent of preexisting lesions were more clearly defined [14–17]. Perhaps the greatest value was realized in the detection and position of sensitive structures relative to the proposed surgical field [18–26]. Manipulation of this data in a Virtual Surgery™ exercise permits the surgeon to predict the potential risks of inadvertent neurovascular impacts or sinus exposures. However, this is but one facet in the decision-making process prior to case acceptance. A recent study by Creasy et al. [27] revealed that 38% of endodontic specialists had poor to fair levels of comfort when mandibular molar surgery was being considered, with more than one-quarter of the respondents also declining to perform apical surgery in the mandibular premolar-molar region as well. Aside from the perceived lack of adequate training in their residencies, the aspects deemed most challenging were access and visualization of the surgical site (somewhat to moderately difficult, 76%) and the creation of the osteotomy (difficult to somewhat difficult, 91%). This reluctance to perform the procedure coupled with the anxiety of potential sensitive structure compromise most often leads to case referral outside the endodontic specialty [27].

A technique that could alleviate these concerns was first proposed and demonstrated by Khoury and Hensher in 1987 [28]. It was dubbed the "bony lid" and was developed for surgical access to mandibular molar root ends. The aim was to gain unprecedented access to these apices while maintaining and preserving the bone volume normally sacrificed during conventional ostectomy techniques. A series of small bur holes through the cortical plate were connected using a chisel, and the lid of bone was harvested and placed in a sterile saline bath. Following the root-end procedures, the lid was replaced, often with little or no additional stabilization. Further refinements of the technique were proposed by Lasaridis in 1991 [29], using a fissure bur to connect the bur holes, and Khoury in 2013 [30] employing a micro-saw to initiate and complete the lid sectioning. In this latter study, all 200 patients healed without infection or complication. The accelerated healing can be explained by several factors: if the graft donor and recipient sites are coincident, there are greater surface contact areas of the lid with the receptor bone, resulting in rapid revascularization via the severed vessels [31]. This ensures that many of the osteocytes and large areas of the lid remain vital [32]. If re-anastomosis of the severed vessels does not occur, the bony lid will repair comparable to a free bone graft due to secondary revascularization and remodeling. Additionally, the reimplanted bone protects the site, controls post-operative hemorrhage, and functions as a biological barrier. This prevents migration of fibroblasts, favoring improved bone regeneration [33].

Although its incorporation into endodontic surgical armamentarium is relatively new, the use of piezosurgery is well documented in the oral maxillo-facial literature [34–39]. When employed at the frequency range of 25–30 kHz, it has the unique property of cutting highly mineralized cortical bone with little or no impact on adjacent soft tissues. This is an especially attractive feature when considering surgical manipulations in close proximity to neurovascular structures [40] or the maxillary sinus [41]. Additionally, the piezoelectric nature of the energy generation is considered safe to use on patients with ICPs (implanted cardiac pacemakers) [42], often a consideration when treating cardiac patients. Contemporary units have sterile solutions delivered to the handpiece via an integrated peristaltic pump, cooling the handpiece, surgical tip, and incised bone surfaces (Fig. 8.1a,b). The combination of light application pressure, diminutive tip profiles, and copious irrigation affords the surgeon the opportunity to execute precision sectioning of bone with unparalleled visibility in a nearly bloodless field [43]. When compared to conventional sectioning instruments, the piezo energized tip caused insignificant vascular disturbances or cellular disruptions in the donor site or harvested lid, facilitating earlier recovery and remodeling [44].

The implementation of piezosurgery would augment the synergy of the SOM and CBCT. Pre-surgical planning and mapping of sensitive structures could produce a blueprint more easily engaged with the precision and tolerance of a piezo-driven instrument. Dimensional control and accuracy are enhanced under higher magnification, and the slender profile of the piezosurgical tips affords an unobstructed view of both the incision cuts of the bony lid and subsequent resection of targeted root apices (Fig. 8.1d). Osteotomy via this technique conserves bone and replacement of the bony lid constitutes an autograft, with the associated benefits of cell and growth factor preservation. It also provides an elevated degree of site protection during the healing phases. Implementation of this technique would address the major concerns of access to the site and enhanced visualization within the crypt that inhibits novice and seasoned surgeons alike. This chapter will chart the progression of the technique, in a case presentation format, from a surgeon-defined site location using in situ measurements, through crude versions of a surgical stent, to the fabrication and use of a precision endodontic surgical stent or PRESS.

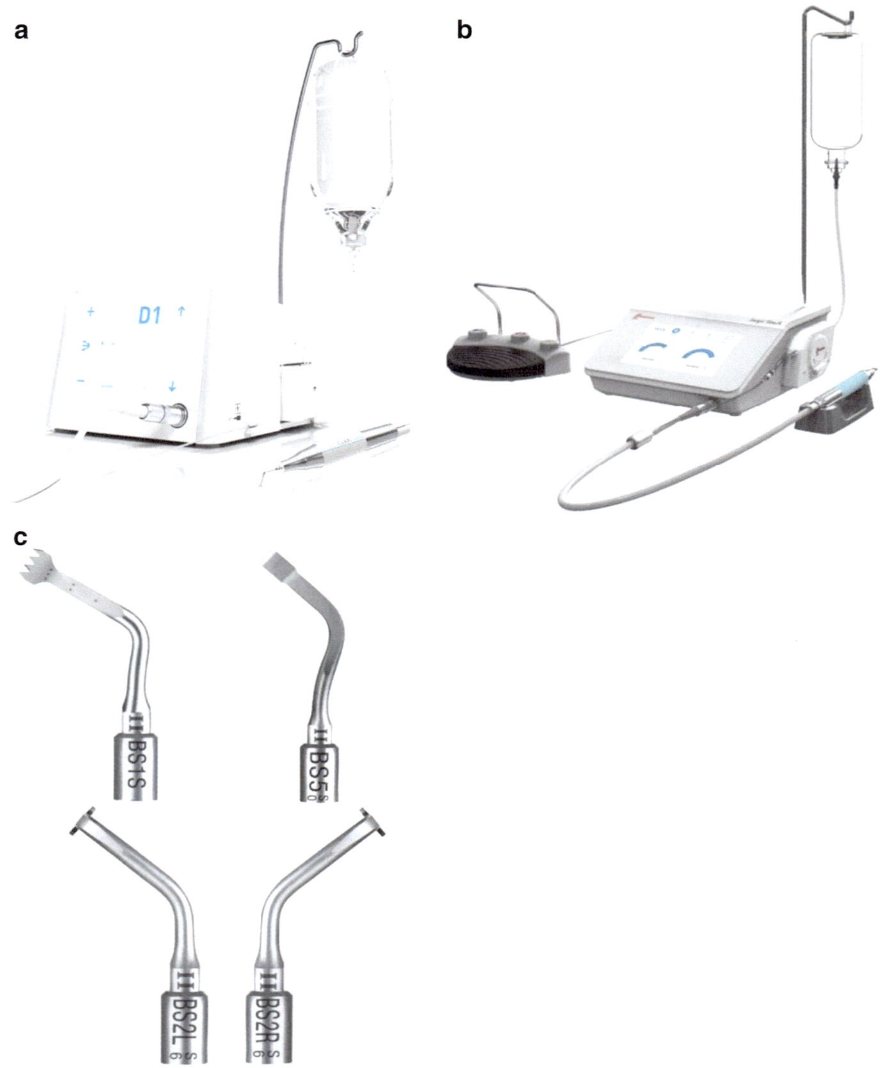

Fig. 8.1 (**a**) Piezo Cube® with peristaltic irrigation and fiber optic light. (**b**) Woodpecker Surgic Touch® Hybrid unit, with dedicated piezosurgical and endodontic power settings. (**c**) Piezosurgery tips (Acteon, Clockwise from top left): BS-1s Piezo Bone Saw tip (straight), BS-5 Piezo scalpel (straight), BS-2l Piezo Bone Saw tip (left bend), BS-2r Piezo Bone Saw tip (right bend). (**d**) Comparison between High Speed HP and Piezo tip for resection in the same surgical site: High Speed HP head obstructs the view of the surgical site, Piezo view is unobstructed. (**e**) Vercellotti study, rabbit calvarium. (Left to right): Bone cut made with Lindemann bone bur, bone cut made with Microsaw; both exhibited debris-filled spaces. The bone cut made with the piezo tip showing debris-free cut site. (Vercellotti T, Majzoub Z, Trisi P, Valente ML, Sabini E, Cordioli G. Histologic evaluation of bone response to piezoelectric, surgical saw and drill osteotomy in rabbit calvaria. (Unpublished data, 1999) (From: *Piezoelectric Bone Surgery; A New Paradigm* Quintessence Publishing, 2020))

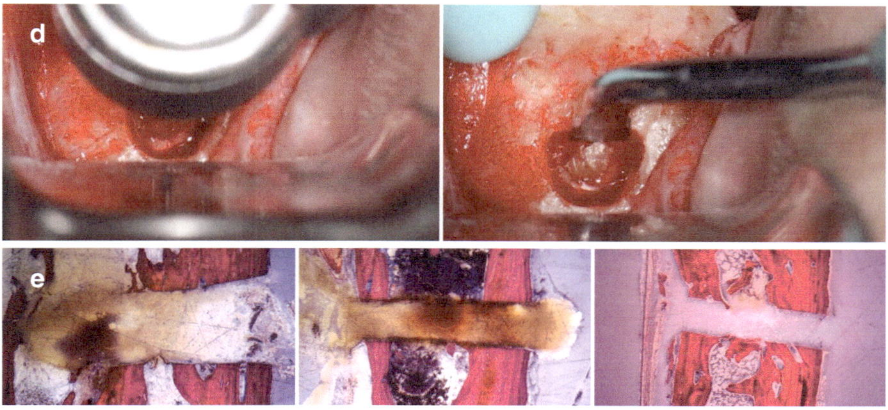

Fig. 8.1 (continued)

8.1 Case Selection/Armamentarium

Radiographic evaluation of the proposed surgical site is a critical first step in the planning process, and the CBCT scan is integral to that assessment [45]. The implementation of the scan in a virtual environment, and the isotropic property of the scan, facilitates accurate measurements of crucial structures such as root length(s), apical width, distances to adjacent teeth/roots, lesion dimensions, and cortical plate thicknesses or defects [7, 46]. It also discloses the location, extent, and proximity of sensitive structures in the vicinity of the proposed surgical location or access corridor [10, 19, 47–49]. Plotting of vertical and horizontal dimensions is visualized in the axial and coronal views, with particular attention to the thickness of the cortical plate at the level of the intended root resection, root apex, and a distance two to three millimeters apical to the physical end of the root. This confirms a cortical bone thickness of at least one millimeter throughout the proposed piezo incisions. Inadequate thickness of the borders of the lid can compromise the integrity of the bone during luxation and harvesting manipulations or stabilization post-replacement [50]. The extent of this three-dimensional compartment should accommodate unhindered access and visualization of the root end(s) and surrounding structures and, by extension, expedite the removal of any pathologic materials in the crypt. If multiple root-end procedures are planned, the integrity of the donor cortical plate is maintained by a single larger lid that is replaced [50] versus multiple separate osteotomies that have been shown to precipitate loss of the associated cortical plate dimension at the site [51].

Traditionally, the dissection of the lid from the cortical plate was achieved with high-speed rotating burs of various configurations [28, 29], shielded microsaw [30], or in combination with ultrasonic instruments [52, 53]. The turn of the century witnessed the debut of the earliest version of the piezosurgical handpiece, termed ultrasonic osteotomes [35]. As the technology and instrumentation evolved and improved, it achieved widespread acceptance and diversity of applications by the mid-2000s [54–58]. The device dedicated for microsurgery in the specialty practice has the capabilities for varied power settings and irrigation flow rates. Using the higher power and flow rate settings, the outlines of the lid are superficially traced with a piezo bone saw tip; the final separating cuts through the cortical plate into cancellous bone are made with a piezo scalpel. The thin profile of the scalpel (0.75 mm), known dimensions (3.5 mm × 5 mm), and micrometric vibrations produce a cut with controlled depth and comparatively smaller gap dimensions. The concomitant irrigation cools and rinses the bone at the site, resulting in significant reduction of microthrombi from heat and osteocyte necrosis. The irrigation fluid, when energized by the tip, produces a cavitation effect that not only cools the site, but clears the surface to enhance visibility as well [43, 44]. The profile of the scalpel tip and the landmarks for depth control allow for an unobstructed view of the cortical surface during the incision, akin to the view afforded with an ultrasonic root-end preparation tip. It also allows for constant monitoring of the depth and direction of the piezo tip, essential in sites where sensitive structures are in close proximity to the operative field. This assumes that the surgeon is adhering to the strict protocols for the dissection: light pressure and continuous movement of the selected piezo surgical tip. Heavy pressure and/or static movement will result in overheating of the bone at that point, thermal shock, and burning of the surface; the same effects are seen with bone burs and microsaws, with similar consequences [44].

Once the lid is harvested and stored for hydration, curettage of the crypt and removal of the lesion is accomplished by traditional means or augmented with piezo inserts at the lowest power settings and reduced flow rates. Using the piezo inserts with irrigation essentially "floats" the lesion in the site, allowing the remaining attachment to be visualized and severed. When the selected root end has been isolated and identified, resection is accomplished with the same piezo scalpel used for the cortical plate cuts. Once the root-end procedures are complete, the lid is reapproximated and stabilized by various means, depending on the degree of support required and potential for post-operative dislodgement. A CBCT scan is exposed at the suture removal visit, serving as a benchmark for post-operative healing and outcome assessment. All patients are recalled at appropriate intervals, with radiographic images to monitor their progress. Conventional radiographs and a CBCT scan are taken at the 12-month post-operative appointment and compared to the earlier images for hard tissue resolution, evaluation, and assessment.

8.2 Case #1: Surgeon-Defined Site Measurement/Location

A 25-year-old woman was referred for evaluation and treatment of tooth #19. She presented with a history of endodontic therapy completed approximately 2 years previously and has had episodes of spontaneous pain for the preceding 3 weeks. The review of systems was normal, and her medical history was non-contributory. Clinical examination of the mandibular left posterior quadrant revealed marked percussion sensitivity of tooth #19 to long axis and right-angle impacts. This tooth was also sensitive to biting, but periodontal probing was within normal limits when compared to the adjacent teeth and the contralateral side. The tooth was restored with a porcelain fused to metal crown and there was no evidence of recurrent decay or marginal leakage. Radiographs revealed root canal therapy had been completed in #19, with slight extrusion of the obturative material in the mesial root. A periapical radiolucency encompassed both apices of #19 but did not extend to any lateral or inter-radicular root surface. Based on the clinical history and radiographic findings, a diagnosis of previous root canal treatment with symptomatic apical periodontitis was determined. Retreatment of tooth #19 was proposed, and the patient presented for treatment the following week. The root canal filling material was recovered from the canals, but patency was achieved only in the mesial root. The therapy was completed on the second visit, and the patient was placed in the recall schedule.

The 6-month recall revealed that the patient's symptoms had returned, and radiographs revealed only slight resolution of the periapical areas (Fig. 8.2a). A CBCT scan was exposed and confirmed a persistent lesion on the distal root apex and slight widening on the mesial (Fig. 8.2b,c). A revision of the previous therapy via root-end surgery was presented and the procedure was explained including risks and alternative treatments. In particular, the dimensions of the cortical plate and depth required for surgical access were described, including the bony lid technique for access to the root ends. The patient understood her options and consented to the surgical procedure.

Informed consent was reviewed and signed the day of surgery and any final questions answered to the patient's satisfaction. The patient was prepped and draped per hospital protocol (split-drape isolation, 0.12% oral chlorhexidine rinse for 30 seconds, 91% isopropyl alcohol swab of exposed facial surfaces) and vital signs (BP/pulse) were obtained and confirmed the health status for the surgical procedure that day (*AEMC protocol*). The patient was anesthetized with 1.75 cartridges of 0.5% bupivacaine (Marcaine™) with 1:2000,000 epinephrine, administered as an IAN block, with 0.25 cartridges of the same anesthetic infiltrated over the mental foramen. After a 10-min delay for onset of signs, the buccal aspect of the cortical plate from the mesial of tooth #20 to the distal of tooth #18 was infiltrated with 1.5 cartridges of lidocaine (Xylocaine™) 2%, with 1:50,000 epinephrine for control of site hemostasis. Following another 5-min pause for anesthetic uptake and confirmation, the surgical procedure was initiated. All microsurgical procedures from incision to flap coaptation/suturing are performed under the surgical operating microscope (SOM).

A full-sulcular incision was made from the distal of tooth #18 to the mesial of tooth #20, with a vertical releasing incision at the mesial line angle of #20 (Fig. 8.2e-dd). A triangular flap was reflected, and the mental nerve/foramen was located, marked with methylene blue dye and isolated via retraction. The site of the lid was determined and a preliminary level for the superior margin of the lid was measured and marked. A shallow score mark in the cortical plate was created using the BS-1 piezo saw tip (Acteon), and the score mark was filled with a compacted piece of gutta-percha. A radiograph was exposed using a parallel technique to minimize parallax errors, and the height/extent of the gutta-percha segment was noted. The length

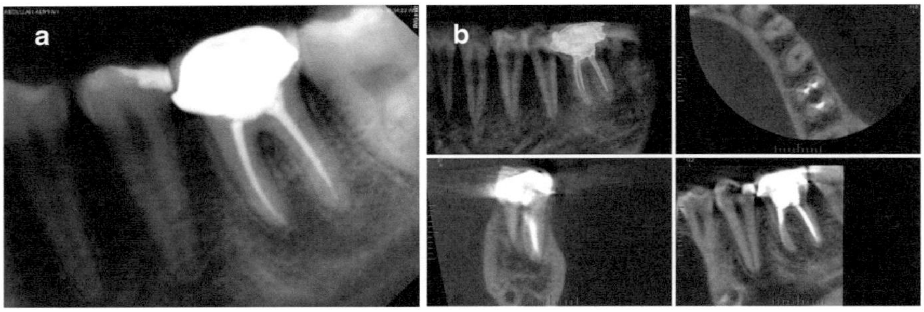

Fig. 8.2 (**a**) Pre-surgical (6-month recall) radiograph tooth #19; planned root-end surgery of the mesial/distal roots. (**b**) Pre-surgical CBCT reveals small areas of less density at both apices of tooth #19 (Unless noted, all 3D images utilize eVolDX, CDT Software, Brazil). (**c**) Coronal views of the mesial root (top) and distal root (bottom) exhibiting the areas of low density at the apices. (**d**) Axial views showing the thickness of the buccal cortical plate in the proposed surgical site. The CBCT view is flanked by the sinus filter (left) and the silicone bone filter (right). (**e**) Periodontal probe measurement to superior lid border. (**f**) Gutta-Percha marker in cortical plate groove (Black arrow). (**g**) Radiograph with Gutta-Percha marker to disclose apical-coronal level (Red arrow). (**h**, **i**) Bony lid outline completed: luxation and delivery with Ruddle curette. (**j**) Isolation of the mesial root apex; repeated for distal. (**k**) Root-end preparation of the mesial root; repeated for distal. (**l**) Micromirror view of completed mesial root preparation including isthmus (yellow arrow). (**m**) Placement of $CaSO_4$ in the crypt to support the replaced bony lid. (**n**) Bony lid replaced; $CaSO_4$ compacted into the bone incisions to stabilize the lid. (**o**) Appearance of the stabilized lid prior to soft tissue closure. (**p**) Immediate Post-surgical radiographs #19. (**q**) Two-week Post-surgical CBCT scan, demonstrating initial dissolution of $CaSO_4$, particularly in the bone incision gaps. (**r**) Two-week Post-surgical CBCT scan, demonstrating initial dissolution of $CaSO_4$, in the mesial gap site (top) and the distal gap site (bottom) using silicone bone filter. (**s**) Two-week Post-surgical CBCT scan: the axial sections exhibit slight remodeling of the lid, especially at the mesial end. Note the bolus of $CaSO_4$ medial to the lid (yellow arrows). Silicone bone filter (left) and sinus filter (right). (**t**) Sagittal and mesial/distal coronal sections reveal the presence of the $CaSO_4$ bolus supporting the lid (yellow arrows) (Sinus filter). (**u**) Two-month Post-surgical CBCT scan, demonstrating complete dissolution of the $CaSO_4$. Note the initial lid remodeling, especially the buccal cortical surface, as compared to 2q. (**v**) Two-month Post-surgical CBCT scan, mesial and distal coronal views. Note the scaffold remodeling of the buccal portion of the lid, the distal is more advanced than the mesial (yellow arrows). (Silicone bone filter). (**w**) Two-month Post-surgical CBCT scan: the axial sections exhibit advanced remodeling of the lid, especially at the mesial end. The bolus of $CaSO_4$ has been resorbed and is being replaced by early bone matrix scaffolding. (**x**) Sagittal and mesial/distal coronal sections revealing the resorption of the $CaSO_4$ bolus and early remodeling of the bony lid buccal surface. (**y**) Twelve-month Post-surgical radiographs exhibiting periapical healing and lid remodeling. (**z**) Twelve-month Post-surgical CBCT scan exhibiting periapical healing and complete reformation of the buccal cortical plate; the original lid is much reduced in size and still undergoing remodeling (Yellow arrow). (**aa**) Twelve-month Post-surgical CBCT scan; axial view. Note the reformed cortical plate over the surgical site. The thinnest portion of the reformed plate coincides with the site of the original lid undergoing remodeling (yellow arrow). (**bb**) Forty-eight month Post-surgical CBCT scan exhibiting final remodeling of the buccal cortical plate (axial and sagittal views). (**cc**) Forty-eight month Post-surgical CBCT scan exhibiting final remodeling of the buccal cortical plate (coronal views, mesial, and distal roots. The lid remnant at the mesial root will continue to remodel or become incorporated in the final cortical plate). (**dd**) Virtual Surgery™ blueprint, outlining cortical plate thicknesses, resection depths, and proposed bony lid dimensions

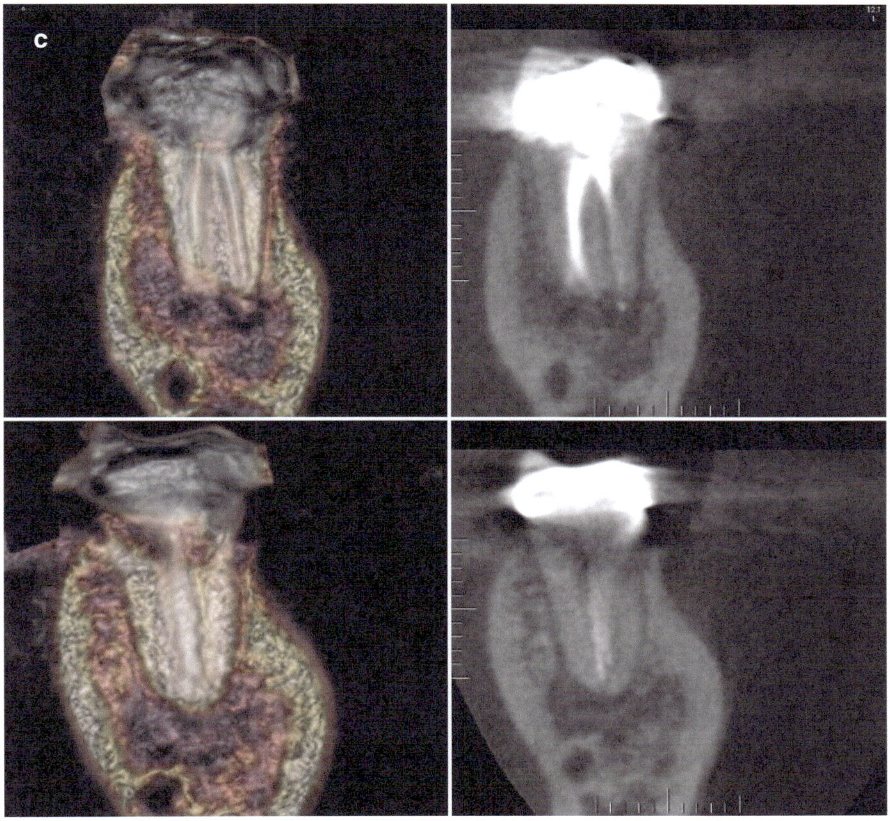

Fig. 8.2 (continued)

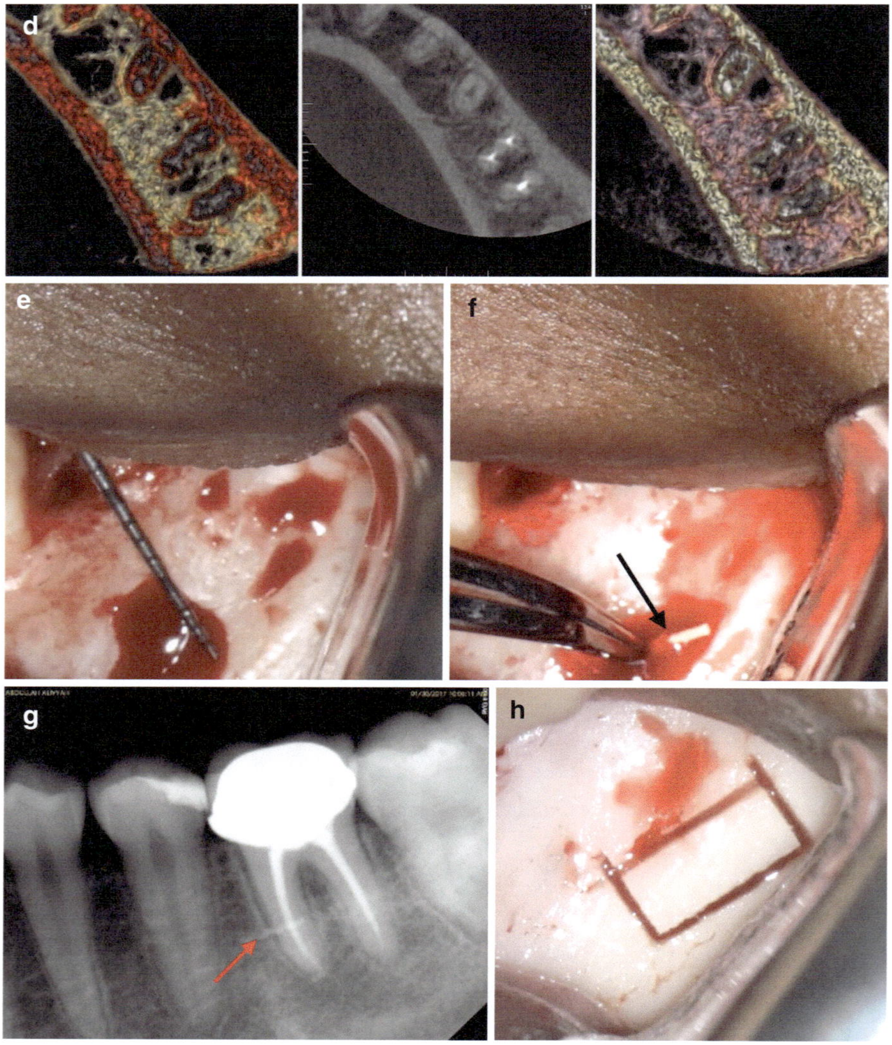

Fig. 8.2 (continued)

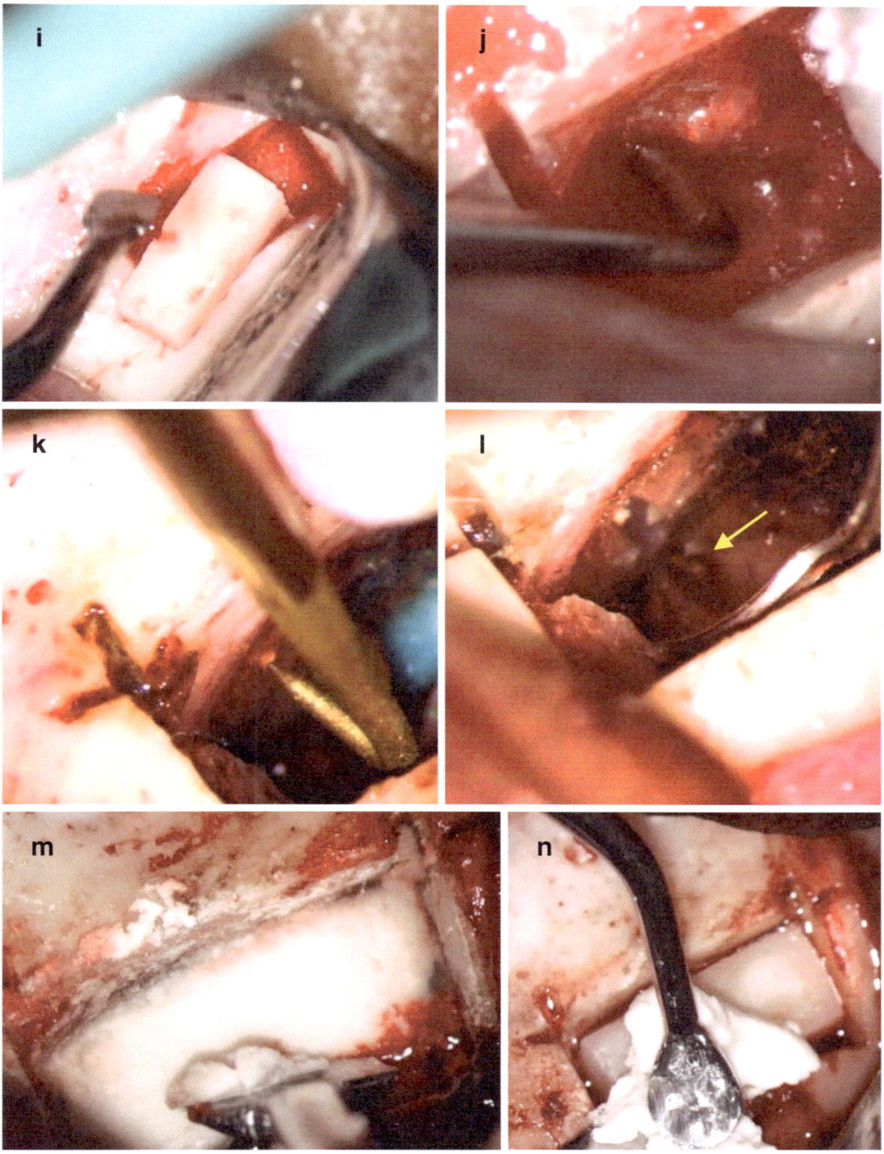

Fig. 8.2 (continued)

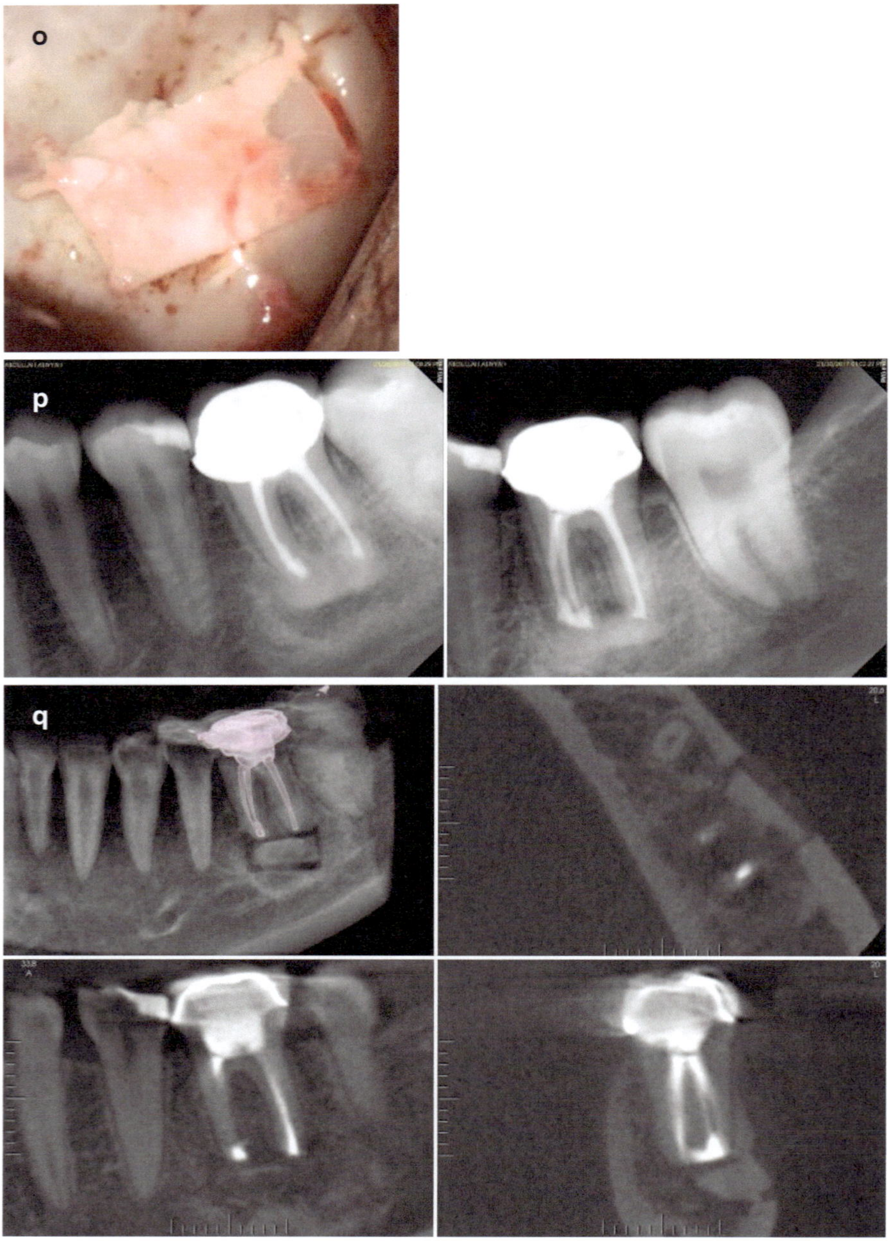

Fig. 8.2 (continued)

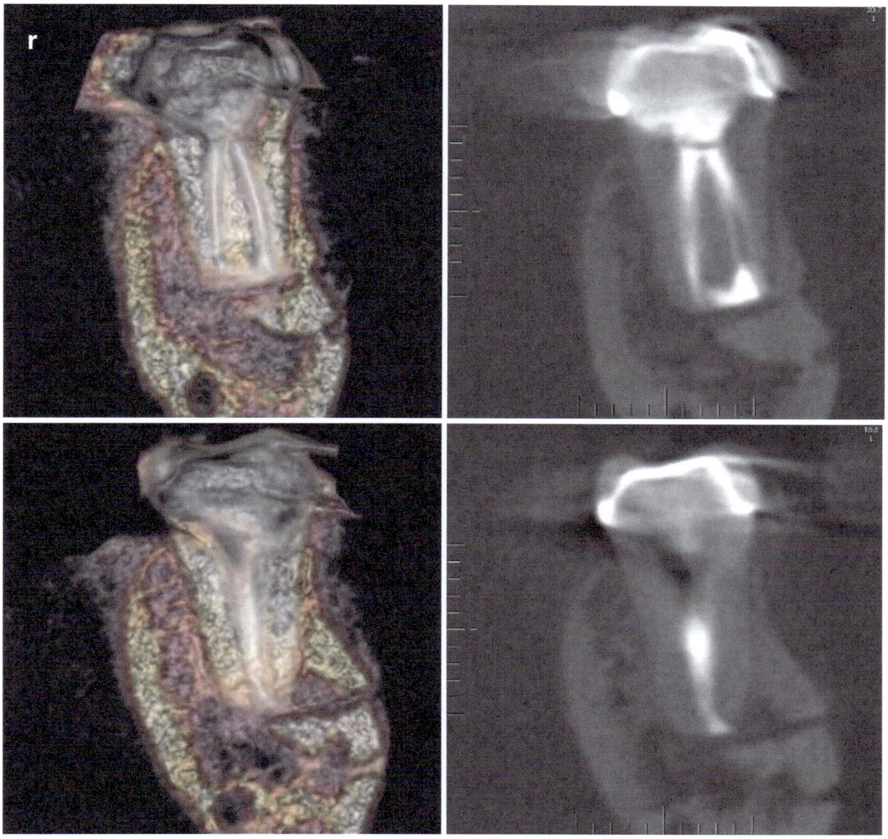

Fig. 8.2 (continued)

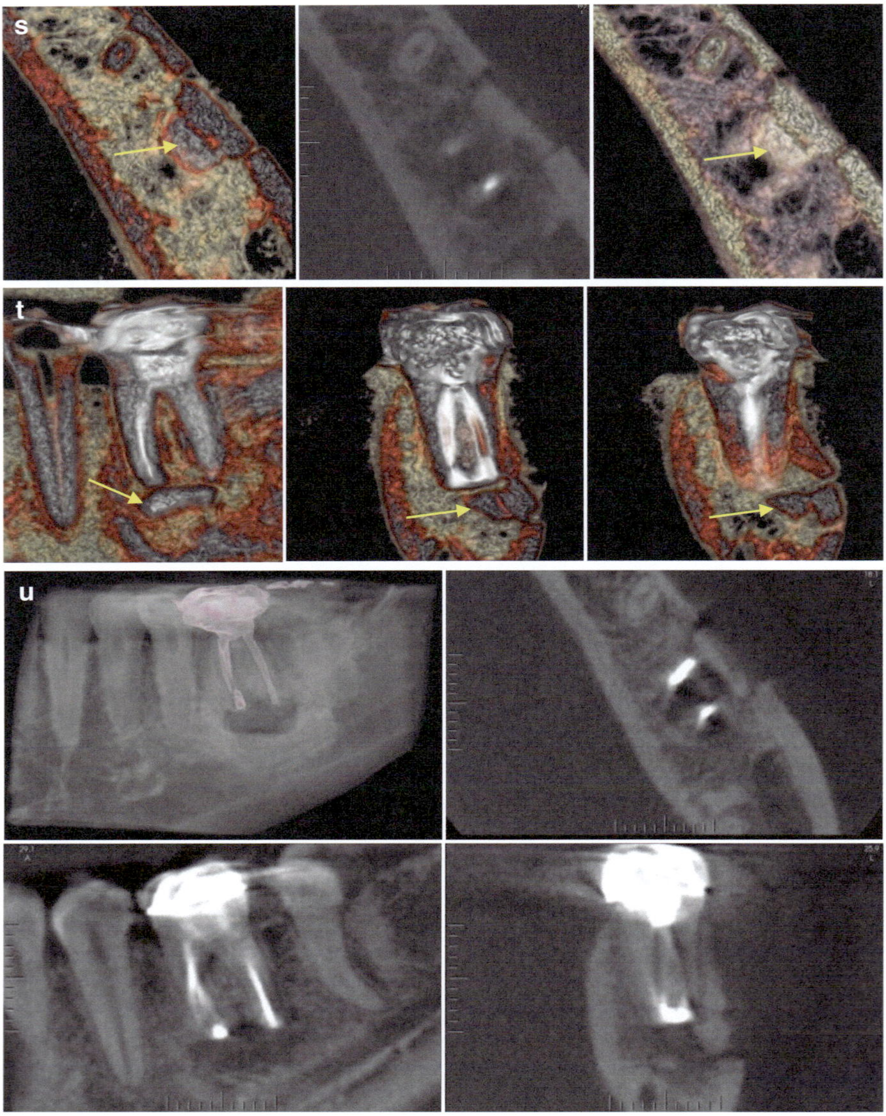

Fig. 8.2 (continued)

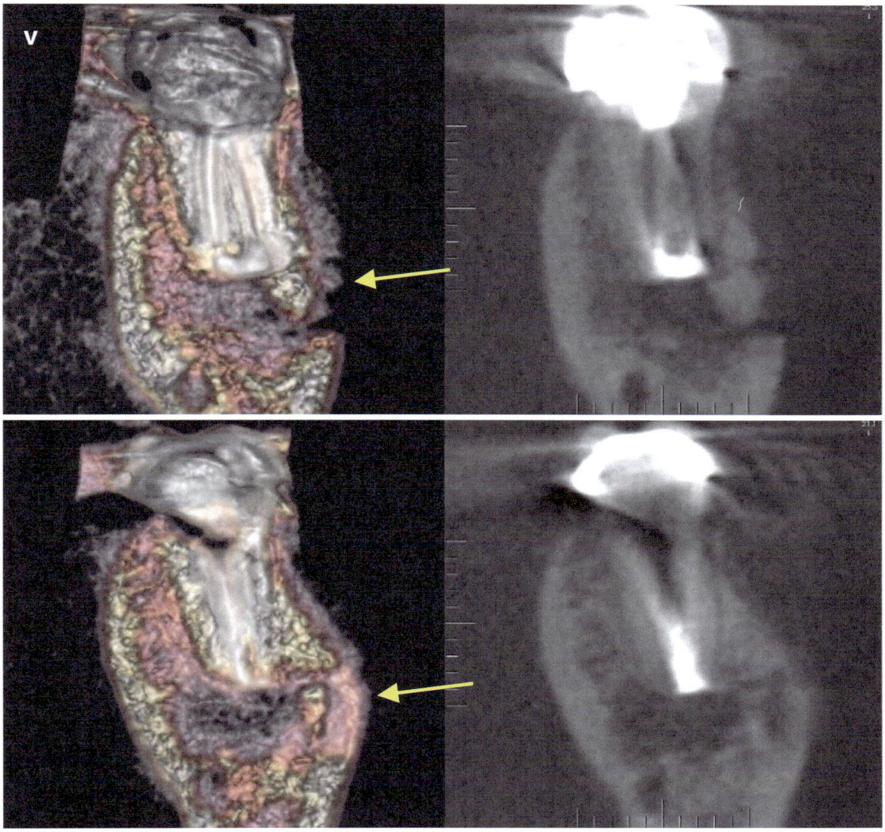

Fig. 8.2 (continued)

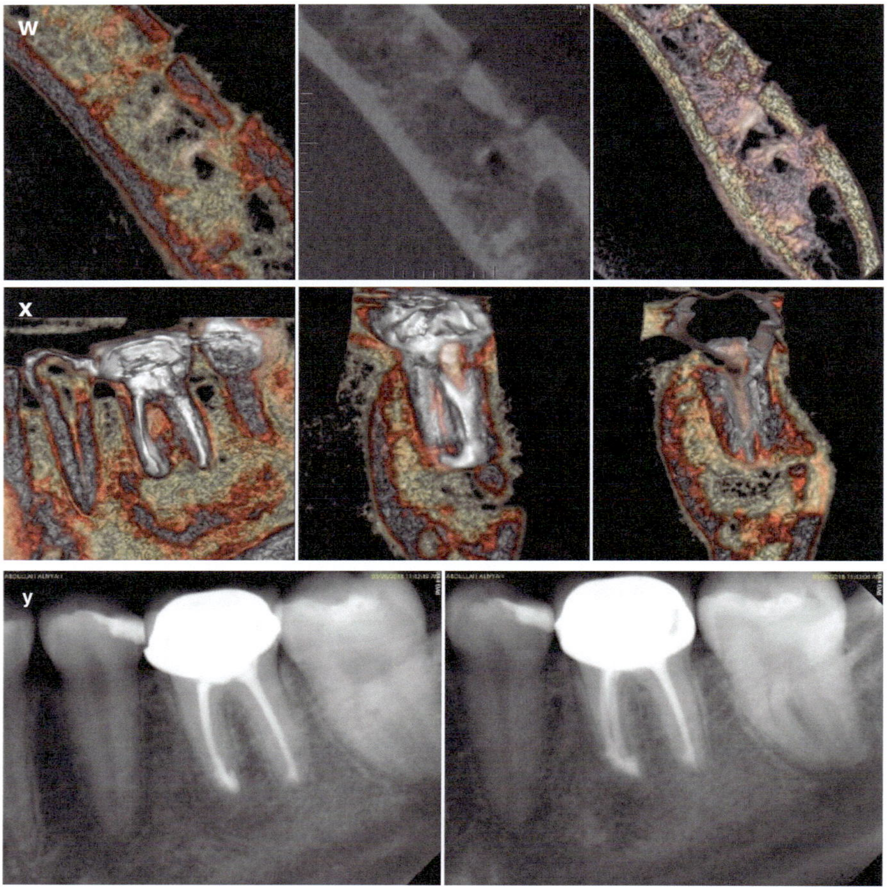

Fig. 8.2 (continued)

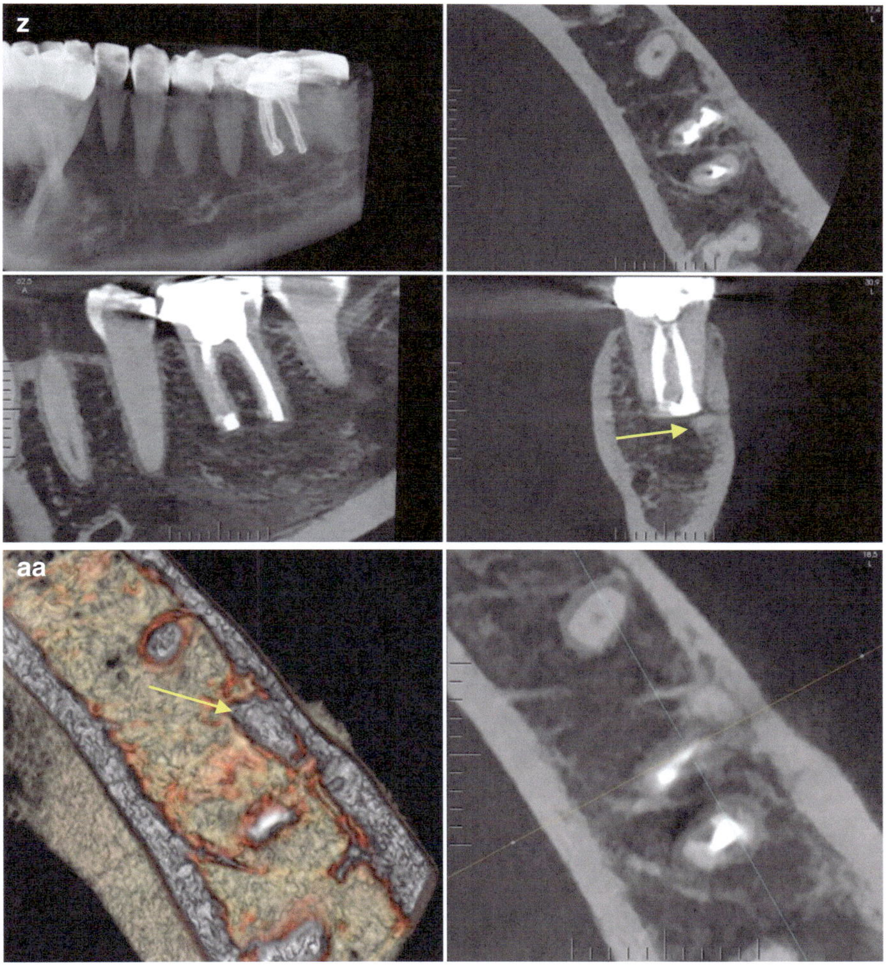

Fig. 8.2 (continued)

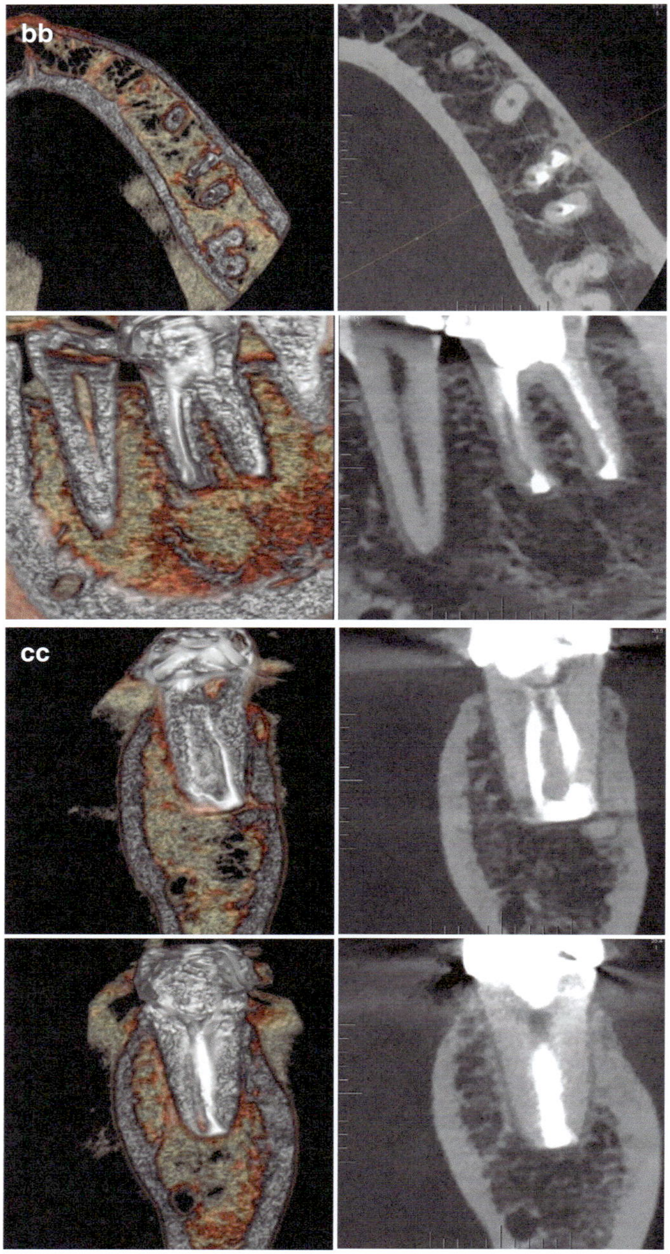

Fig. 8.2 (continued)

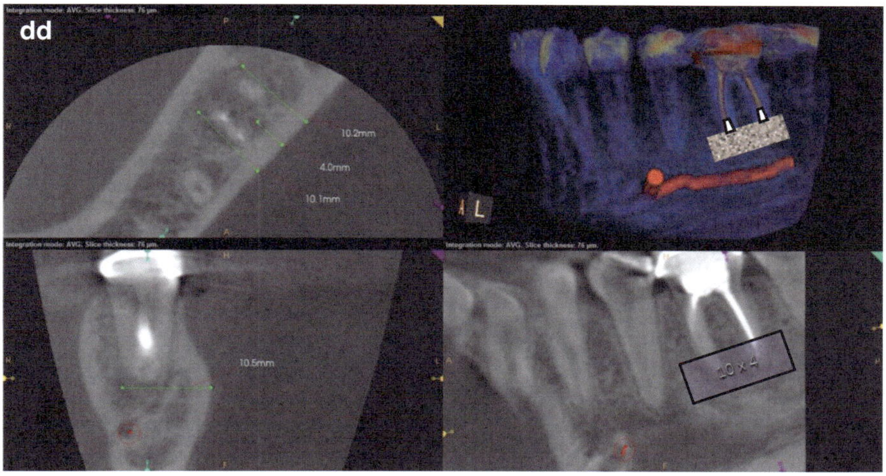

Fig. 8.2 (continued)

of the gutta-percha segment was known, and this facilitated the calibration and accuracy of all the subsequent measurements. The adjustments to apical-coronal heights/ angles on both roots were made relative to the score mark on the cortical plate, and the outline of the lid was plotted according to the Virtual Surgery™ blueprint. The initial outline of the lid boundaries was made using the BS-1 piezo saw tip (Acteon) to a depth of 1.5 mm, with a final separation incision using the BS-5 piezo scalpel tip (Acteon) with copious irrigation. (As the surgeon gains experience, the use of the saw tip can be minimized to just imprinting the sawtooth marks on the cortical plate with activation, and then the surgeon "connecting the dots" using the piezo scalpel. The result is a much narrower incision in the bone and improved adaptation of the lid post-operatively.) When transition through the cortical plate into cancellous bone was realized circumferentially in the lid incisions, an elevating instrument (Ruddle curette) was inserted into the superior and inferior cuts and luxated alternately until the underlying bone was fractured and the lid was dislocated and delivered from the site. The lid was examined for any incomplete or "green stick" fractures and placed into a sterile basin containing 0.9% sterile saline (normal) for hydration until replacement. The mesial and distal root apices were located and isolated, and any hard/soft tissues removed to enable resection. A biopsy of the soft tissue lesion attached to the distal root apex was harvested and sent to the Oral Pathology service. The mesial and distal root apices were resected (2.5 mm and 3.0 mm, respectively) using the BS-5 scalpel tip with copious irrigation and reduced power. The resected surfaces were examined for extent and completeness using low and high powers with direct and indirect means. The resected root ends were prepared using ultrasonic root-end preparation (USREP) tips (KiS 4D, 5D Dentsply Sirona) and the preparations examined with micromirrors for extent and centering. The preparations were filled with BC putty (Brasseler) applied with a MAPS triple angle tip. The excess material was removed from the cavosurface of the preparations, and a radiograph exposed to confirm placement and compaction of the root-end fillings (REF). Calcium sulfate (Ace Surgical) was mixed and placed into the depth of the crypt, allowed to set, and carved back to a depth to support the lid. The lid was removed from the sterile bath and replaced into the site with its former orientation. The incision gaps were sealed with additional amounts of calcium sulfate to seal and stabilize the lid. The soft tissue flap was coapted and allowed to re-perfuse with hydration for approximately 5 min. Closure was achieved with interrupted 6/0 Vicryl sutures in the interdental papilla and vertical release incision sites. Prescriptions for an antibiotic (amoxicillin 500 mg TID) and NSAIDs (ibuprofen 400 mg every 5–6 h) were supplied, as well as post-operative instructions for diet and hygiene. A telephone call that night found the patient resting comfortably, and she presented 5 days later for suture removal. Healing was uneventful, and the post-operative instructions were reinforced. She subsequently presented for periodic recalls, with the last post-surgical recall at 48 months, revealing the site completely resolved in the 2D and 3D imaging and the patient remaining asymptomatic.

8.3 Case #2: Vacuformed Stent with Imprinted Gutta-Percha Fiducial Markers

A 24-year-old woman was referred for evaluation and treatment of tooth #20 prior to prosthetic restoration with a new crown. She presented with a history of endodontic therapy completed approximately 3 years previously and the tooth was restored with a fiber post and PFM crown. The crown became dislodged and lost 2 months before and has had episodes of spontaneous and biting pain for the last 3 weeks. A review of systems was normal, and her medical history was non-contributory. Clinical examination of the mandibular left posterior quadrant revealed elevated percussion sensitivity of tooth #20 to long-axis and right-angle impacts. This tooth was also sensitive to biting, but periodontal probing was within normal limits when compared to the adjacent teeth and the contralateral side. The crown preparation was exposed, but the core buildup material appeared well sealed without evidence of recurrent decay or marginal leakage. Radiographs (Fig. 8.3a) revealed root canal therapy had been completed in #20, with a large post terminating in the middle third of the root. A slight widening of the apical PDL space was noted on the periapical radiographs but did not appear to extend coronally along the root surface. CBCT (Fig. 8.3b) revealed the apex of tooth #20 to be situated 2.5 mm lingual to the mental nerve and at the same apico-coronal level as the foramen. Based on the clinical history and radiographic findings, a diagnosis of previous root canal treatment with symptomatic apical periodontitis was determined. Retreatment of the tooth was considered but then disregarded because of the dimensions of the existing root canal filling and post diameter. Surgical revision was proposed, and the risk/benefits of the procedure were outlined and explained, especially the risk of paresthesia. The patient agreed to the surgical procedure and a mandibular alginate impression was taken for fabrication of a study model. This model became the foundation in the production of the stent. The tray used for the impression was border molded with

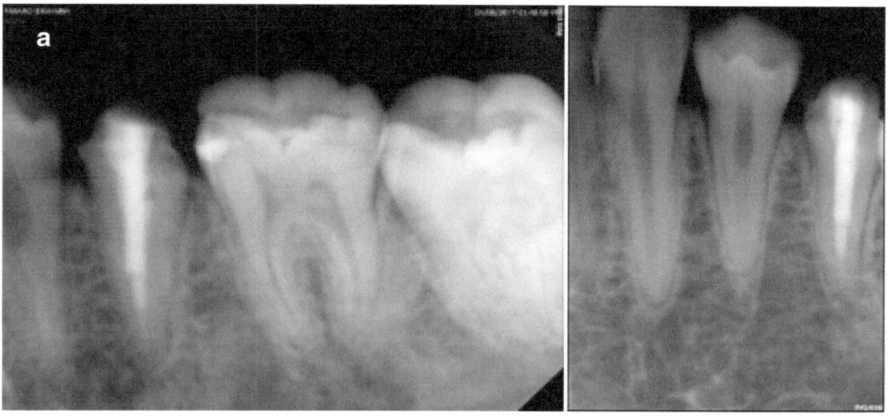

Fig. 8.3 (**a**) Pre-surgical radiographs of tooth #20; temporary crown absent. (**b**) Pre-surgical CBCT image of tooth #20 detailing the thickness of the cortical plate and the proximity of the apex to the Mental Nerve (Carestream Software). (**c**) Study model with the vacuformed stent in place. Small segments of gutta-percha have been secured on the vertical flange corresponding to landmark measurements derived from the scan. (**d**) CBCT image taken with the stent in place, revealing the position of the fiducial markers in the sagittal and axial views. Pre-surgical sagittal view is merged with the scan for comparison. (**e**) CBCT image taken with the stent in place; the red line corresponds to the primary resection level, the yellow line to the secondary level. Approximately 3.2 mm of the apex is to be removed (Green arrow). (**f**) Axial and sagittal views with a stent in place (silicone bone filter). The outline and dimensions of the lid are represented by the red rectangle. (**g**) Realistic rendering (eVolDX) showing superimposed fiducial markers and proposed bony lid dimensions (Black rectangle). (**h**) Reflected buccal flap; stent in place, Mental Nerve stained with methylene blue dye. (**i**) Bone saw tip marking the distal margin of the bony lid outline. (**j**) Measuring the distance from the Mental Foramen to the superior border of the lid. (**k**) Marking the superior lid border with the bone saw tip. (**l**) Bony lid outline complete. (**m**) Bone scalpel tip incising the mesial lid cut through to the cancellous bone; tip slightly angled to produce a beveled cut. (**n**) Inferior lid border incised to cancellous bone depth; superior border to buccal root surface only. (**o**) Lid harvested, buccal root surface exposed (Black arrow). (**p**) Coronal root resection initiated 1 mm apical to the superior lid border incision. (**q**) Coronal and apical root resections complete. Primary segment can be seen in osteotomy (Black arrow). (**r**) Resected primary root segment harvested; apical root tip segment delivered via curette. (**s**) Micromirror view of the resected root surface. (**t**) Ultrasonic root-end preparation after keyhole relief for tip clearance. (**u**) Crypt filled with a small segment of CollaPlug. (**v**) Bony lid replaced; incision cuts to be grouted with $CaSO_4$. (**w**) Immediate Post-surgical radiographs from two angles. (**x**) Two-week Post-surgical CBCT scan showing stable lid position and dissolution of the $CaSO_4$ from the bony incision sites. (**y**) Two-week Post-surgical CBCT scan, axial and sagittal views with silicone bone filter (left) and the sinus filter (right). Lid position and CollaPlug presence confirmed. (**z**) Two-week Post-surgical CBCT scan, coronal views showing lid position and proximity to the Mental Foramen/Nerve (Silicone bone and sinus filters). (**aa**) Realistic rendering showing the actual lid dimensions/position (top) and sagittal section. The green arrow represents the inferior lid border and the red arrow the superior border of the Mental Nerve; distance is 0.7 mm

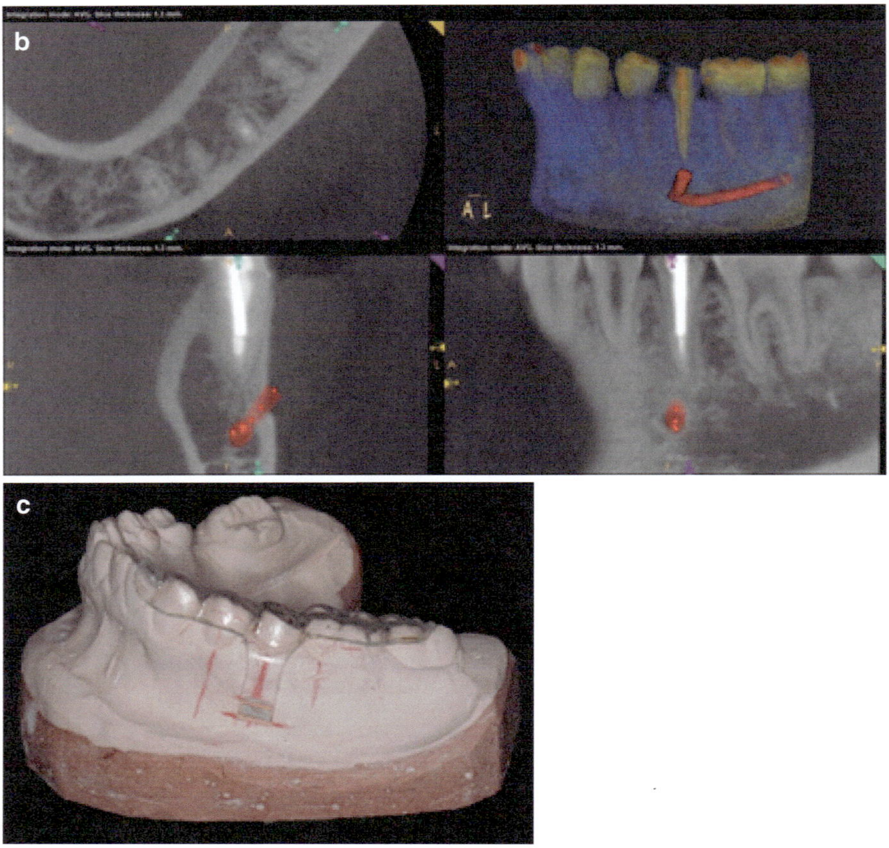

Fig. 8.3 (continued)

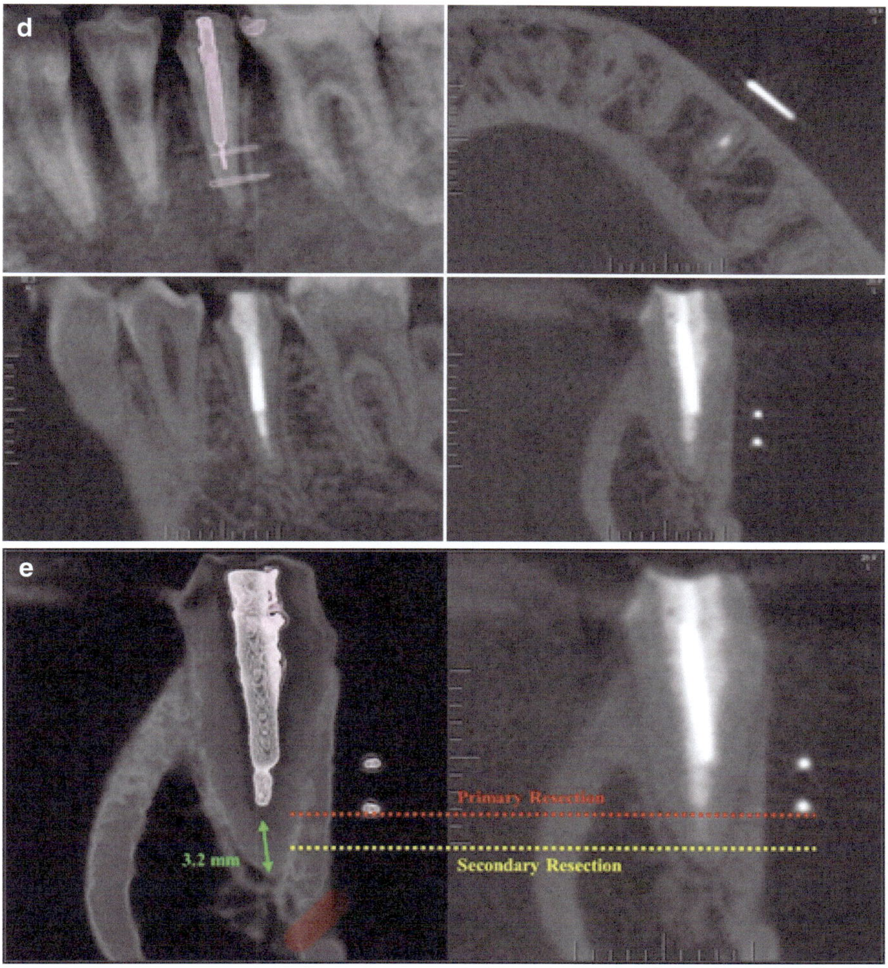

Fig. 8.3 (continued)

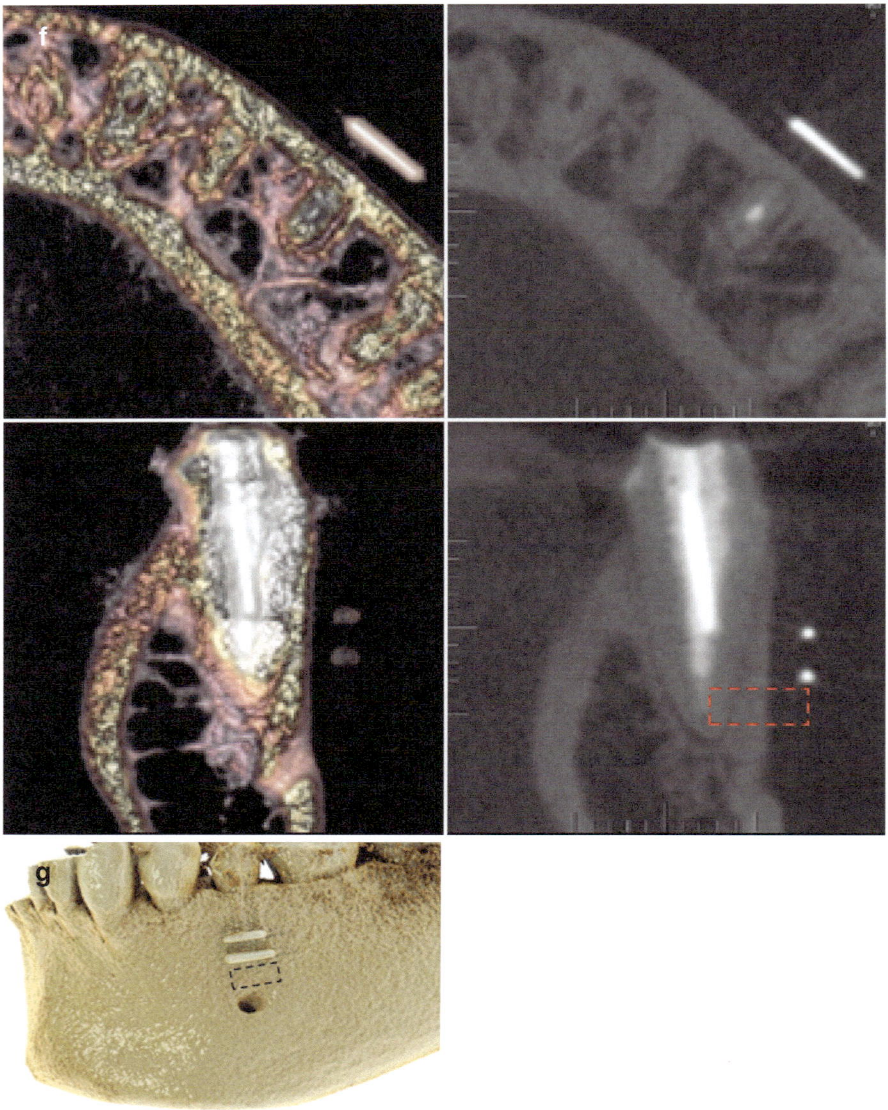

Fig. 8.3 (continued)

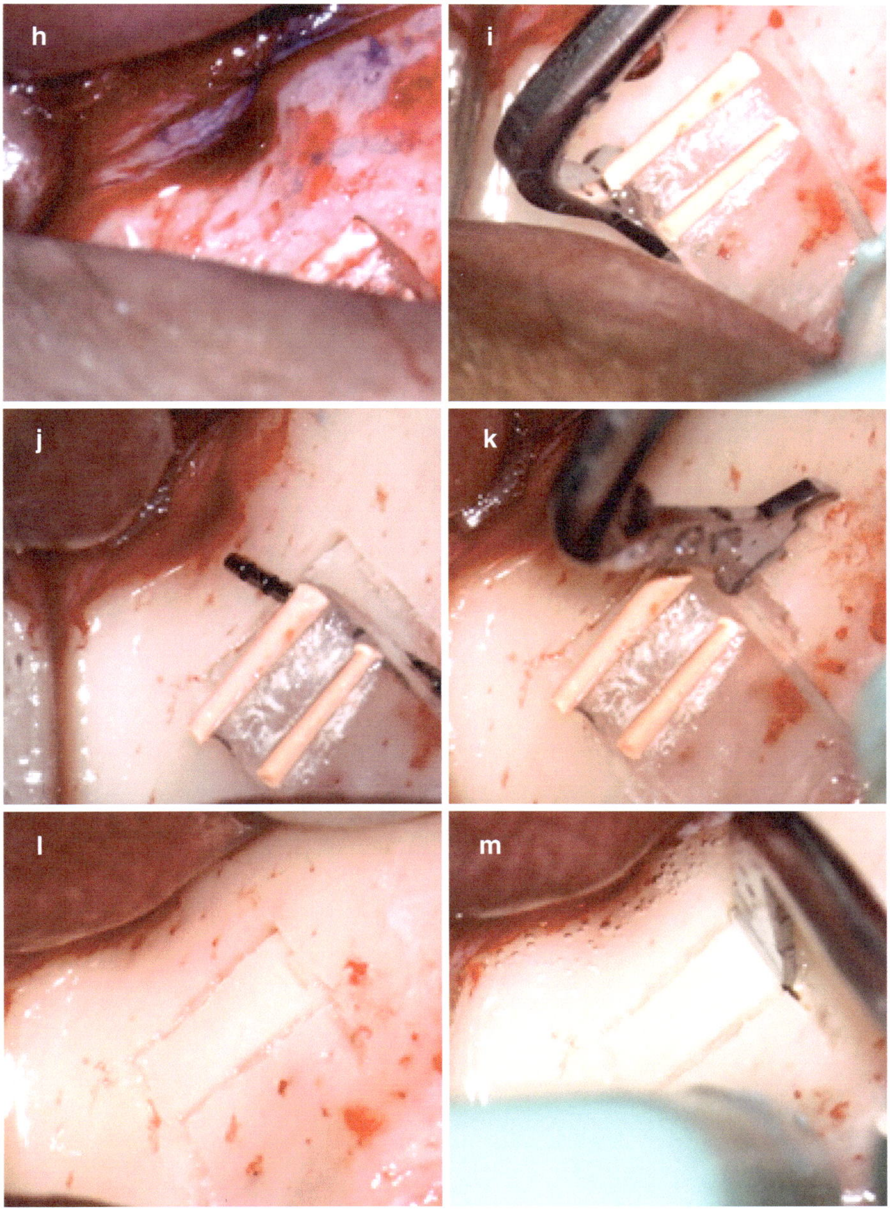

Fig. 8.3 (continued)

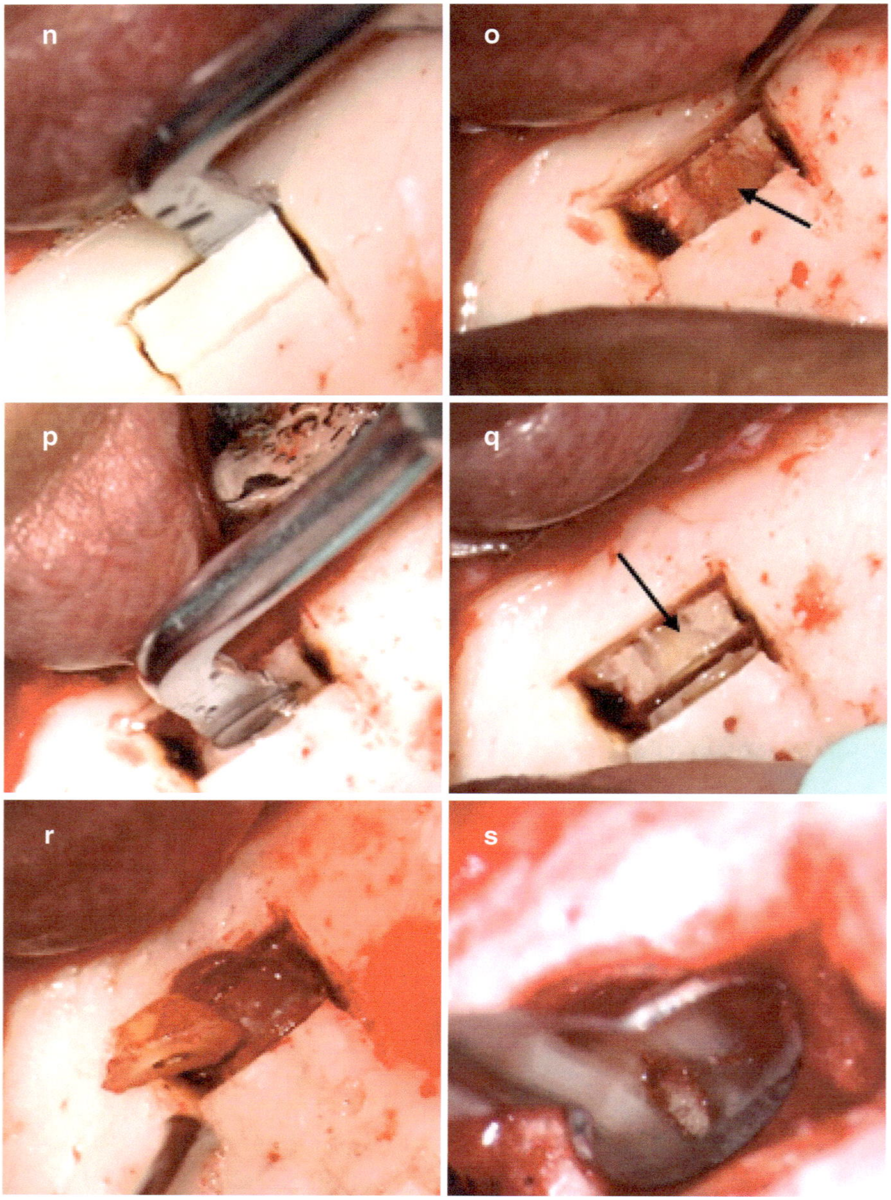

Fig. 8.3 (continued)

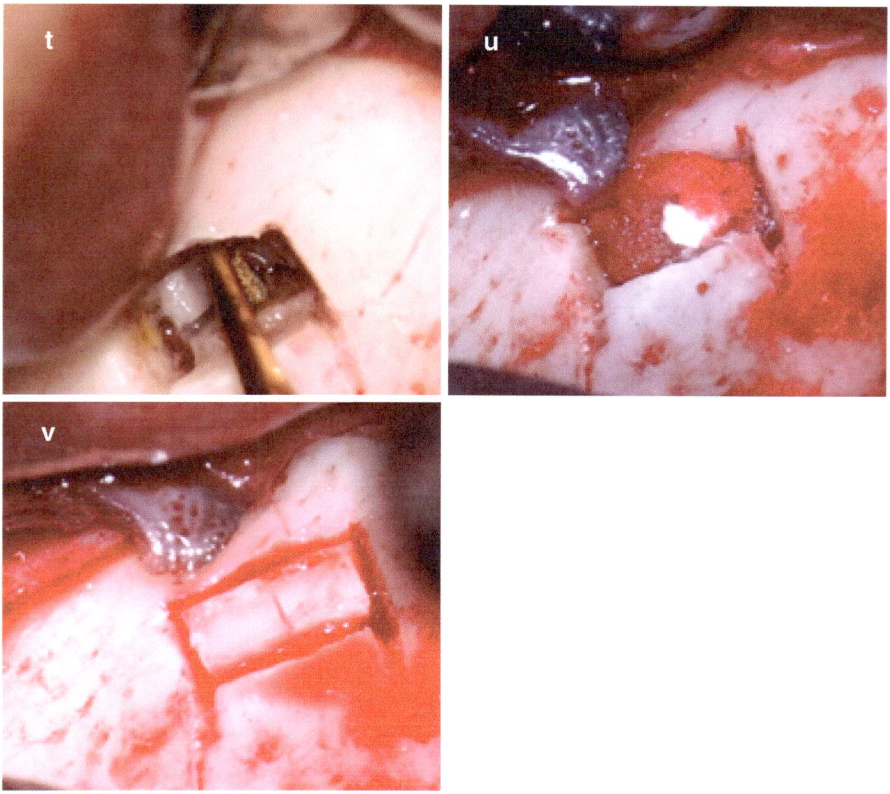

Fig. 8.3 (continued)

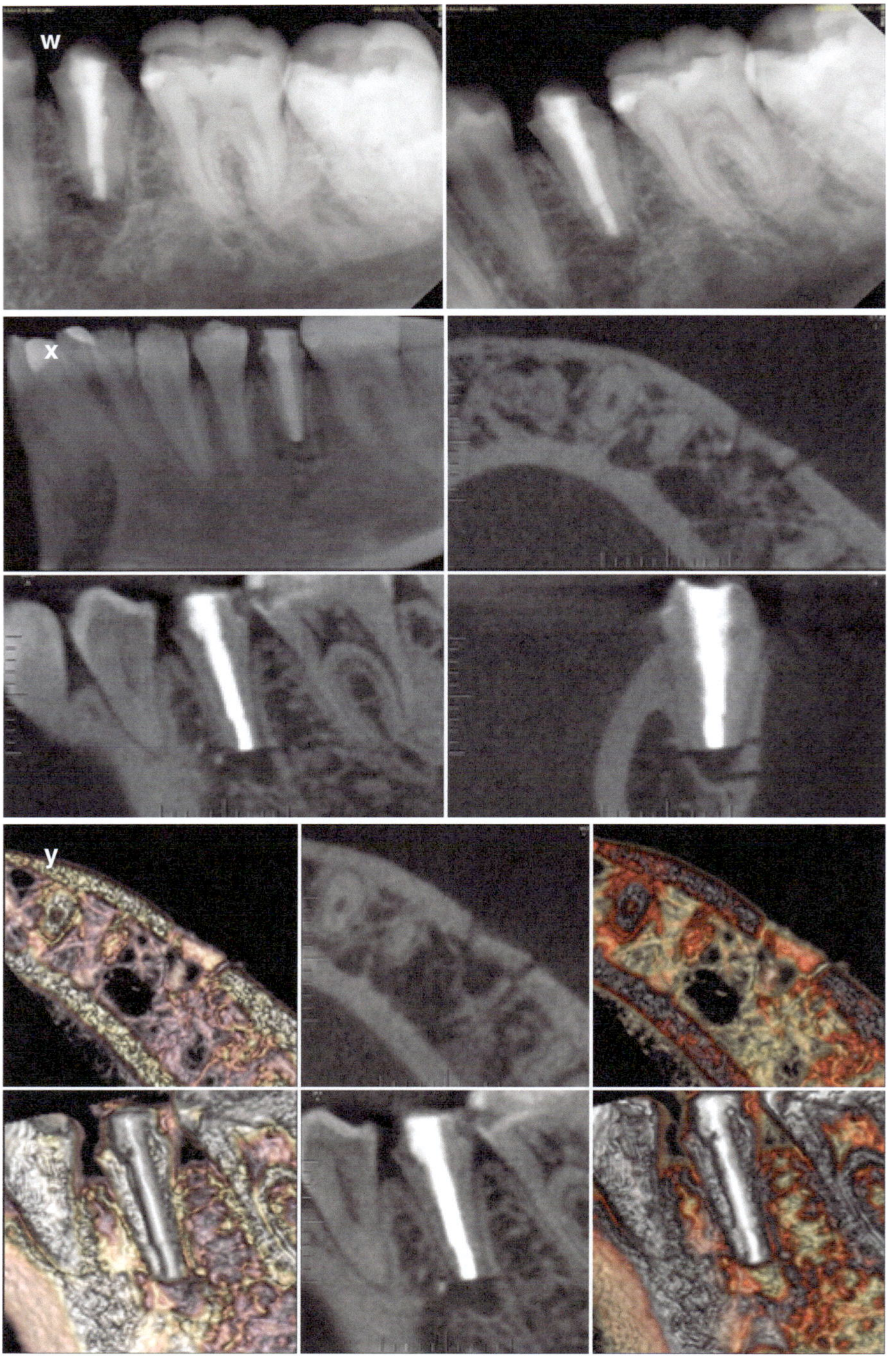

Fig. 8.3 (continued)

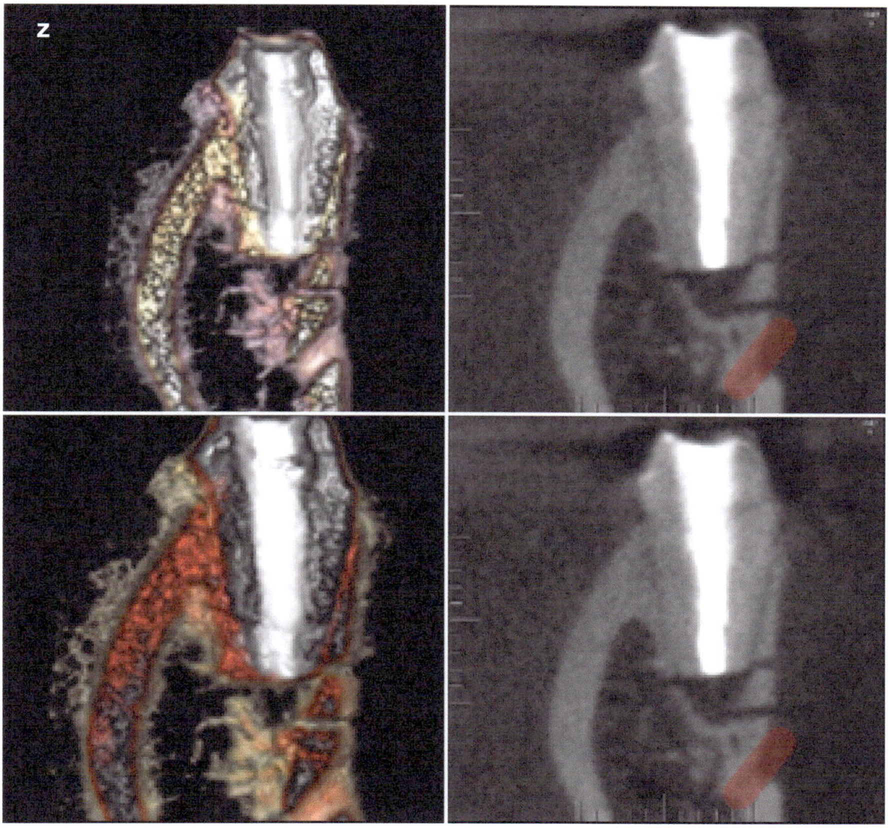

Fig. 8.3 (continued)

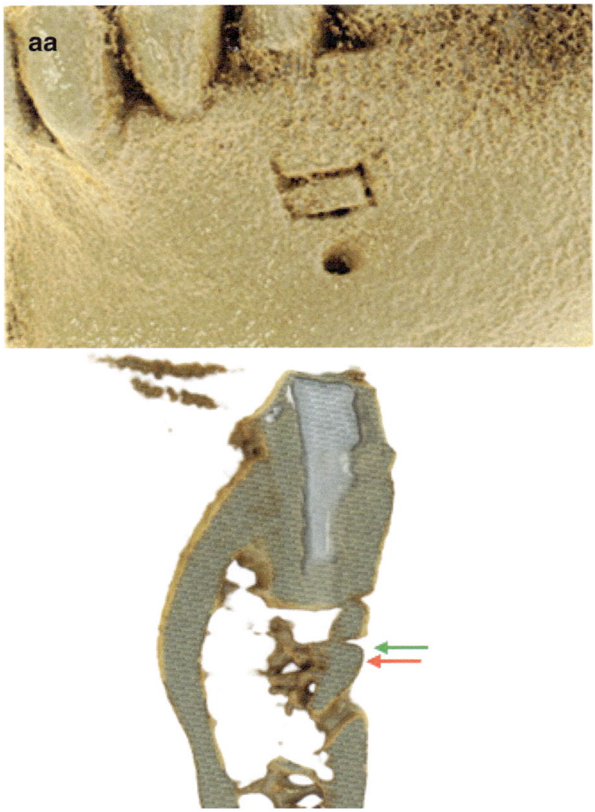

Fig. 8.3 (continued)

wax ropes to extend the flange of the tray apically over the mental foramen, effectively stretching and thinning the buccal gingival tissues covering the cortical plate. This would ensure that the flange of the stent would be as closely approximated to the surface of the bone as possible.

The CBCT scan was used to construct a Virtual Surgery™ blueprint, detailing the distances of the apex to the terminal end of the post, the available root structure for resection and root-end preparation, the distances of the root surfaces to the mental nerve, and the thickness of the cortical plate in the proposed surgical location. A surgical stent thickness (0.60) plastic sheet was heated and vacuformed over the model and cut back to seat over the occlusal surfaces of teeth #18–23, with an apical extension leg 6 mm wide over the root of #20. Using the coronal views of the scan, measurements of the distance from the buccal CEJ to the apical end of the fiber post, existing gutta-percha obturation, and radiographic apex were plotted on the stone model. These landmarks were visualized through the clear extension leg of the fabricated stent on the model, and, using small pieces of gutta-percha bonded to the extension, the terminal ends of the post and gutta-percha were transferred and fixed to the stent (Fig. 8.3c). The patient was then scanned with the stent fully seated, effectively transferring the radiographic markers to the scanned image (Fig. 8.3d,e).

The axial view revealed the mesio-distal extent and dimension of the proposed window was centered on the root and of sufficient length to facilitate the piezo incision. The coronal view revealed the superior marker corresponded to the terminal end of the post and the inferior marker to the apical extent of the gutta-percha filling. Lastly, the sagittal view confirmed the mesio-distal margins of the proposed window and angle of the root resection (Fig. 8.3f,g). A revised blueprint was conceived based on the unique requirements of the surgical access. A conventional 3 mm resection of the apex would leave insufficient room for an adequate root-end filling; hence, a 2.5 mm resection level was selected and designated as the primary resection level. This level would correspond to a line 1 mm apical to the superior lid margin. A secondary resection level, corresponding to the inferior level of the lid piezo incision, was also plotted (Fig. 8.3e). This "split-resection" technique would allow for complete removal of the resected apex without unduly enlarging the lid access and compromising the integrity of the mental nerve and foramen. Finally, the coronal level of the piezo incision would be the level of the inferior marker, and this would be a shallow (1 mm) bone cut to avoid impacting the root surface. Once the lid was harvested, the primary resection would be initiated 1 mm apical to this shallow incision and continued to complete the root resection. During the pre-surgical appointment, any final questions were answered to the patient's satisfaction, informed consent was reviewed and signed, and the surgical appointment scheduled.

Informed consent was reviewed the day of surgery and any final questions answered to the patient's satisfaction. The patient was prepped according to AEMC protocol outlined in the previous case and medical competency confirmed. The patient was anesthetized with 1.75 cartridges of 0.5% bupivacaine (Marcaine™) with 1:2000,000 epinephrine, administered as an IAN block, with 0.25 cartridges of the same anesthetic infiltrated over the mental foramen. After a 10-min delay for onset signs, the buccal aspect of the cortical plate from the mesial of tooth #21 to the distal of tooth #19 was infiltrated with 1.5 cartridges of lidocaine (Xylocaine™) 2%, with 1:50,000 epinephrine for control of site hemostasis. After another 5-min pause for anesthetic uptake and confirmation, the procedure was started. All microsurgical procedures from incision to flap coaptation/suturing were performed under the SOM.

A full-sulcular incision was made from the distal of tooth #18 to the mesial of tooth #21, with a vertical releasing incision at the mesial line angle of #21 (Fig. 8.3h–t). A triangular flap was reflected, and the mental nerve/foramen was located, marked with methylene blue dye and isolated via retraction. Once the retraction was stabilized, the stent was inserted, and complete seating verified. The mesial and distal margins of the lid incisions were lightly scored with the BS-1 piezo saw tip (Acteon) using the edges of the stent as a guide. The inferior/secondary lid incision was measured, according to the blueprint, and lightly scored with the same tip. The level of the superior lid incision was marked on the cortical plate adjacent to the guide edges at the mesial and distal aspects before the guide was removed.

Retraction was reestablished and the piezo incisions were completed using the BS-5 piezo scalpel tip (Acteon). The mesial and distal incisions extended coronally beyond the level of the superior score line to accommodate the movement of the scalpel tip and angled to form a pair of converging bevels to create a "keystone" effect to the lid. This would serve to index the lid during the re-approximation phase and limit submergence. All the incisions were performed until the cancellous bone level was breached; the exception was the superior incision, which was intentionally shallow to avoid damaging the root surface. The result was a lid that measured 3.5 mm × 6 mm and was delivered without complication from the site and stored as outlined in the previous case. The buccal surface of the root was identified, the level of the primary resection was marked 1 mm apical to the superior lid edge, and resection at that level completed with the BS-5 tip. The secondary resection was initiated during the piezo incision of the inferior lid boundary and was now completed using the same scalpel tip. A small ball diamond piezo tip (CE-1, Acteon) was used to expose the 0.5 mm apex by discreetly removing the overlying bone and the two sections of resected root apex were luxated and delivered from the crypt. The resected root surface and harvested root section were examined for completeness and evidence of root fracture. The vertical working dimensions of the access were less than 3 mm by design, inhibiting insertion of the USREP tip. This situation was remedied by using the side of the tip to create minimal vertical relief without compromising the lid boundaries. The root end was prepared without further incident and the preparation filled with BC putty (Brasseler) applied with a MAPS triple angle tip. The excess material was removed from the cavosurface of the preparation and examined with a micromirror and a radiograph exposed to confirm placement and compaction of the root-end filling. A 4 mm × 4 mm section of collagen (CollaPlug™, Ace Surgical) was inserted into the resected root void and allowed to be infiltrated with blood. The lid was removed from the sterile bath and replaced into the site with its former orientation. The lid was minimally stabilized with small amounts of calcium sulfate in the superior and inferior piezo incisions, leaving the beveled surfaces open for perfusion. Radiographs from different angles confirmed the density/placement of the root-end filling and the position of the bony lid (Fig. 8.3w). The soft tissue flap was coapted and allowed to re-perfuse with hydration for approximately 5 min. Closure was achieved with interrupted 6/0 Vicryl sutures in the interdental papilla and vertical release incision sites. Post-operative medications and instructions followed the same protocol as in the previous case and a telephone call that night found the patient resting comfortably. Healing was uneventful and she presented 5 days later for suture removal. A CBCT scan 2 weeks post-surgically verified the dissolution of the calcium sulfate and stable location of the bony lid with excellent approximation (Fig. 8.3x-a).

8.4 Case #3: Single Root/PRESS, Fabrication, and Root-End Surgery

A 14-year-old female was referred for evaluation and treatment of tooth #8. The patient admitted to a history of asthma triggered by allergies, for which she has a prescription inhaler (Montelukast™) and is allergic to ibuprofen. Her past dental history disclosed an impact trauma to her maxillary anterior teeth when she was younger, resulting in a crown fracture of undetermined extent in tooth #8. The tooth was restored with a PFM crown, but the patient complained of the short clinical length and dark margins. A clinical examination confirmed the short crown and discolored margins on tooth #8, but the remaining soft tissue findings were unremarkable. Radiographs (Fig. 8.4a) revealed a periapical lesion at the apex of tooth

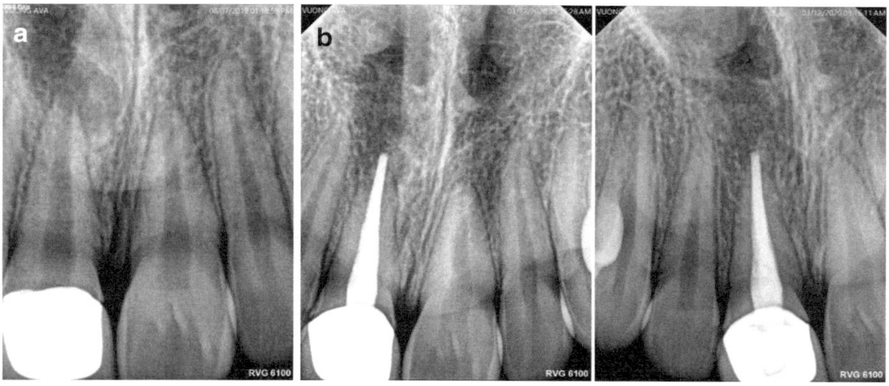

Fig. 8.4 (**a**) Pre-operative radiograph tooth #8; immature apex, periapical lesion. (**b**) Post-operative radiographs; extent/density of obturation, lesion persistent. (**c**) Pre-surgical CBCT scan showing the location and extent of the lesion. Note the more dense object palatal to the apex. (**d**) Pre-surgical CBCT scan, axial view with silicone bone/sinus filters. Note the position of the apex and thickness of the facial cortical plate. (**e**) Pre-surgical CBCT scan, sagittal and coronal views with silicone bone/sinus filters. Note the size and position of the apical areas of less density and the thickness of the facial cortical plate. (**f**) Tissues reflected, PRESS positioned according to the index and stable. (**g**) Marking the inferior lid border/apical resection level with the straight scalpel tip. (**h**) Bony lid incisions completed through root apex and into cancellous bone to depth. (**i**) Elevation and delivery of the intact bony lid. (**j**) Visualization through window; exposed root apex and lesion (Black arrow). (**k**) Apex resection is confirmed by separation of the apical section from the root. (**l**) Resected root apex section harvested. (**m**) Ultrasonic root-end preparation initiated. (**n**) Root-end preparation complete; root-end filling with MTA (white). (**o**) CollaPlug placed into crypt to support repositioned lid (Black arrow). (**p**) Bony lid repositioned in the original orientation. (**q**) Grouting the bone incisions with $Ca(SO)_4$. (**r**) Immediate Post-surgical radiographs from two angles; faint outline of bony lid evident. (**s**) Two-week Post-surgical CBCT scan demonstrating $Ca(SO)_4$ dissolution in the bone incision sites. (**t**) Two-week Post-surgical CBCT scan showing (top to bottom) axial, sagittal, and coronal views of the surgical site. Note the position of the bony lid, extent of the osteotomy, and density of the root-end filling. (**u**) Twelve-month Post-surgical radiograph demonstrating complete resolution of surgical site. (**v**) Twelve-month Post-surgical CBCT scan demonstrating complete reformation of buccal cortical plate and cancellous regeneration. Bony lid incision outlines are no longer evident. (**w**) Twelve-month Post-surgical CBCT scan showing (top to bottom) axial, sagittal, and coronal views of the surgical site. Note the normal axial profile of the facial cortical plate and reformation of the cancellous bone around the apex

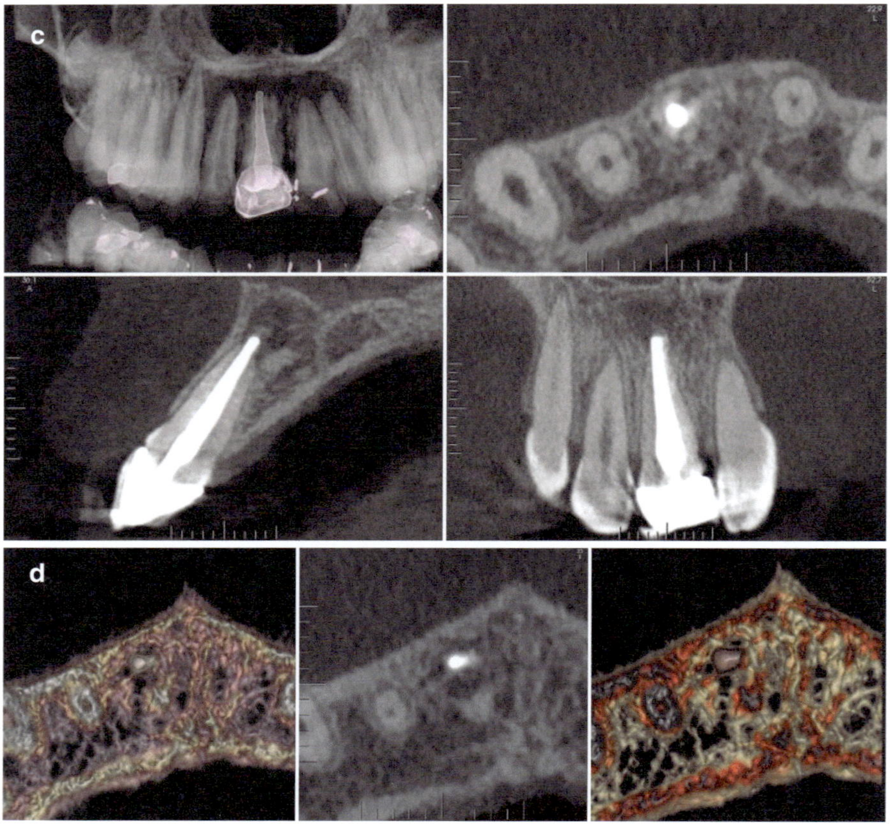

Fig. 8.4 (continued)

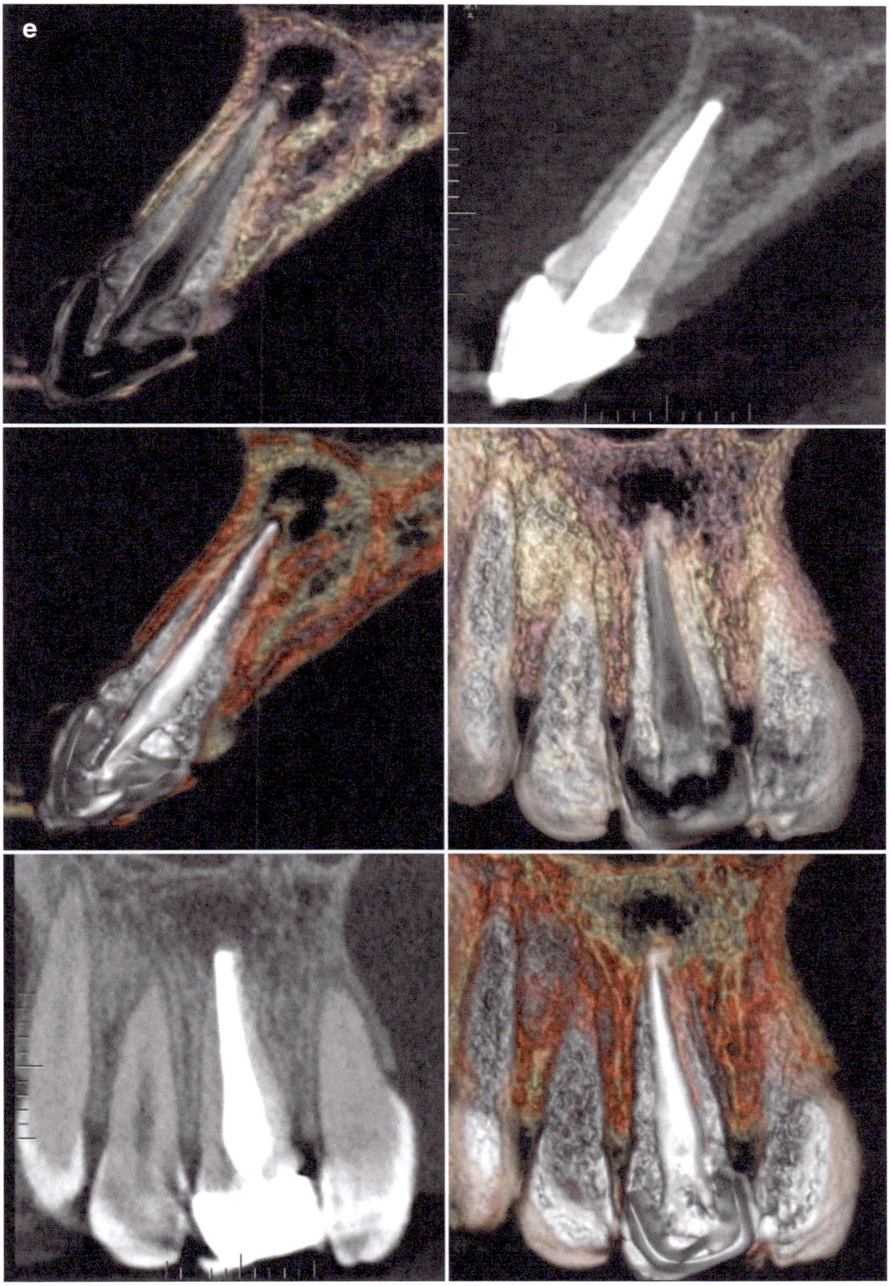

Fig. 8.4 (continued)

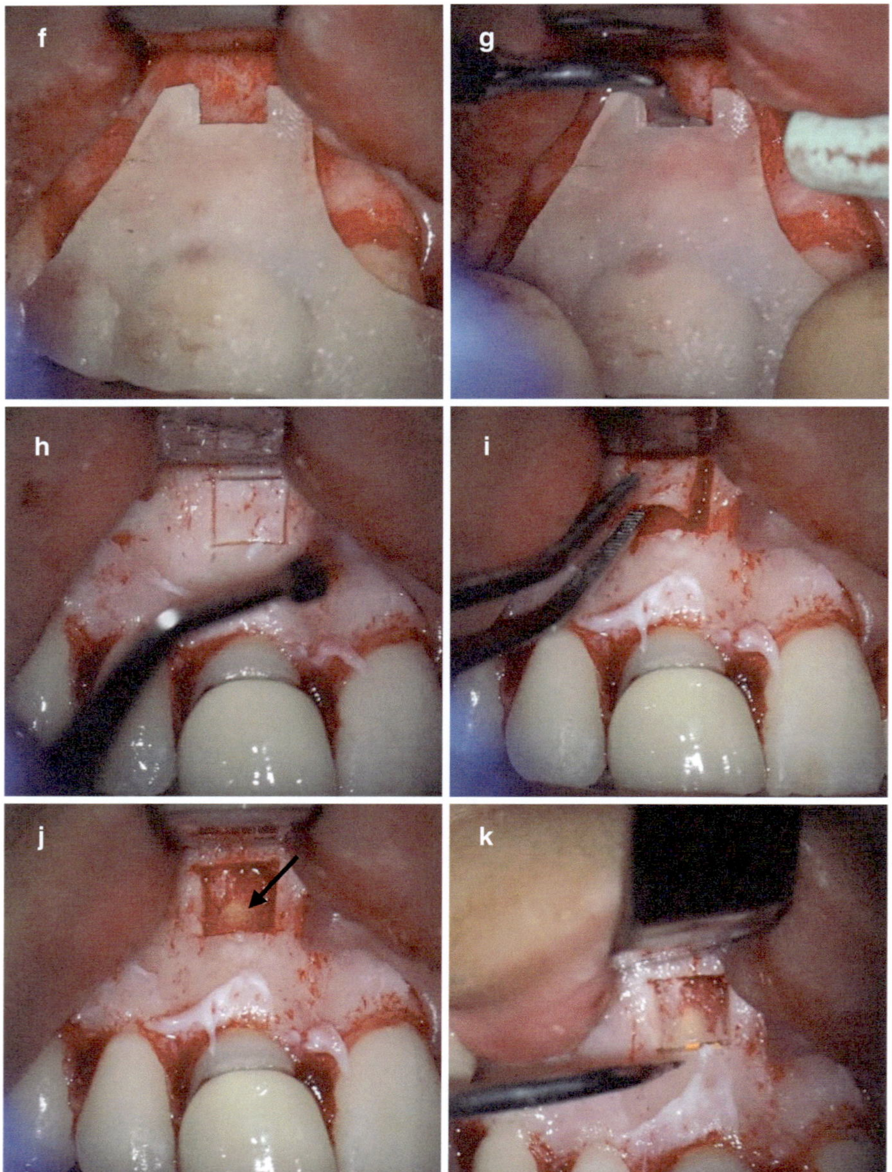

Fig. 8.4 (continued)

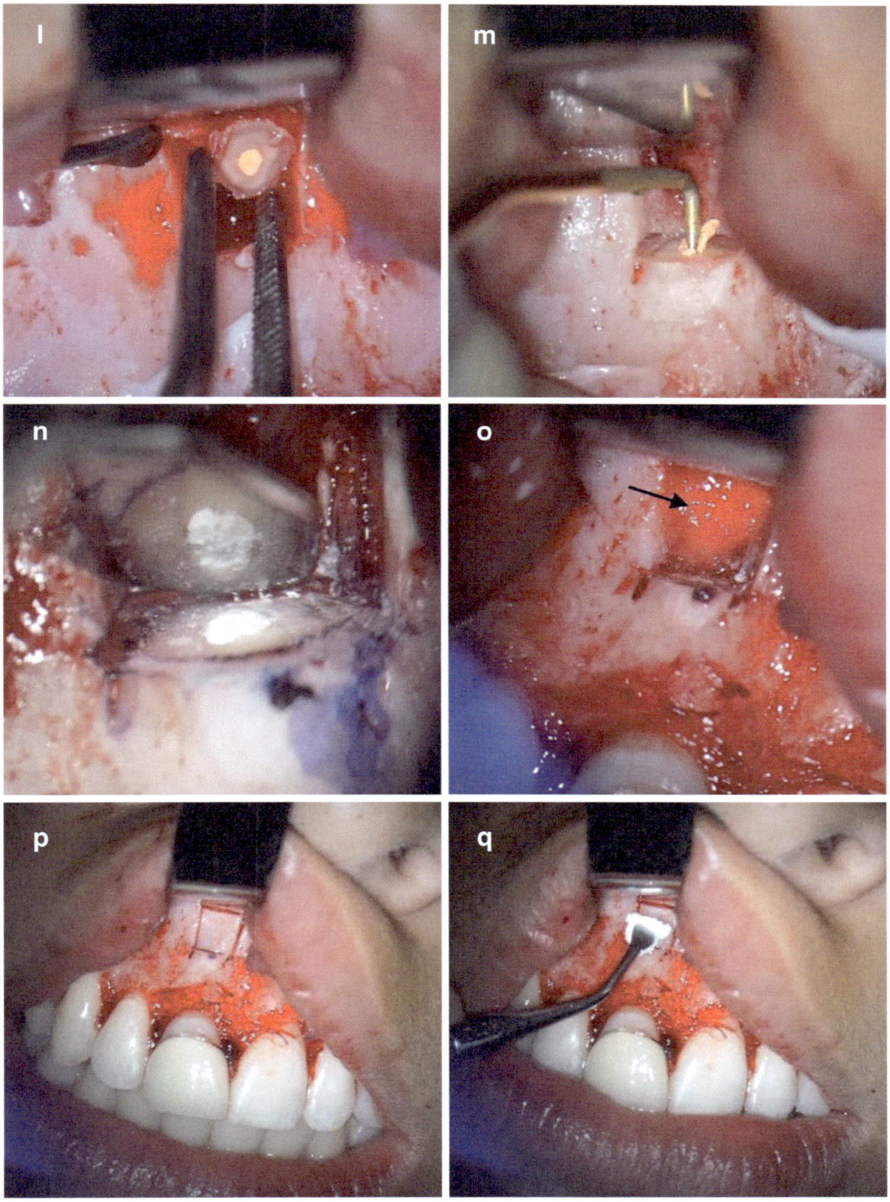

Fig. 8.4 (continued)

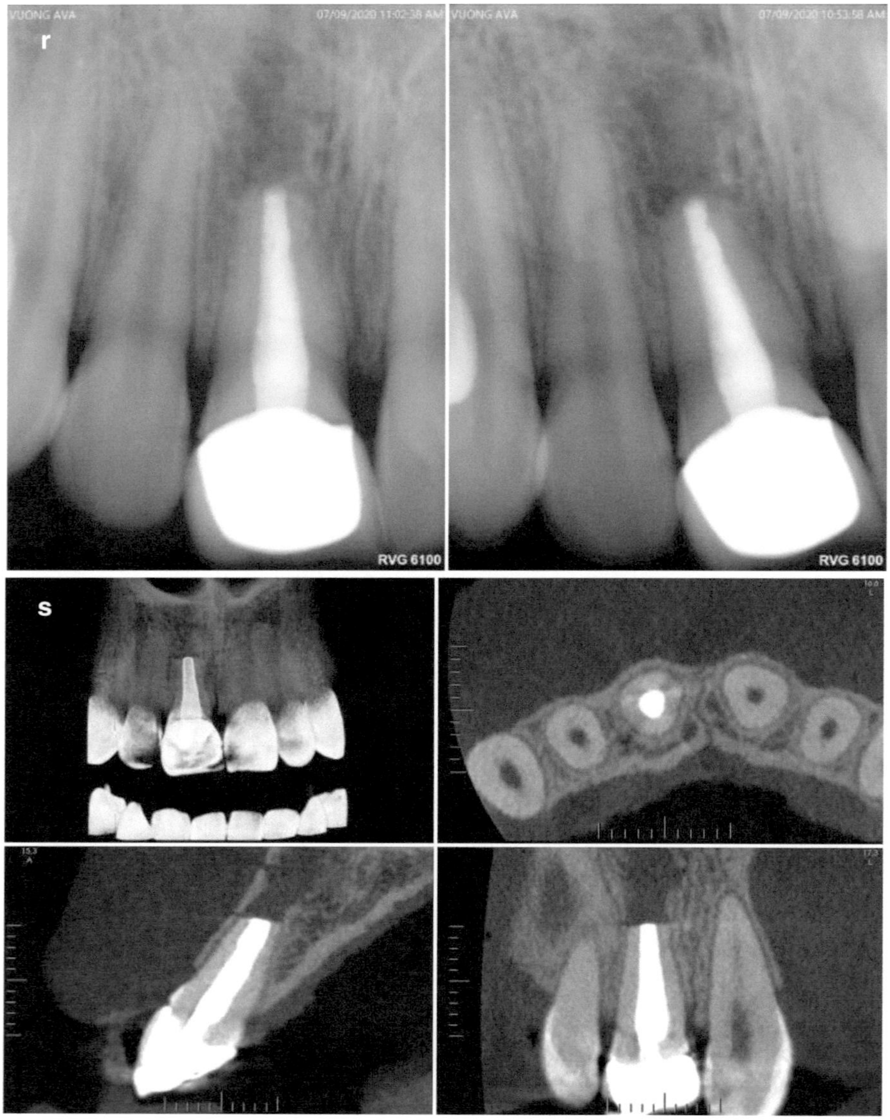

Fig. 8.4 (continued)

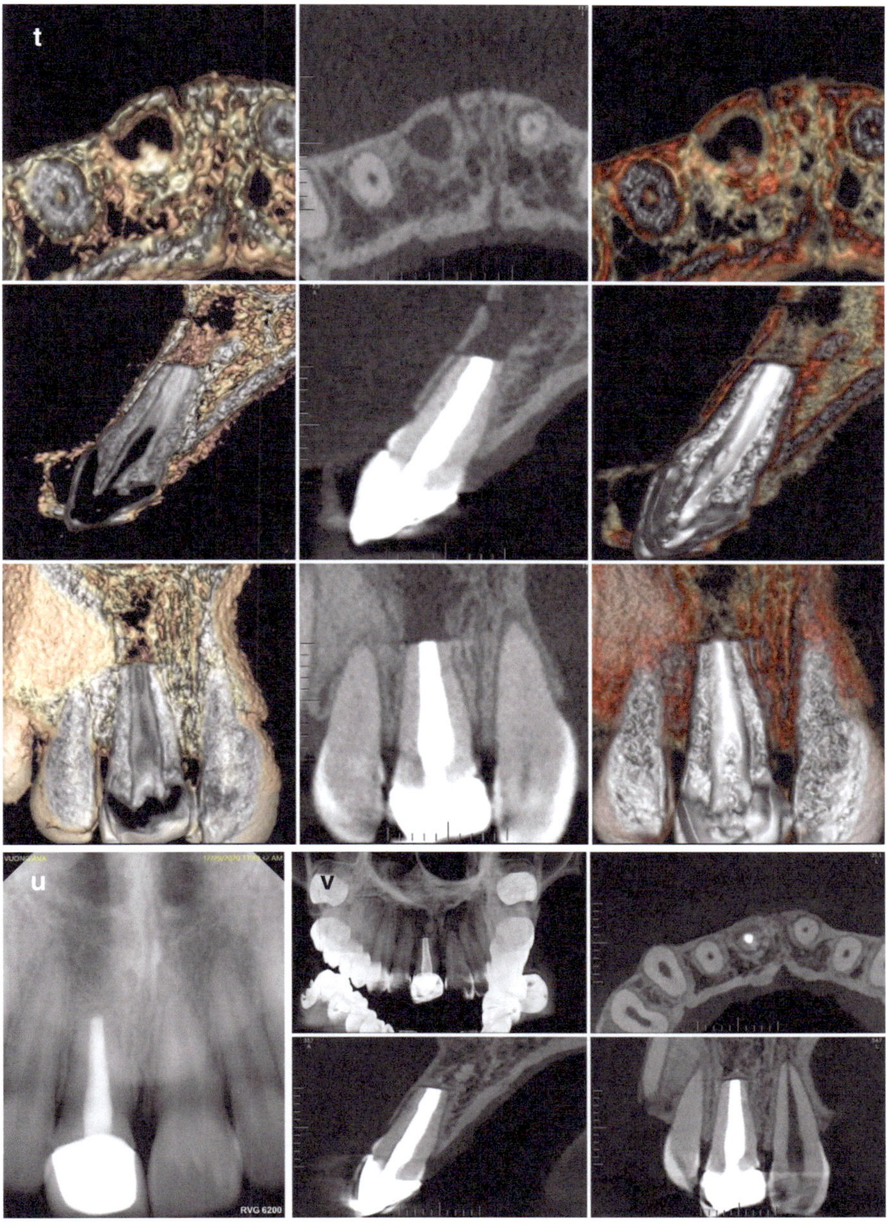

Fig. 8.4 (continued)

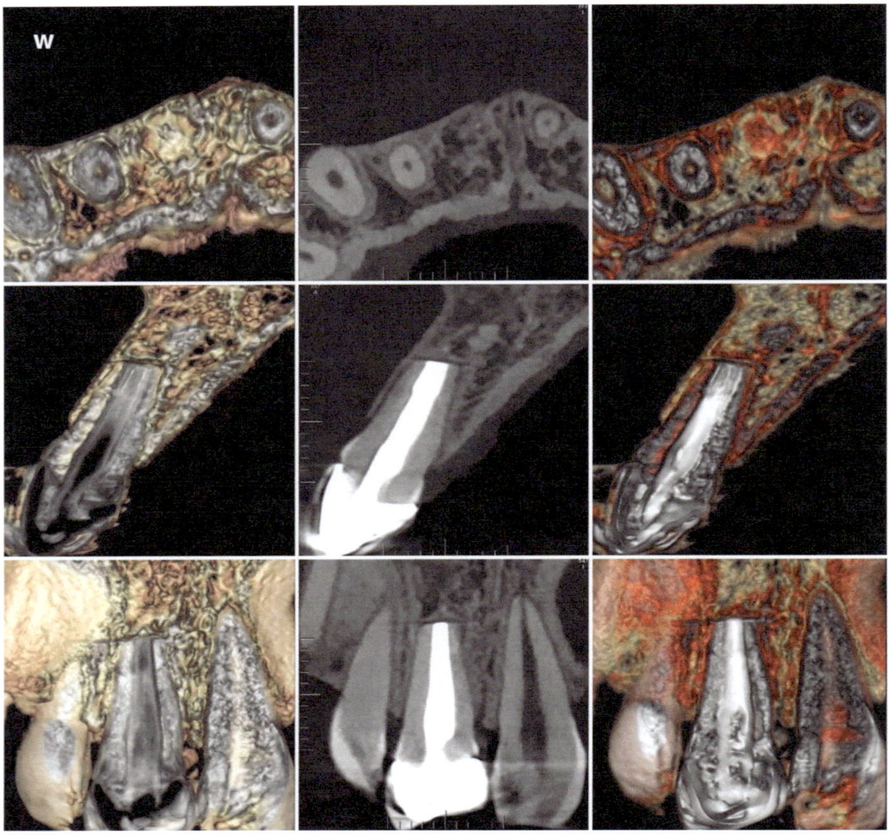

Fig. 8.4 (continued)

#8, with evidence of arrested apical development regarding canal size and foramen constriction. A CBCT scan disclosed a 5 mm × 5 mm lesion at the apex of #8, but it had not yet compromised either cortical plate. There was also evidence of irregular resorption of the apex, with one site close to perforating the canal space. The diagnosis was determined to be pulp necrosis with asymptomatic apical periodontitis. The treatment plan included non-surgical RCT with calcium hydroxide and new prosthetic when completed. Informed consent included the probable need for surgical revision due to the resorption and questionable integrity of the apical seal, but this would be evaluated later post-treatment. The patient and guardian understood her options and consented to treatment.

The therapy was completed in 2 visits, separated by 30 days, but the obturation resulted in the material flush with the radiographic apex (Fig. 8.4b). The apical seal was uncertain, and the patient was instructed to return in 6 months for re-evaluation. The recall full-arch scan (Fig. 8.4c–e) demonstrated slight resolution of the lesion, but the patient had become increasingly sensitive to biting and had periods of spontaneous discomfort. The treatment plan was revised to add surgical revision of the previous therapy. The patient and guardian understood the risks and benefits of the root-end surgery and consented to the procedure. Due to the age of the patient and desire to conserve as much of the cortical plate as possible, a precision endodontic surgical stent (PRESS) was planned. The full-arch scan had already been taken in anticipation of this outcome and a full-arch maxillary impression of the arch was captured, with extension of the tray borders to stretch and thin the apical mucosa around the apex of #8. The model generated from this impression was scanned using a 3Shape Trios® scanner and software to generate an STL file. This, along with the DICOM file of the full-arch scan, would be imported into the Blue Sky Bio® (Libertyville, IL) planning program to construct the surgical guide. The planning and construction of this guide is illustrated in Fig. 8.5a–k and will be briefly outlined here.

The program is opened with the tab "surgical guide" selected. The DICOM file of the full-arch scan is imported, and the volume image is adjusted for axis planes and cropped to remove unwanted portions. The captured STL (stereolithography or standard tessellation language) file is then imported and aligned with the 3D model using various menu selections. The alignment process involves the selection of teeth in the STL file and matching teeth in the panoramic-like image representation of the 3D scan. At least six teeth must be matched and evenly distributed to ensure an accurate rendering of the STL superimposition on the 3D model. Once the alignment is verified by cycling through the axial and coronal views, the alignment is confirmed, and planning can begin.

The tooth is selected and isolated in the "Tangential 3" mode and the apex visualized at the selected site of the resection. The slices to the left and right are plus or minus 1 mm, so it simplifies the bracketing. A custom pin (1 mm × 19 mm) is selected from the implant dropdown menu, and it is positioned so that the inferior plane of the pin is even with the proposed plane of resection. (If the planning is for a mandibular tooth, then it would be the superior plane of the pin.) The markings at the perimeter of each slice window are in 1 mm increments (program default) and the length of the pin is long enough to index with these markings. Therefore, starting at the apex of the tooth, it becomes a simple and accurate process to navigate the pin's position to match the selected level of resection. The angle of the pin is also adjusted to reflect the resection angle in the facial-palatal direction and, in the axial view, the mesio-distal direction as well. Once the pin's position is determined, it is locked to prevent accidental misalignment. The surgical window guide is added by right clicking on the merged 3D-STL image and positioning the window to match the custom pin's position and angle in the coronal view and centered on the pin in the axial view. The size of the window is adjusted to suit the site requirements, in this case 5 mm wide by 4 mm high and 20 mm deep. The depth assures that the operator can visually match the angle of the pin in the coronal view. Lastly, the transparency of the window and STL image is adjusted so the underlying

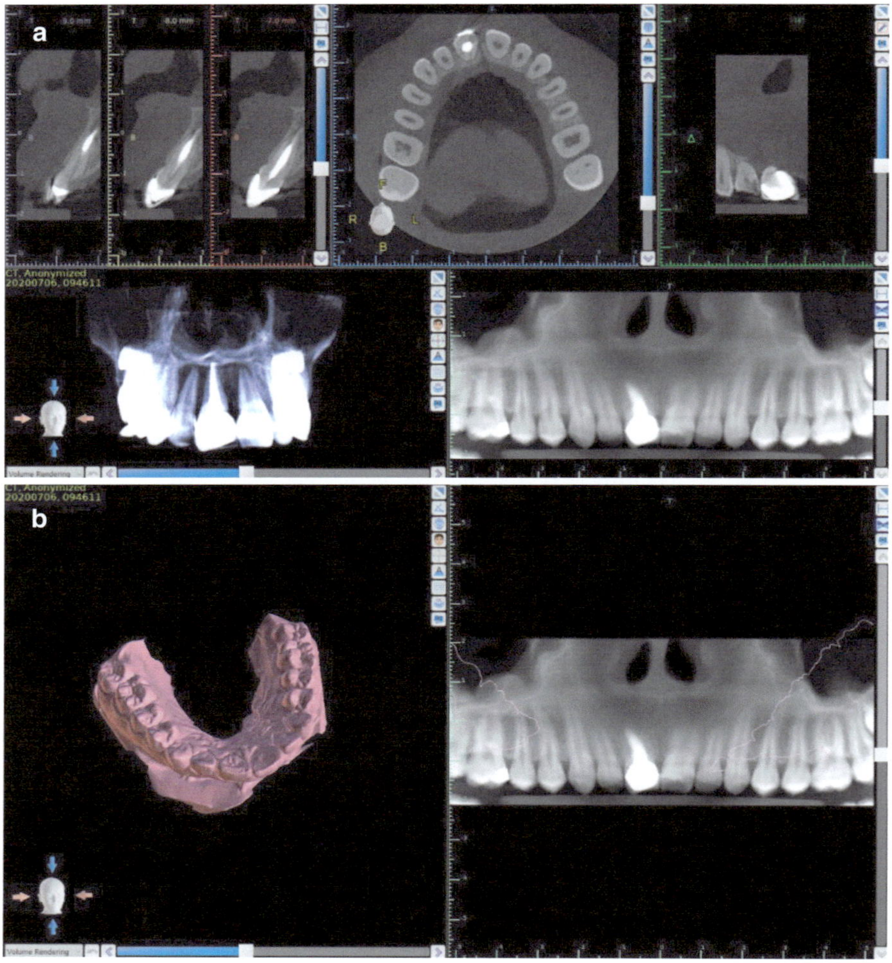

Fig. 8.5 (**a**) Importation of CBCT volume; Tangential 3 selected for planning. (**b**) Importation of selected arch STL file. (**c**) Selection of matching teeth/crowns on STL image and panographic image. (**d**, **e**) Custom pin selected; positioning for height/depth and angle of resection in coronal and axial views in merged images. (**f**) Adding resection window and adjusting for width and height of proposed bony lid. (**g**) Positioning the resection window for correct angulation in all three axes. (**h**) Resection window transparent to verify angulation with respect to guide pin. (**i**) Freehand outline of proposed stent from facial and palatal aspects to verify extent and locations of stent margins. (**j**) Final stent rendered and radiographic image selected to verify location and adaptation of stent prior to fabrication. (**k**) Final stent outline (blue) and soft tissue (pink) overlays superimposed onto sagittal and axial scan views. Stent to bone distance: 0.93 mm

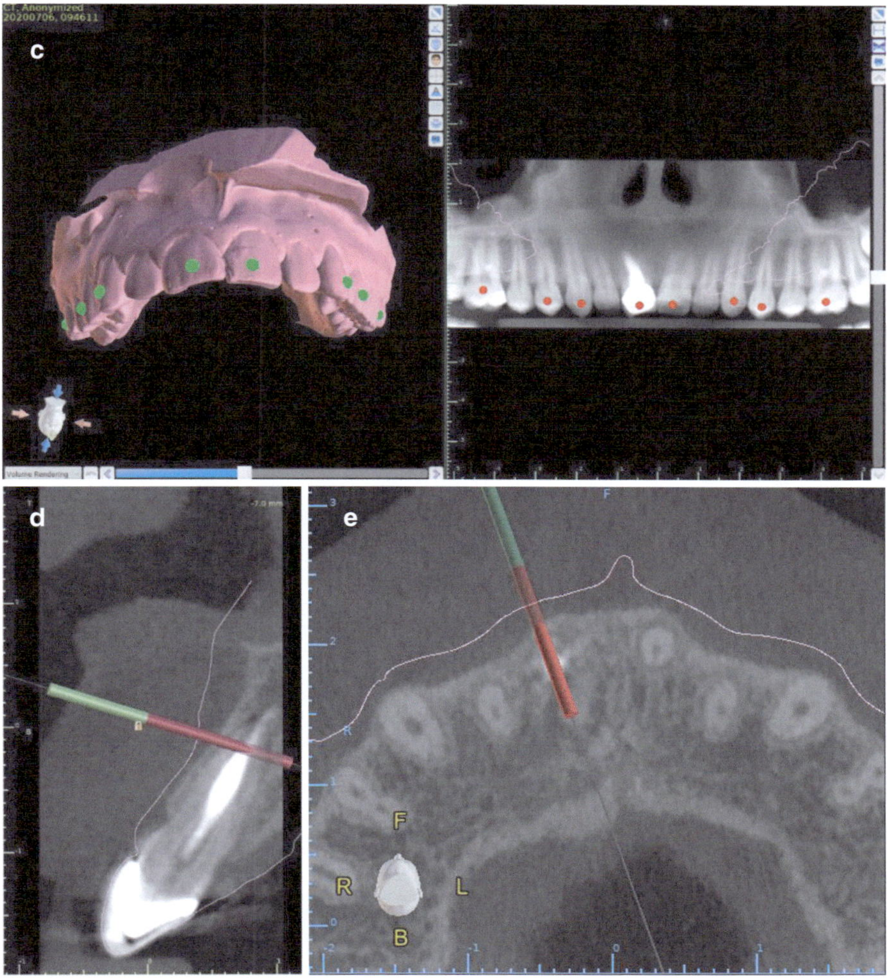

Fig. 8.5 (continued)

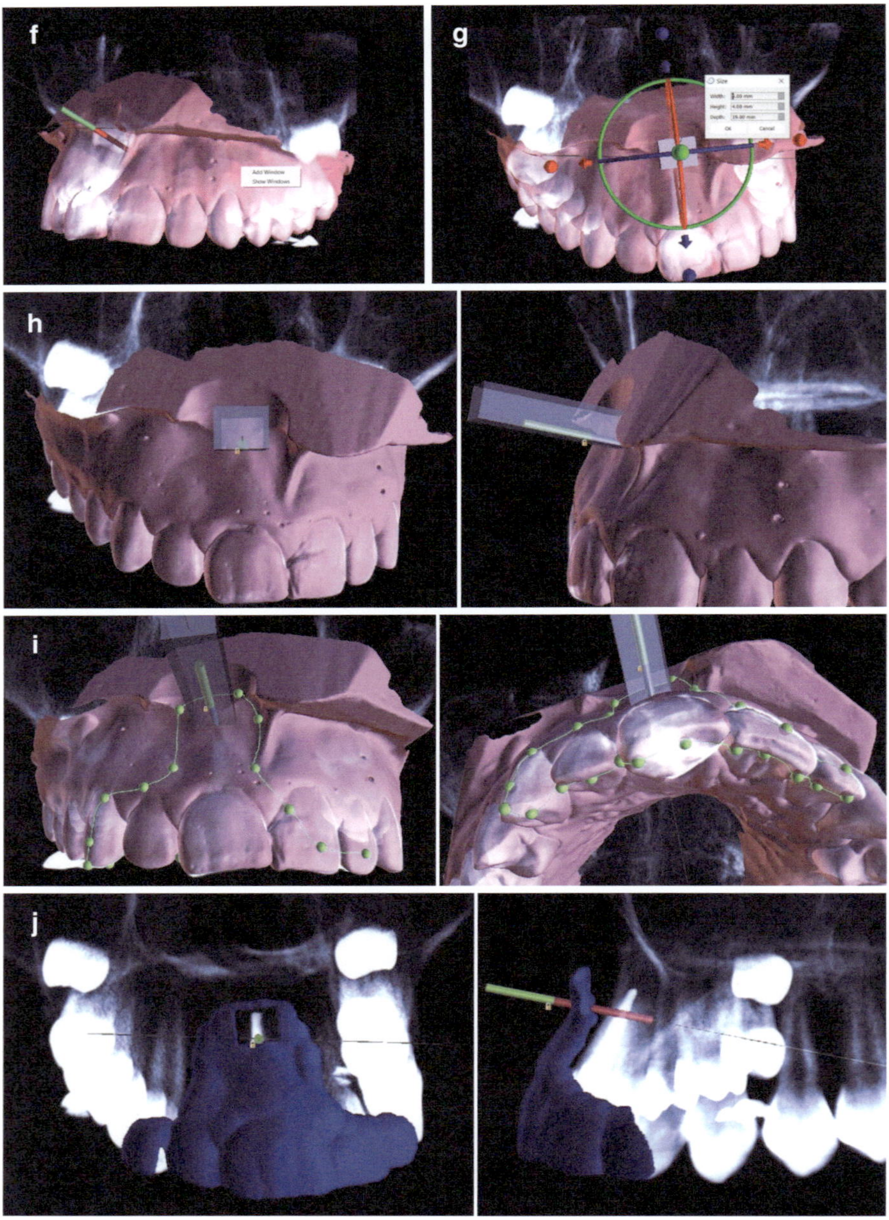

Fig. 8.5 (continued)

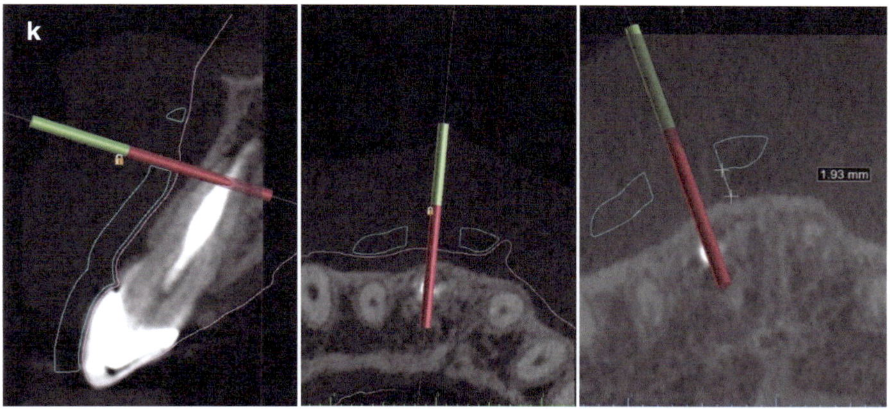

Fig. 8.5 (continued)

radiographic image of the tooth can be seen, and the mesio-distal angle of the window is adjusted to reflect the correct resection angle in this plane. The window angles and placement are verified then locked into place as well. The guide fabrication tab is selected, the correct arch chosen, and the outline of the guide is traced using the computer cursor. After tracing, the edit button is selected, and the operator can adjust the position of the tracing as needed. When satisfactory, the edit is verified and the create guide button is selected. The program generates the guide according to the planned outline, and the finished guide is displayed and ready for production. Once the guide is approved and saved, an STL file of the guide is created and can be exported to the printer for fabrication.

On the day of surgery, the guide adaptation was verified clinically prior to the commencement of the procedure. The informed consent was reviewed with the patient and guardian, and the patient prepared according to the AEMC protocol. The patient was anesthetized with 1.5 cartridges of 0.5% bupivacaine (Marcaine™) with 1:2000,000 epinephrine, administered above the apices of teeth # 6, #8, and #10 using slow infiltration technique. After a 10-min delay for onset signs, the facial aspect of the cortical plate from the mesial of tooth #6 to the distal of tooth #10 was infiltrated with 1.5 cartridges of lidocaine (Xylocaine™) 2%, with 1:50,000 epinephrine for control of site hemostasis. The interdental papilla on the palatal aspect of these teeth was infiltrated with small increments of the same anesthetic as well. After another 5-min pause for anesthetic uptake and confirmation, the procedure was started. All microsurgical procedures from incision to flap coaptation/suturing were performed under the SOM.

A full-sulcular flap was incised and raised from the distal of tooth #6 to the mesial of tooth #10, with a vertical release at the distal of #6 (Fig. 8.4f–w). The flap was retracted and secured to minimize impingement, and the stent was inserted and stabilized. The outline of the lid was marked on the cortical plate with a series of indents from the BS-1 saw tip, then the stent was removed, and the piezo incisions were completed with the BS-5 scalpel tip. The incised lid was luxated and delivered from the site without complication and stored in a sterile basin containing 0.9% sterile saline (normal). The root apex was readily visible, and the resection level corresponded to the inferior level of the piezo incision border. The apex was resected using the BS-5 tip and harvested from the crypt. A small lesion (3 mm × 4 mm) was also curetted from the site and conserved for biopsy. The resected surface was examined under low and high powers for extent and completeness using micromirrors and indirect vision. The USREP was performed with a ProUltra 2 USREP tip (Dentsply Sirona) and the preparation examined for extent and residual RCF material. The preparation was filled with BC putty, delivered with a MAPS hook tip, condensed, and carved to the preparation cavosurface. The final root-end filling was examined with direct and indirect vision, and a radiograph exposed to verify extent and placement. A small segment of collagen (CollaPlug™, Ace Surgical) was inserted into the resected root void to support the lid and allow for blood infiltration. The lid was repositioned without incident and the perimeter piezo incision cuts grouted with a small amount of calcium sulfate. The soft tissue flap was coapted and allowed to re-perfuse with hydration for approximately 5 min. Closure was achieved with interrupted 6/0 polypropylene sutures in the interdental papilla and 6/0 Vicryl sutures in the vertical release incision sites. Post-operative medications and instructions followed the same protocol as in the previous case and a telephone call that night found the patient resting comfortably. Healing was uneventful and she presented 5 days later for suture removal. A CBCT scan exposed at the 2-week post-surgical visit revealed the calcium sulfate dissolved from the lid spaces and the lid stable and in the appropriate position (Fig. 8.4s,t) . The 12-month post-surgical CBCT scan revealed complete resolution of the surgical site and remodeling of the bony lid borders to render them indistinguishable from the surrounding cortical plate (Fig. 8.4v,w).

8.5 Case #4: Multiple Roots/ PRESS, Root-End Surgery

This 56-year-old female was referred for evaluation and treatment of tooth #30. The patient admits to a history of hyperlipidemia, for which she has a prescription (Ezetimibe™), but reports no other medications or drug allergies. Her past dental history disclosed multiple endodontically treated teeth in the quadrant with varied completion timelines. Tooth #30 has had a history of non-surgical retreatment 2 years previously, and the tooth is percussion, palpation, and biting sensitive. Radiographs reveal periapical lesions on the mesial roots of #30 and #31 and widening of the PDL space on the distal root of #30 (Fig. 8.6a). There is evidence of a screw post in the distal canal of #31, and the obturations in all roots appear to be incomplete. A CBCT scan reveals an atypical canal anatomy of the mesial root of #30 and evidence of a misdiagnosed distolingual canal in the distal root (Fig. 8.6b–d). There was also a large low-density lesion encompassing both apices of tooth #31. Based on the clinical and radiographic findings, it was proposed that tooth #31 be retreated non-surgically and a surgical revision be performed on #30. This decision was based upon the history of previous retreatment of #30. A second

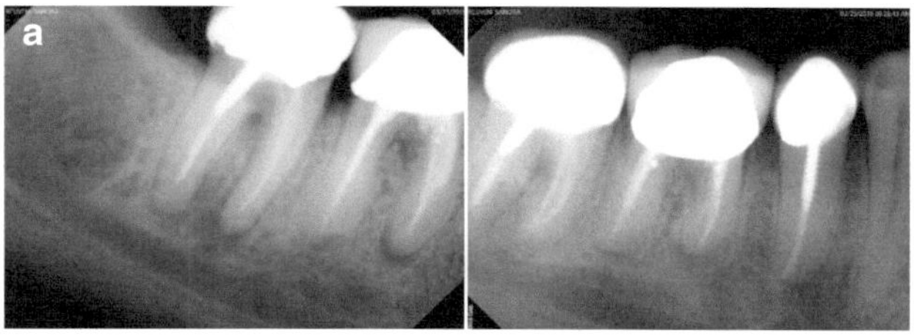

Fig. 8.6 (**a**) Pre-surgical radiographs of tooth #30; Root-end surgery planned for the mesial and distal roots. (**b**) Pre-surgical CBCT scan showing areas of low density on both molar apices and dissimilar apical contours of the mesial root of tooth #30. (**c**) Pre-surgical CBCT scan, axial (top) and sagittal (bottom) views with silicone bone/sinus filters. Note the thickness of the buccal cortical plate, areas of low density and asymmetry of the mesial root (yellow arrow) (**d**) Pre-surgical CBCT scan, mesial (top) and distal (bottom) roots with silicone bone/sinus filters. Note the asymmetry of the mesial root and the unfilled DL canal (yellow arrow) (**e**) CBCT Virtual Planning for height/depth of resection, as well as dissimilar angles for each root end. Average cortical plate thickness: 2.5 mm. (**f**) Tissue reflected and PRESS seated completely. Initial outline with the bone saw started at the mesial border of the bony lid (**g**) Outline complete (dotted line is the inferior border). PRESS is removed. (**h**) Bony incisions are completed with the straight scalpel tip through the cortical plate to the approximate planned resection depth (**i**) Luxation and delivery of the intact bony lid; stored in 0.9% (Normal) saline. (**j**) Resection completed on the distal root with the straight scalpel tip. (**k**) Harvest of the distal root apex intact. (**l**) Inspection of the resected distal root surface with the micromirror. (**m**) Inspection of the partial resection of the mesial root; the mesial longitudinal apical half remains intact. (**n**) Removal of the distal longitudinal apical half of the mesial root from the underside of the lid. (**o**) 1 mm mesial extension of the window to enable access to the remaining half of the mesial root apex. (**p**) Resection completed on the mesial root with the straight scalpel tip. (**q** Elevation and harvest of mesial longitudinal apical half of the root. (**r**) Inspection of both stained resected root surfaces; pictured is the distal revealing missed DL canal. (**s**) Inspection of both root-end preparations prior to root-end filling; pictured is the mesial showing the isthmus. (**t, u**) Inspection of the distal and mesial root end fillings (White MTA). (**v**) Repositioning the bony lid; CollaPlug in distal portion of the crypt. Note the gap at the mesial from the expansion of the osteotomy to access/harvest the remaining longitudinal segment of the mesial root. (**w**) Delivering $CaSO_4$ to the mesial gap with a graft syringe. (**x**) Final grouting of the remaining incision gaps with $CaSO_4$. (**y**) Immediate post-surgical radiographs. (**z**) Two-week Post-surgical CBCT scan showing the position of the lid and graft materials in the crypt. (**aa**) Two-week Post-surgical CBCT scan showing the position of the lid (silicone jaw rendering) and axial section with the same filter. Note the position of the bony lid and mesial gap filled with $CaSO_4$ (yellow arrow). (**bb**) Two-week Post-surgical CBCT scan, axial (top) and sagittal (bottom) views with silicone bone/sinus filters. Note the alignment of the bony lid with the buccal cortical plate and the density of the $CaSO_4$ (mesial) and Colla Plug (distal). (**cc**) Two-week Post-surgical CBCT scan, mesial (top) and distal (bottom) roots with silicone bone/sinus filters. Note the alignment of the bony lid with the buccal cortical plate and the density of the $CaSO_4$ (mesial) and Coll aPlug (distal). (**dd**) Two-month post-operative radiograph taken at the completion of #31 retreatment showing evidence of the lid borders remodeling. (**ee**) Twenty-four month post-surgical recall radiographs demonstrating remodeling and healing of the surgical site and resolution of the retreatment of tooth #31. (**ff**) Twenty-four month Post-surgical CBCT scan demonstrating remodeling and healing of the surgical sites as well as the retreatment of #31. (**gg**) Twenty-four month Post-surgical CBCT scan, axial (top) and sagittal (bottom) views with silicone bone/sinus filters. Note the complete incorporation of the bony lid with the buccal cortical plate and the density of the cancellous bone. (**hh**) Twenty-four month Post-surgical CBCT scan, mesial (top) and distal (bottom) roots with silicone bone/sinus filters. Note the complete incorporation of the bony lid with the buccal cortical plate and the density of the cancellous bone. (**ii**) Forty-eight month Post-surgical CBCT scan demonstrating remodeling and healing of the surgical sites. Tooth #31 was diagnosed with a vertical root fracture 2 months previously and was extracted. Note the density of the buccal cortical plate over the surgical sites (axial view). (**jj**) Forty-eight month Post-surgical CBCT scan, axial (top) and sagittal (bottom) views with silicone bone/sinus filters. Note the complete incorporation of the bony lid with the buccal cortical plate, thickness of the bone over the surgical sites, and the density of the cancellous bone. (**kk**) Forty-eight month Post-surgical CBCT scan, mesial (top) and distal (bottom) roots with silicone bone/sinus filters. Note the thickness of the buccal cortical plate and evidence of slightly thicker deposition as compared to the pre-surgical CBCT sections (**d**)

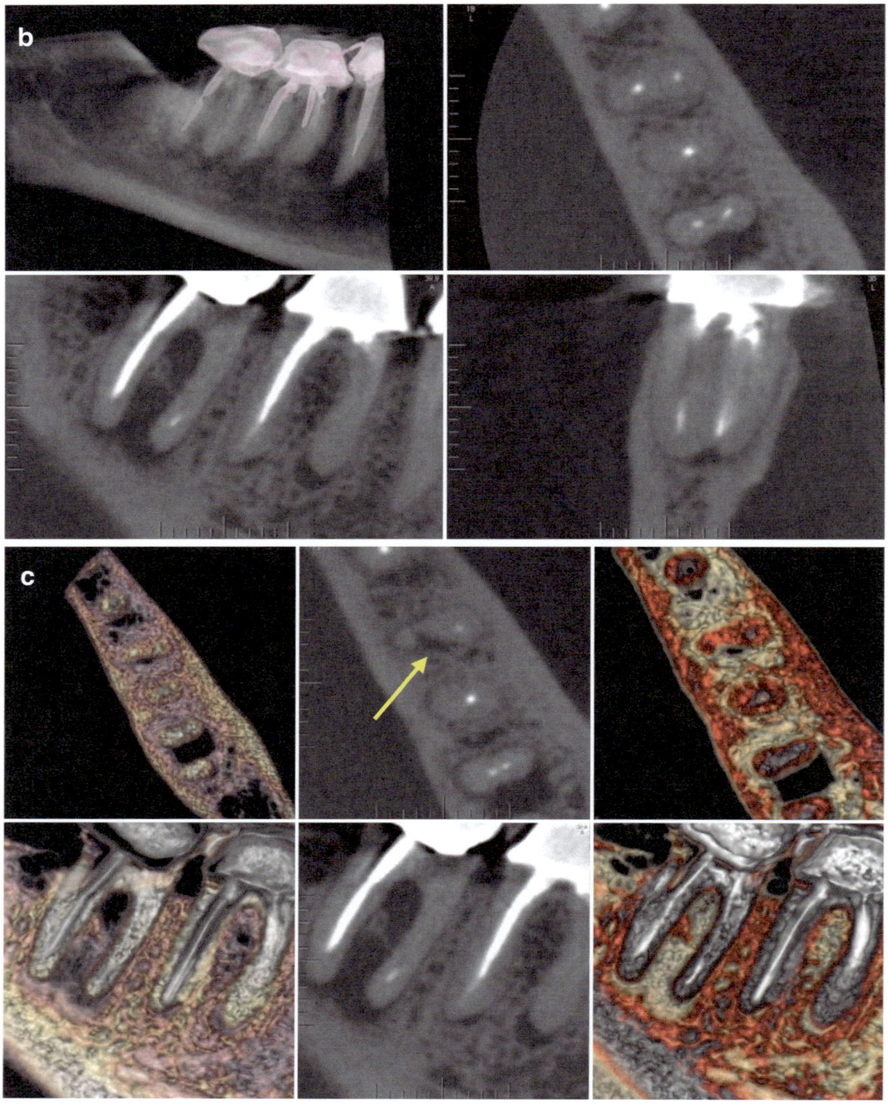

Fig. 8.6 (continued)

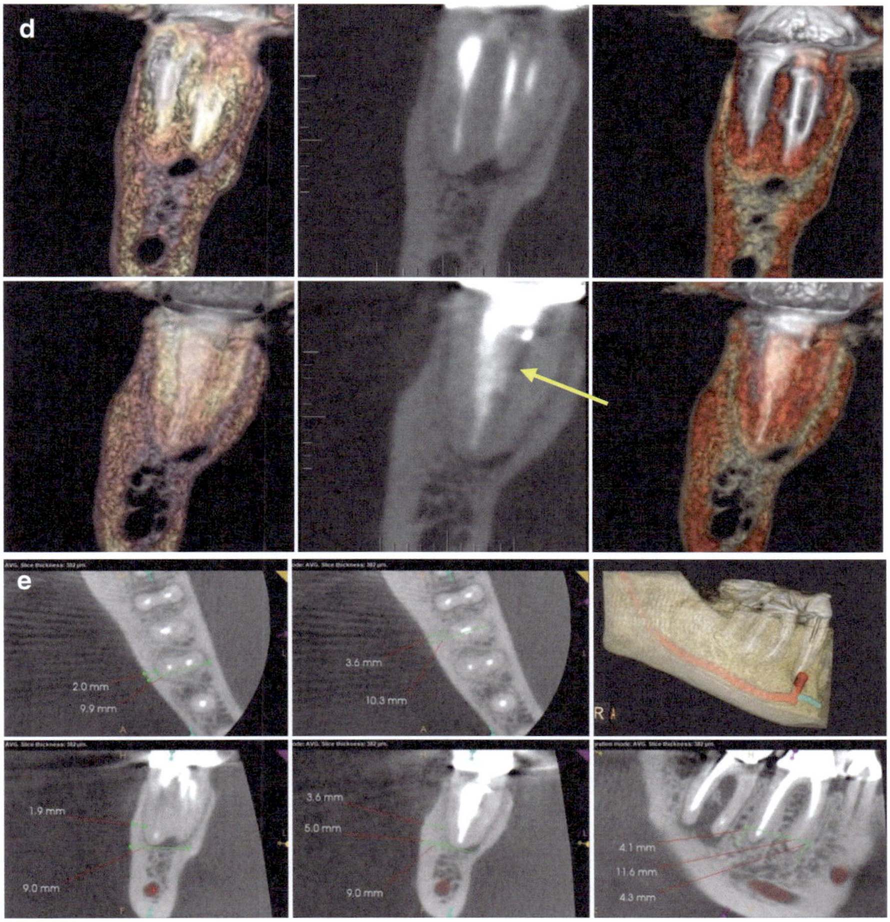

Fig. 8.6 (continued)

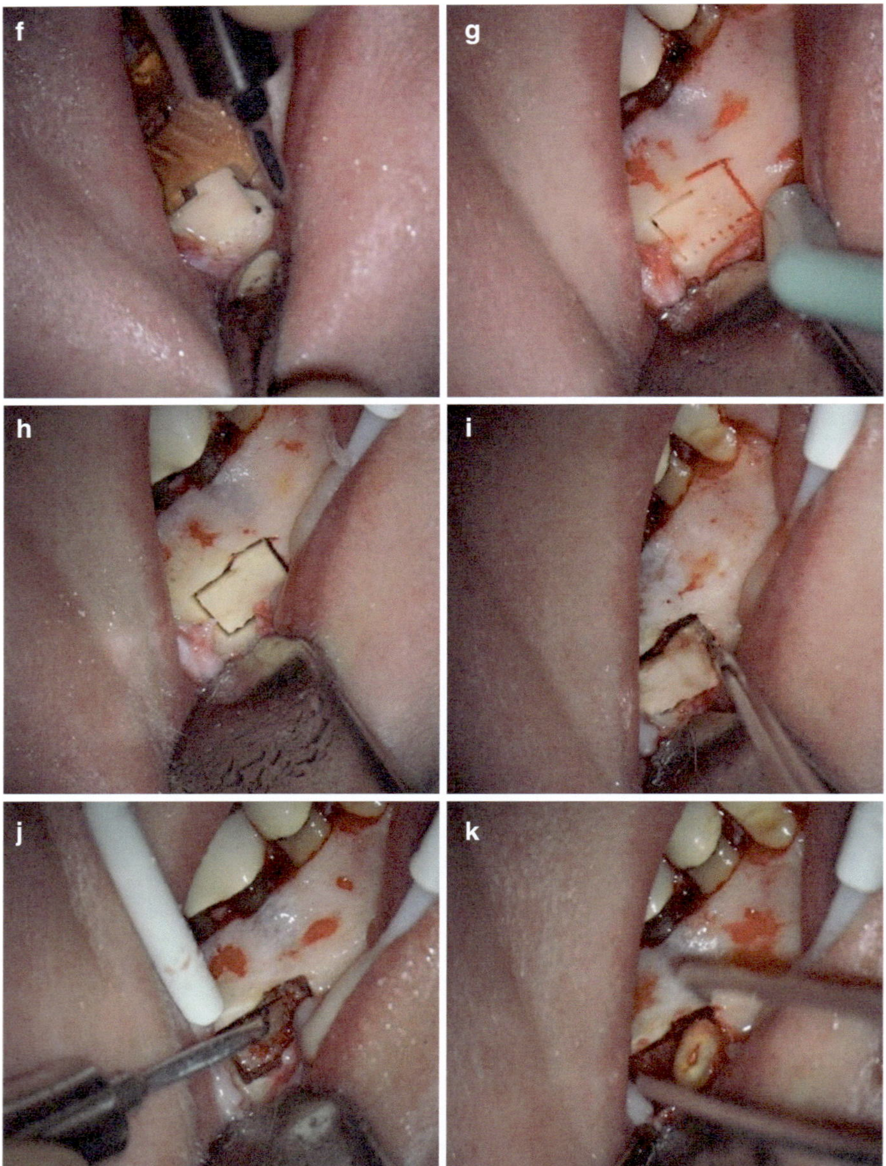

Fig. 8.6 (continued)

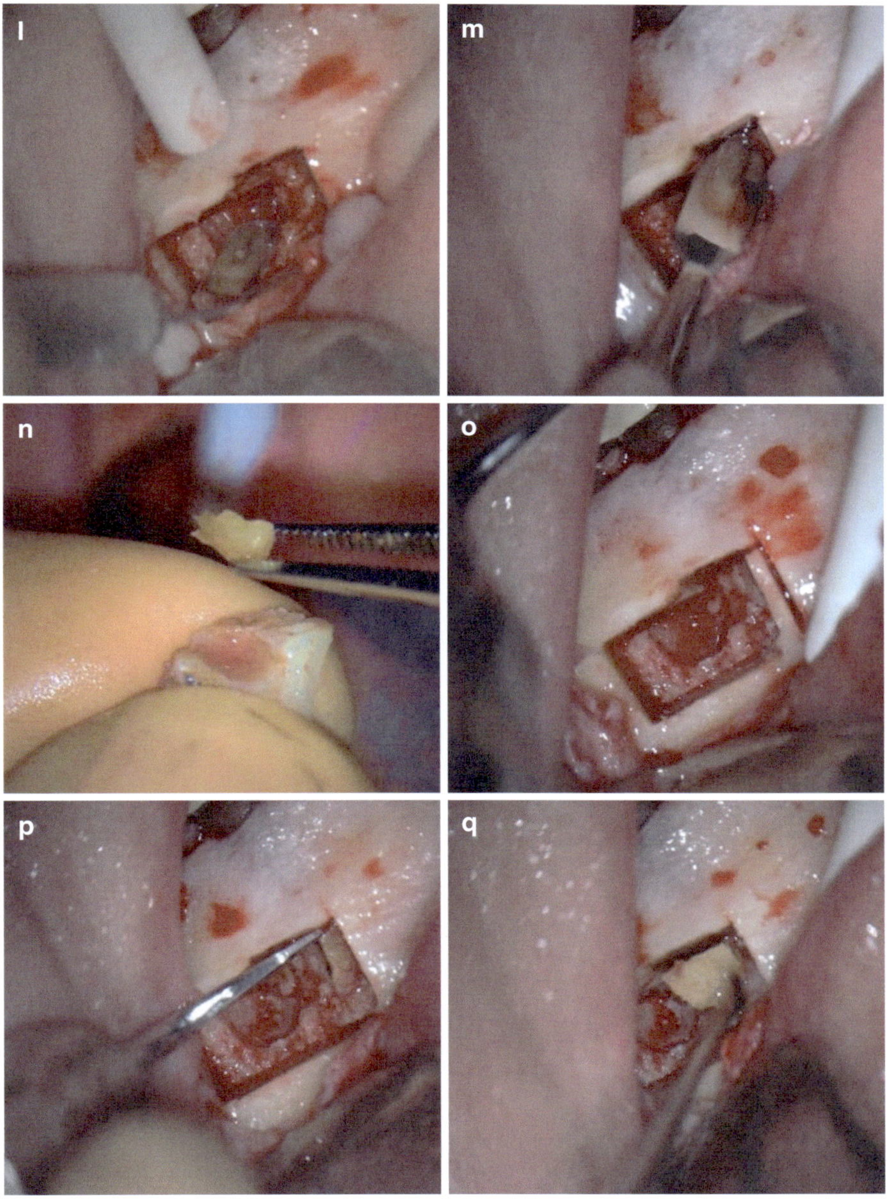

Fig. 8.6 (continued)

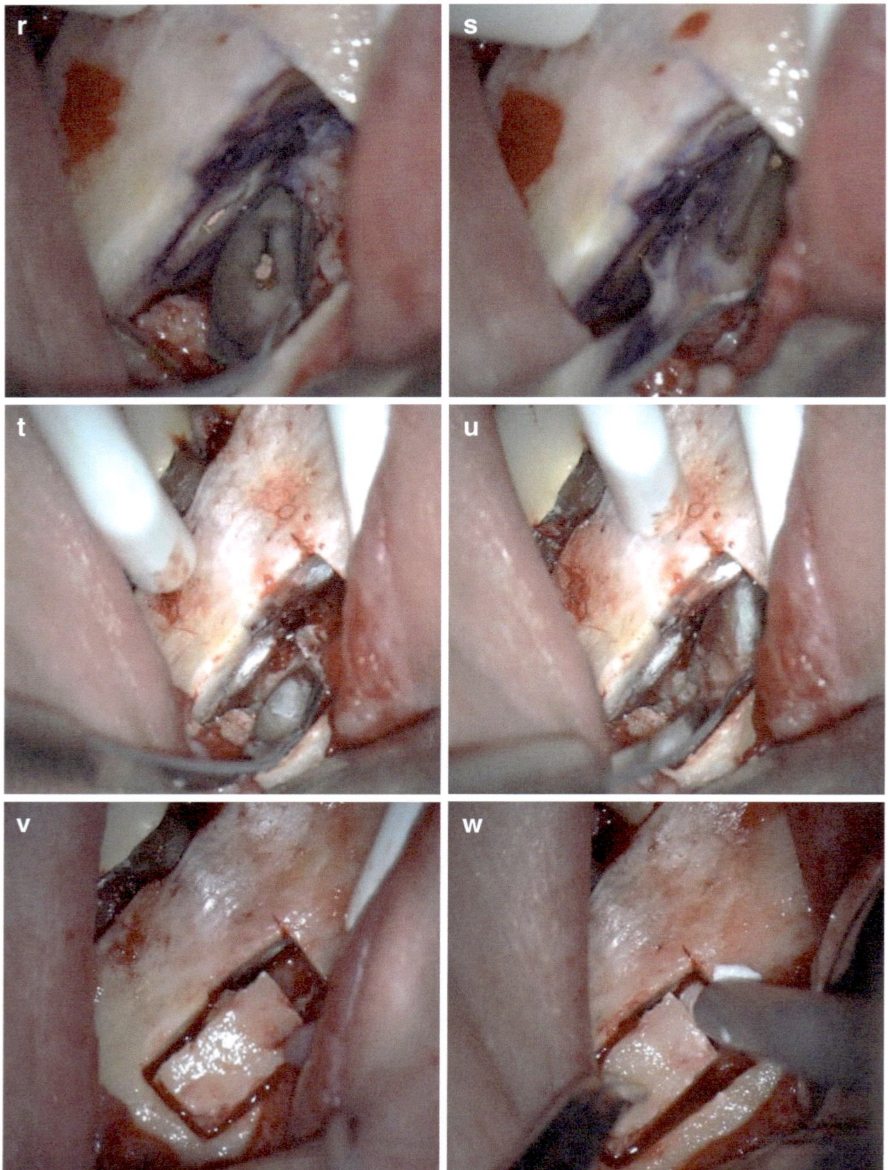

Fig. 8.6 (continued)

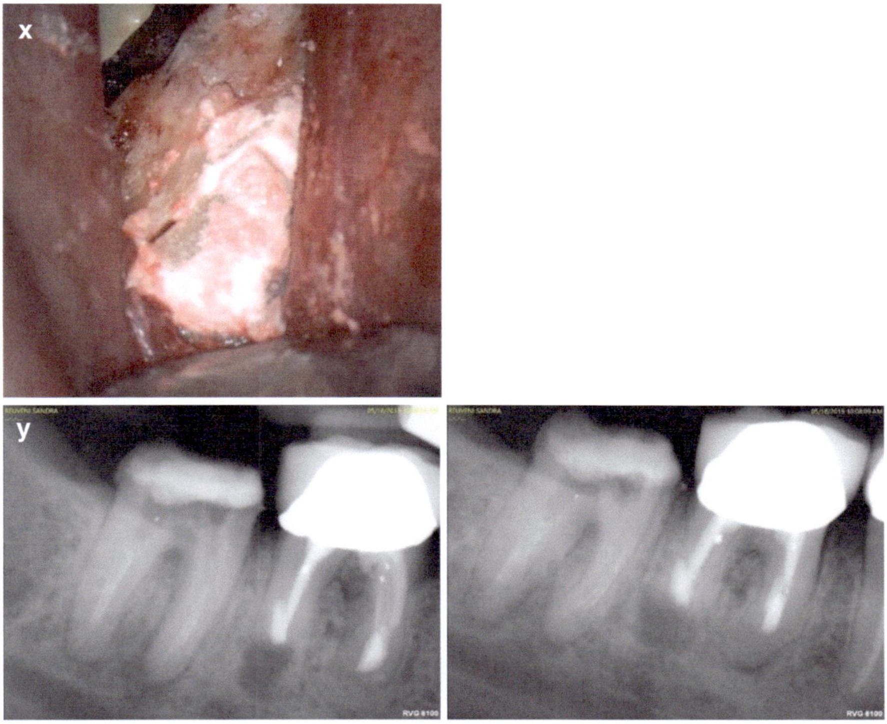

Fig. 8.6 (continued)

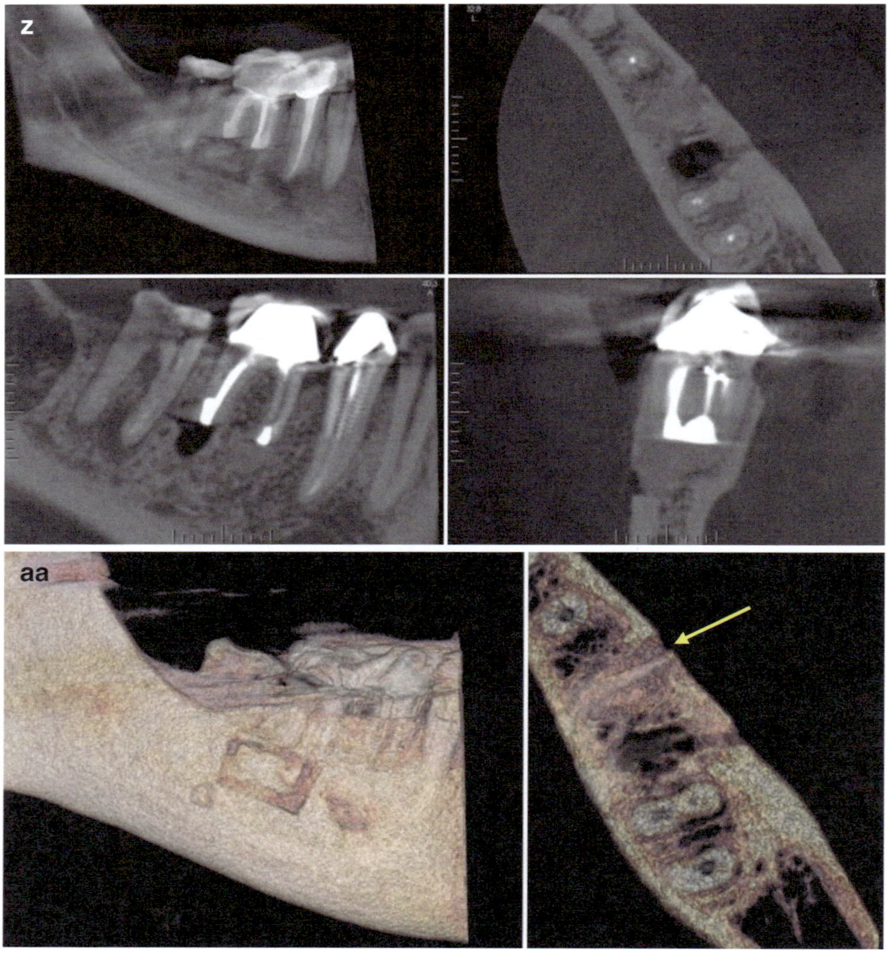

Fig. 8.6 (continued)

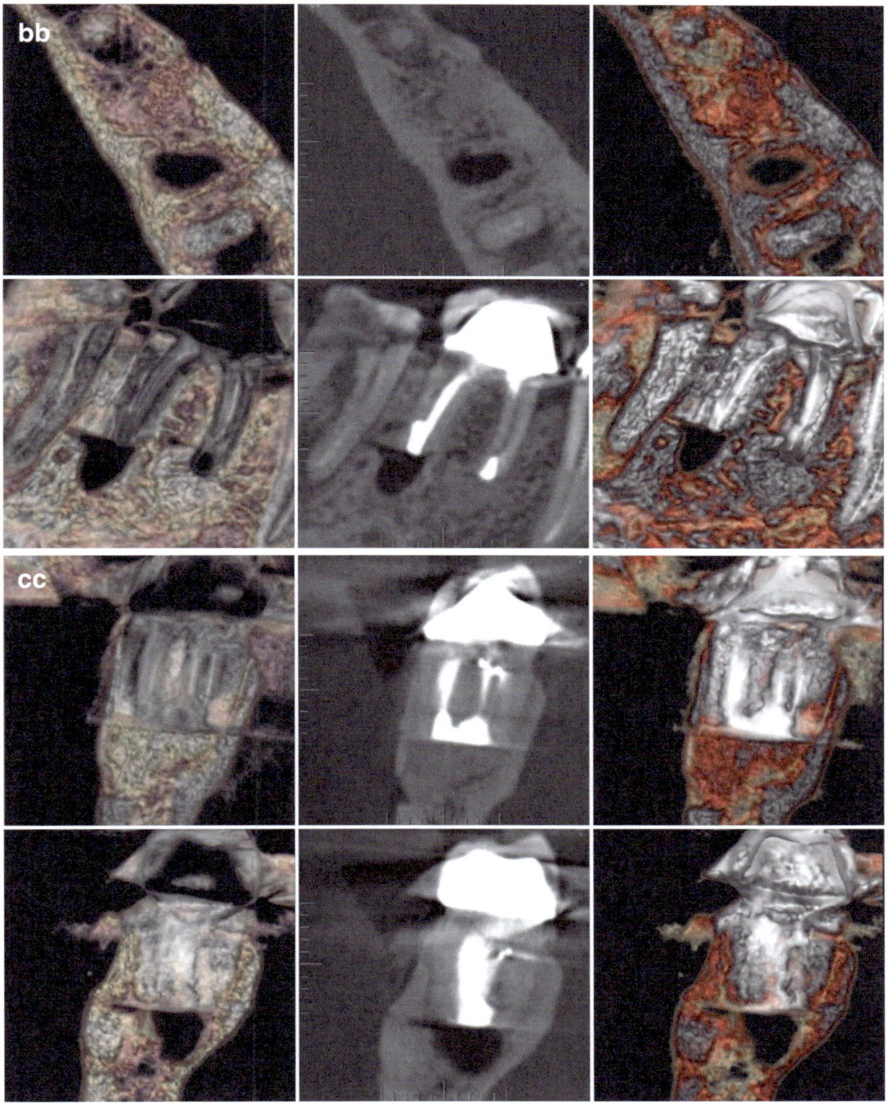

Fig. 8.6 (continued)

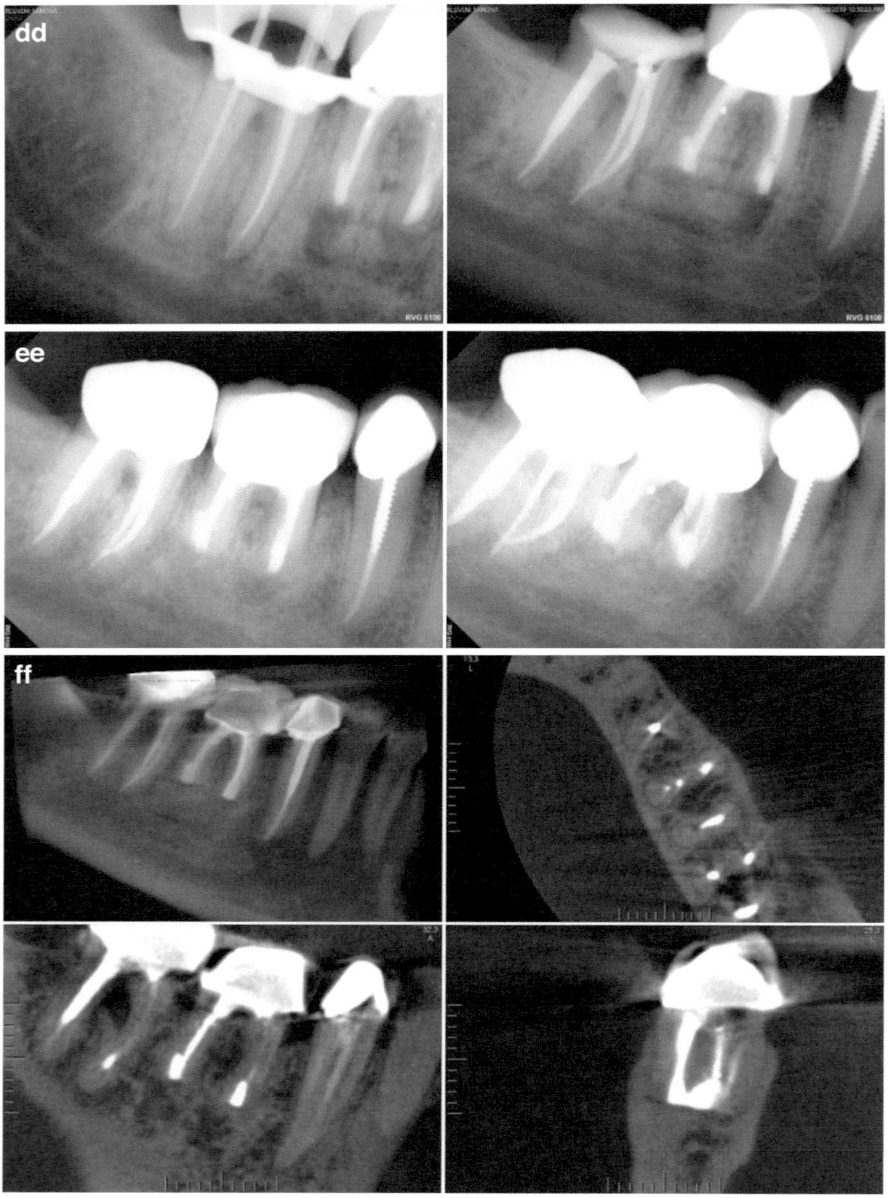

Fig. 8.6 (continued)

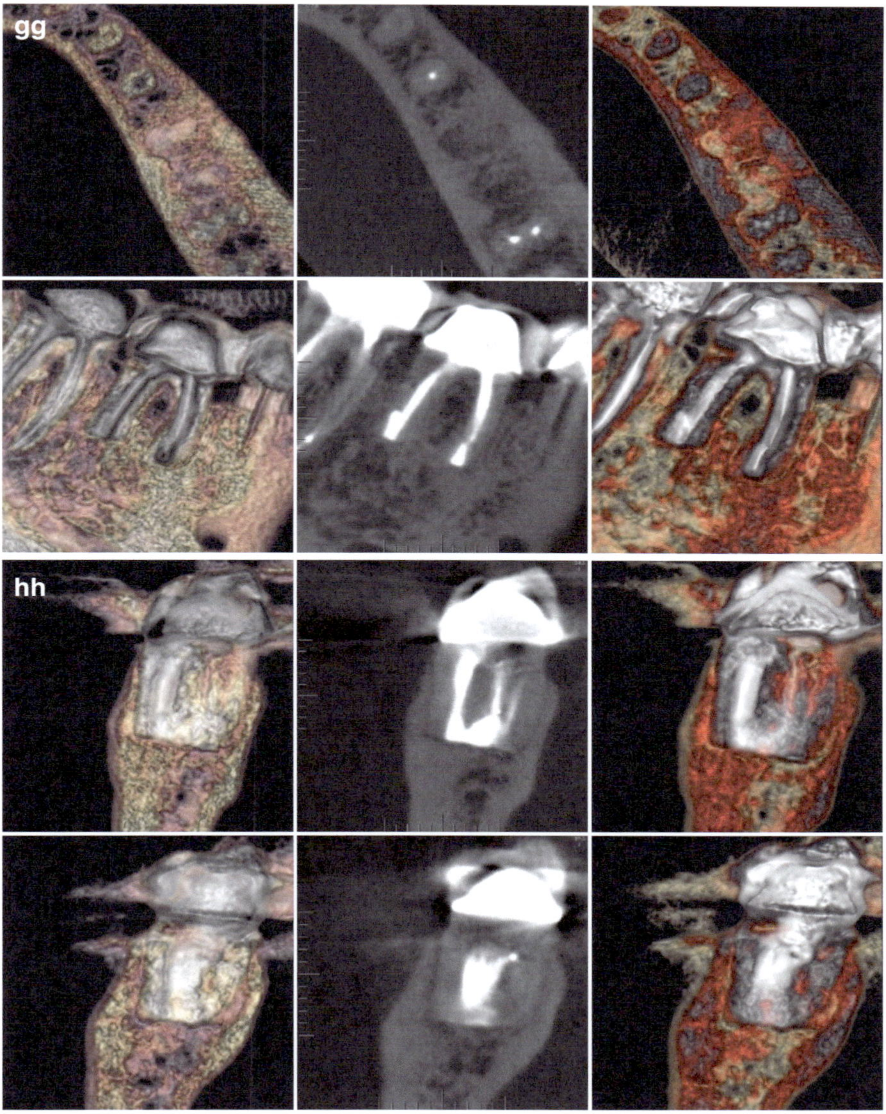

Fig. 8.6 (continued)

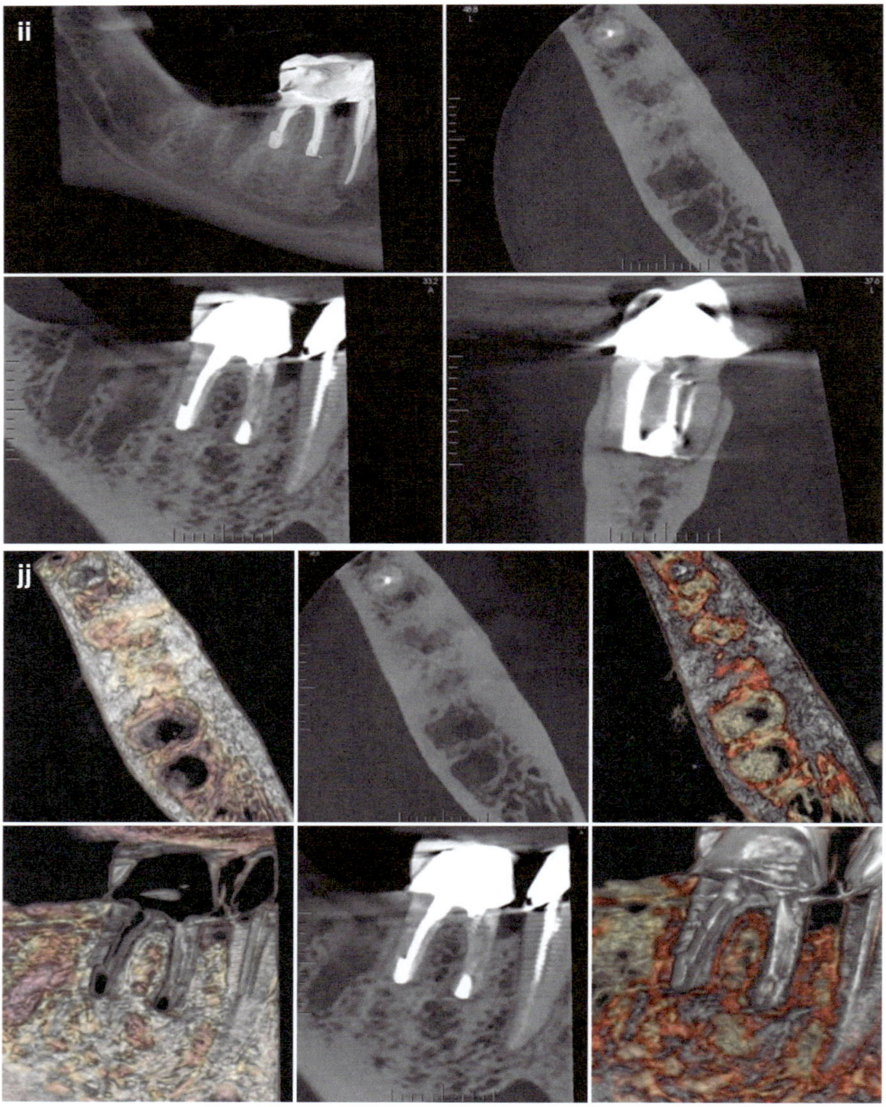

Fig. 8.6 (continued)

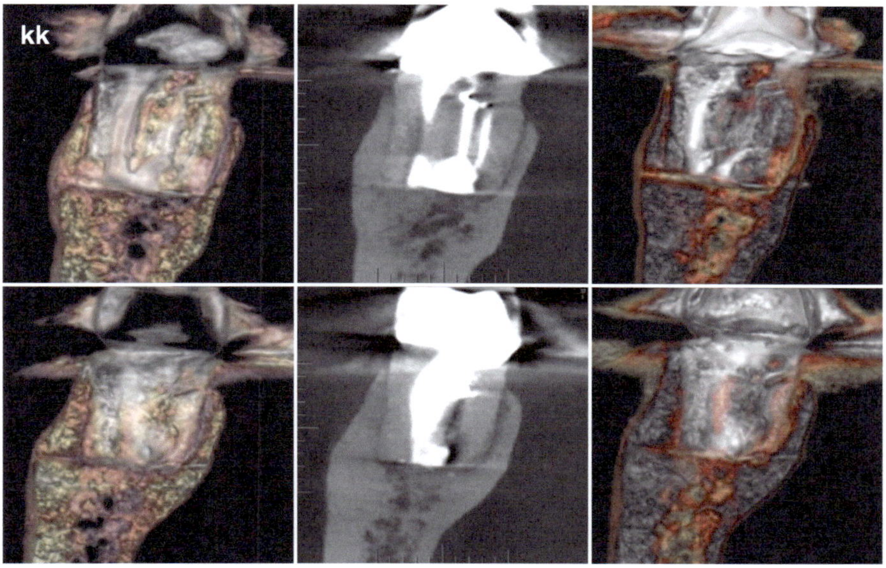

Fig. 8.6 (continued)

retreatment could possibly further weaken the root structure during discovery and harvesting, with a new access compromising a crown that appears to be well sealed and in proper function. The patient consented to the surgical intervention, desiring to preserve the existing crown and leave it undisturbed.

A full-arch CBCT scan of the mandible was exposed and a full-arch impression, with the same buccal extension protocol as the previous case, was taken of the same arch as well. The finished model was scanned with the iTero as in the previous case, and the final STL file was imported into the BSB software containing the mandibular arch DICOM (Fig. 8.7a–j).

The two files were merged as in the previous case and axes arranged to begin the planning manipulations. The sequential steps involved were identical with the previous case, with one notable exception: there are two separate guide pins at two different levels with two surgical window guides inserted to reflect the differing angles of resection. The Virtual Surgery™ plan with the appropriate measurements is illustrated in Fig. 8.6e. This contrasts with the initial case (Case #1) that essentially had confluent levels and angles of resection of the mesial and distal root apices. Once the levels and angles of resection were verified for each root, the guide outline was drawn and virtually rendered. The final design was again verified by adjusting the transparency of the virtual guide and viewing the apices through the surgical windows. The apices appeared centered in their respective windows, and the guide was finalized for production.

On the day of surgery, the guide adaptation was verified clinically prior to the commencement of the procedure. Notation was made of the difficulty in retraction and custom retractors were added to the surgical armamentarium. The informed

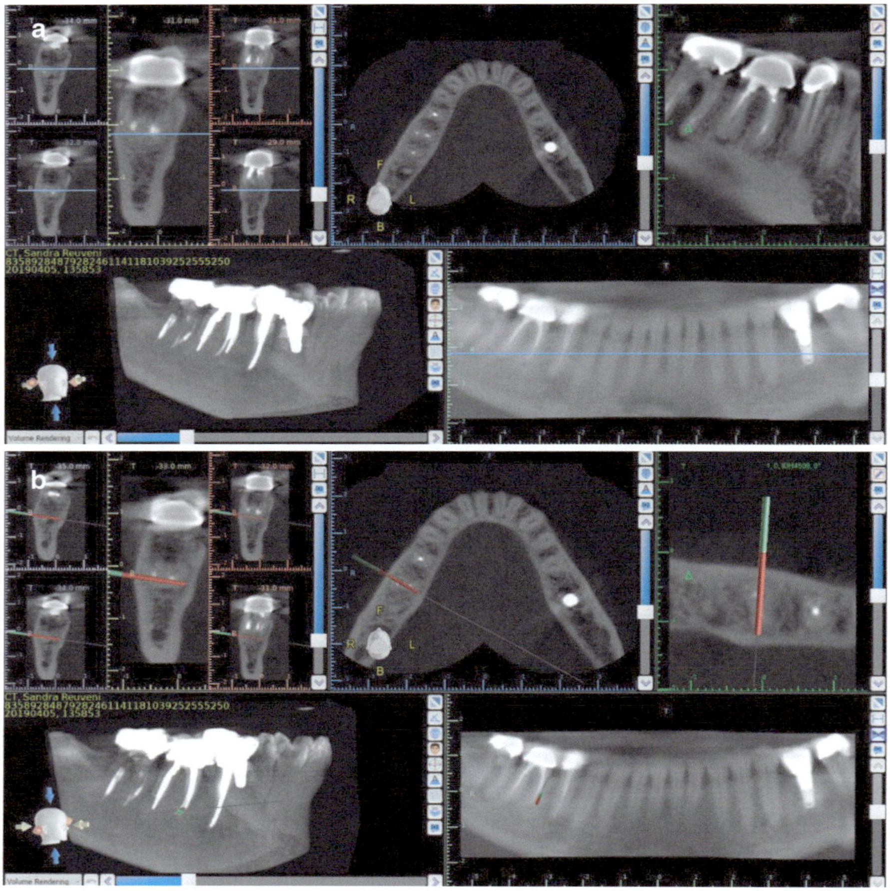

Fig. 8.7 (**a**) Importation of CBCT volume; Tangential 5 selected for planning. (**b**) STL file imported, merged, and hidden; custom guide pin positioned for mesial root resection. (**c**) Guide pins positioned for mesial and distal root resections with respect to height, depth, and angle. (**d**) Resection windows selected and positioned on the respective apices and angled to reflect the dissimilar angles of each root resection. A stent seating window is positioned over the crown to confirm correct in situ positioning. (**e**) STL image revealed (pink line) and proposed stent rendered. (**f**) Proposed stent radiographic overly with windows removed to confirm the relationship of the stent window levels with the respective apex. (**g**) Final virtual stent showing guide pin position preserved. (**h**) Final PRESS on model demonstrating complete seating of the stent. (This is also confirmed by the patient prior to scheduling the procedure.) (**i**) Final PRESS in transparent pink. (**j**) Detail of PRESS showing dissimilar resection angles and levels

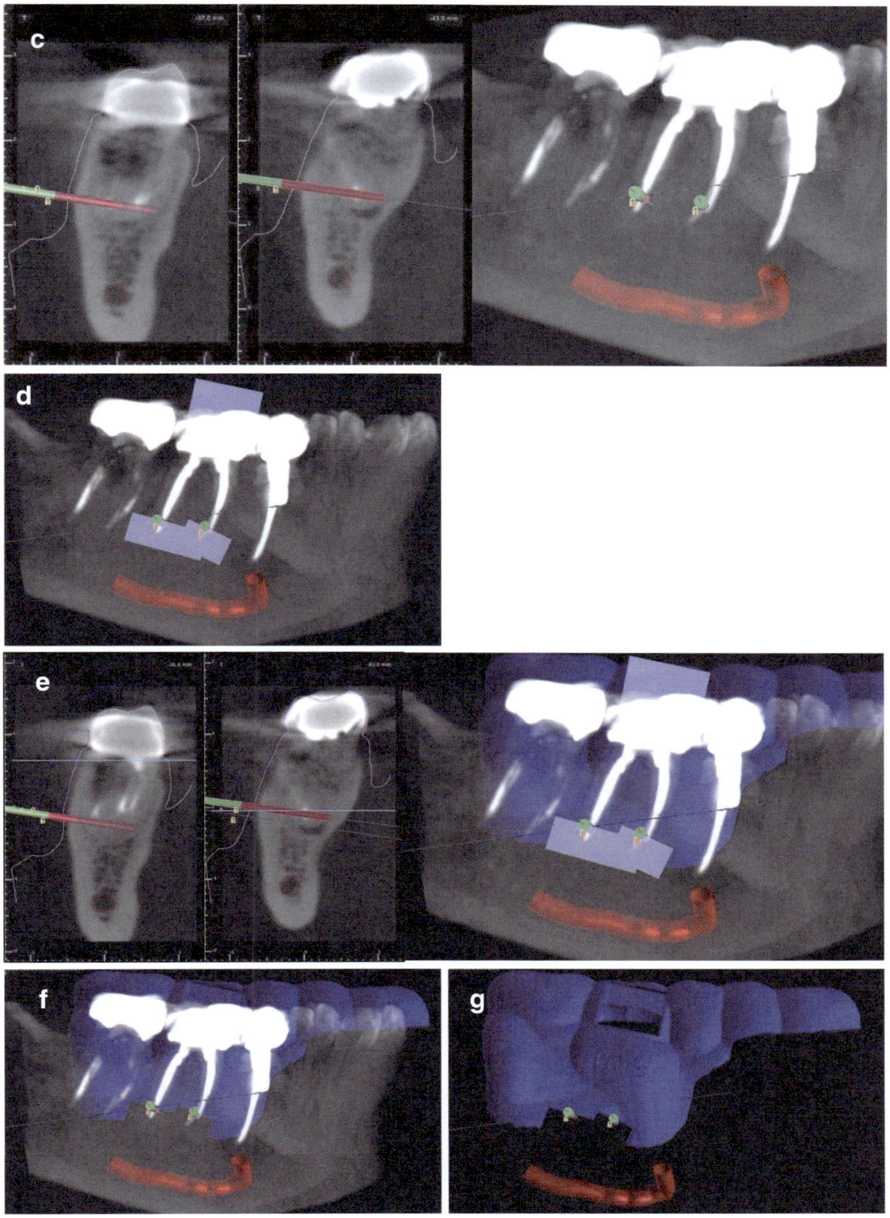

Fig. 8.7 (continued)

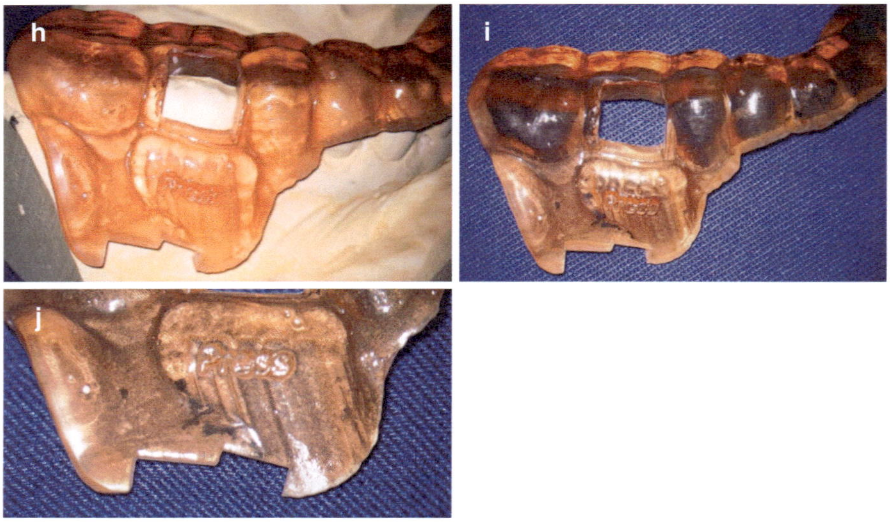

Fig. 8.7 (continued)

consent was reviewed, and the patient prepared according to the AEMC protocol. The patient was anesthetized with 1.75 cartridges of 0.5% bupivacaine (Marcaine™) with 1:2000,000 epinephrine, administered as an IAN block, with 0.25 cartridges of the same anesthetic infiltrated over the mental foramen. After a 10-min delay for onset signs, the buccal aspect of the cortical plate from the mesial of tooth #28 to the distal of tooth #31 was slowly infiltrated with 1.5 cartridges of lidocaine (Xylocaine™) 2%, with 1:50,000 epinephrine for control of site hemostasis. After an additional 5-min pause for anesthetic uptake and confirmation, the surgery commenced. All microsurgical procedures from incision to flap coaptation/suturing were performed under the SOM.

A full-sulcular incision was made from the mesial of tooth #28 to the mesial of tooth #31, with a vertical releasing incision at the mesial line angle of #28 (Fig. 8.6f-kk). A triangular flap was reflected and the mental nerve/foramen located, marked with methylene blue dye, and isolated via retraction. The stent was placed, full seating verified, and soft tissue retraction stabilized. The outlines of the windows were transferred onto the cortical plate with the BS-1 saw tip. But instead of scoring the bone, the tip was lightly pressed onto the bone and momentarily activated; this produced a series of dot impressions on the plate that replicated the boundary of the windows. Once all the dimensions were transferred, the stent was removed, retraction reestablished, and the site stabilized. The BS-5 piezo scalpel tip was used to lightly trace the trail of impressions on the plate, and, when all the margins of the lid were connected, the incisions were completed with copious irrigation. The mesial and distal incisions were angled to converge medially to create the keystone effect, but the stock angles of the piezo tips and soft tissue interferences (lip and corner of the mouth) constrained the execution of the correct angle in these vertical incisions, especially the mesial. When transition through the cortical plate into cancellous bone was realized circumferentially, the lid was carefully elevated as in the previous cases. It was examined for any incomplete or "green stick" fractures and placed into a sterile basin containing 0.9% sterile saline (normal) for hydration until replacement. The mesial and distal aspects of the lid were beveled, but the mesial wall of the lid contained the distal half of the mesial root. It had been resected at the selected level and angle, but the mesial incision was over-beveled and transected the root in the buccal-lingual dimension. An additional 1 mm of bone was removed at the mesial border of the lid, allowing access to the remaining portion of the root. The mesial root resection was completed without further difficulties with the BS-5 tip with copious irrigation and reduced power. The distal root apex, already partially resected from the lid incisions, was removed as well, and both apices examined at low and high powers for extent and completeness of resection. The soft tissue lesions from both root ends were harvested and sent to the Oral Pathology service for evaluation. The resected root ends were prepared using ultrasonic root-end preparation (USREP) tips (KiS 4D, 5D Dentsply Sirona) and the preparations examined with micromirrors for extent and centering. The preparations were filled with BC putty (Brasseler) applied with a MAPS triple angle tip. The excess material was removed from the cavosurface of the preparations, and a radiograph exposed to confirm placement and compaction of the root-end fillings (REF). A slight deviation was observed in the distal REF, but, given the difficulty in access and angulation secondary to the soft tissue influences, it was deemed acceptable. A small segment of collagen (CollaPlug™, Ace Surgical) was inserted into the resected root void at the distal for support and blood infiltration. The lid was removed from the sterile bath and replaced into the site with its former orientation, but the gap created by the additional bone resection at the mesial portion of the lid created concern for post-operative stabilization. A more stable base for that portion of the lid was fashioned by injecting calcium sulfate (Ace Surgical) into the gap and underlying crypt, employing a grafting syringe for delivery. The material set without disturbance and the excess carved back to the surface of the plate. The smaller incision gaps were sealed with additional amounts of calcium sulfate to surface seal and stabilize the lid. The soft tissue flap was coapted and allowed to re-perfuse with hydration for approximately 5 min. Closure was achieved with interrupted 6/0 polypropylene sutures in the interdental papilla and 6/0 Vicryl in the vertical release incision sites. Prescriptions for an antibiotic (amoxicillin 500 mg TID) and NSAIDs (ibuprofen 400 mg every 5–6 h) were supplied, as well as post-operative instructions for diet and hygiene. A telephone call that night found the patient resting comfortably, and she presented 5 days later for suture removal. Healing was uneventful, and the post-operative instructions were reinforced. A post-surgical small FOV scan revealed the lid in the correct orientation, with the calcium sulfate in the mesial root location and collagen void in the distal (Fig. 8.6z-cc). The REPs were well centered and spanned the isthmuses in the mesial and distal root ends. Retreatment of #31 was initiated 6 weeks post-surgery and completed 2 months post-surgery. Post-surgical recall at 24 and 48 months (Fig. 8.6ee-kk) reveals complete resolution of the surgical sites and remodeling of the bony lid borders. What is of particular interest is that the position of the lid buccal to the surgical sites appears to be thicker than the preoperative presentation; this is not unusual and has been observed in other bony lid cases as well.

Although the bony lid technique is not employed in every microsurgical procedure, it has proven invaluable in those instances where cortical plate thickness and posterior location of the surgical site pose operational challenges. The lid can be designed to include the selected root apex/apices and alleviate lesion harvesting without compromising the regeneration of the site. The size of the lesion and, associated with it's removal, the dimension of the osteotomy is an important prognostic factor when evaluating the potential outcome of a procedure. Investigators agree that small crypt proportions ≤ 10 mm in diameter present better outcomes [59–62], with one author reporting that the depth of the crypt was an important factor in the healing as well [63]. The repositioning of the lid post-surgically essentially diminishes the crypt volume to the space occupied by any lesion and the void of the resected root end. The replacement also constitutes an autograft, with all the benefits of viable cells and growth factors. Autogenous grafts are still considered the standard for osseous defect reconstruction because they provide the three basic factors for bone remodeling: osteoinductive molecules, a proper scaffold, and osteogenic cells [64, 65]. However, contrary to particulate autogenous grafts, these lids are subject to some delay in their reintroduction into the recipient site, so their extra-oral handling and storage requires careful consideration. The variables of most importance are time, temperature, and storage media. An ex vivo study [66] evaluated these parameters, employing freshly harvested cortical blocks that were subjected to different test combinations, then fixed, sectioned, and examined for the presence of osteoblasts. Aside from autologous blood, the most effective storage media was normal saline at room temperature for less than 2 h, an observation in agreement with previous studies [67, 68]. Using the same parameters, Rocha [69] observed the viability of osteocytes in replanted calvarium bone segments. The segments were harvested with trephines under copious irrigation and either air-dried for 30 min or stored in saline or platelet-poor plasma (PPP) for the same amount of time prior to replantation. After 28 days the segments were explanted and prepared for histologic assessment. Those segments stored in ambient air for 30 min had significantly greater numbers of empty lacunae and decreased bone graft areas when compared to the saline or PPP groups. The absence of cells in the graft will most likely not interfere with osteoconduction [70], but it negatively influences osteoinduction and increases bone resorption [70, 71] beyond the normal remodeling.

These cell populations can also be impacted by the device employed for creating the cortical incisions. Mouraret observed that the cell density was higher at the piezo cut bone edge when compared to the bur cut edges, and a greater percentage of viable osteocytes were attached to the lacunae in the piezo cut graft versus the bur [72]. Significant structural differences were noted by Maurer, comparing osteotomies created with a bone bur (Lindemann), microsaw, or piezo tip. The cancellous bone surfaces created by the rotating or oscillating instruments were either partially or completely destroyed, with bone debris occluding the cancellous spaces. By contrast, the surfaces created by the piezo tip preserved the delicate cancellous features with no debris accumulation [44]. This accumulated debris may present a mechanical obstacle for centrifugal blood supply of the graft [73], inhibiting perfusion and potential cell viability.

The frequency of the vibrations and the micromovements of the tips create a cavitation effect [74], essentially aerosolizing the sterile irrigating solution. The result is a nearly bloodless surgical field [36, 38, 75] with unparalleled visibility [56, 76–78], permitting accurate and precise incisions in the site [79, 80]. Care must be exercised with the application and force of the selected tip on the bone or surface being resected. We are keenly aware in endodontics of the damaging effects of prolonged ultrasonic applications and the generation of damaging thermal changes in the bone [81]. Although the use of appropriate pressure and constant movement minimize the risk of overheating, in-depth or prolonged cutting sequences and regular interruptions of the bone incision are prudent to avoid overheating [82]. An adjunct benefit is realized when performing root-end resections or refinements with the scalpel tip. The thin silhouette of the tip offers an unobstructed view of the level and angle throughout the process, enhancing the precision and control within the crypt. This is especially imperative in locations where sensitive structures are coincident in the site; the surgeon can approach them with a degree of confidence due to the selective cutting properties of the instrument and unobtrusive nature of the handpiece.

The use of a stent for guided endodontic microsurgery with a piezoelectric delivery system was first presented in 2017 by Strbac [83], but failed to gain popularity for several reasons. The planning software (coDiagnostiX, Dental Wings, Montreal, Quebec, CA) was cumbersome to use and poorly adaptable to microsurgical orientations. Stent fabrication requires multiple scans for different file types (STL, DICOM) and either in-house fabrication or access to an outside dental lab. Training in the surgical technique is not universally available, and the basics of the computer software skills are available online but focused on endosseous implant applications. These drawbacks are also inherent with targeted endodontic microsurgery (TEMS) where stents are fabricated to guide hollow trephines of various dimensions to the selected root-end sites [84]. This technique will also allow for harvesting of a bone "plug" but can suffer the same complications of instrument misapplication, i.e., thermal, or mechanical damage to the bone. In addition, the trephined portal may be inadequate for root-end manipulations and require enlargement [85] or the crescent-shaped resection profile of the root end created by the trephine needs to be leveled with a bur [86]. Finally, the TEMS guide must remain in place and stable throughout the entire surgical procedure to ensure the accuracy of the access and resection. In certain scenarios that may present a significant challenge regarding retraction and introduction of the trephine. By contrast, once the lid outline(s) is transferred to the cortical surface, the stent is removed, and the surgical access reverts to the demands of conventional surgical isolation and retraction.

One of the universal disadvantages of piezosurgery cited is the slow cutting rate [34, 36, 55, 87, 88] although this tends to decrease with operator experience [36]. This is especially true in cases presenting with thick cortical plates, where the penetration pressures should be light with copious irrigation, and in concert with occasional pauses, to ensure against thermal damage. The benefit in those cases is the retention of the autologous bone for regeneration and site protection. Coupled with a precision endodontic surgical stent (PRESS), only the planned dimension of bone is discreetly removed, eliminating indiscriminate enlargement. A corollary disadvantage that has been cited is the damage to adjacent teeth because of the lid dimensions [89]. This may be true if the bony lid is attempted freehand, relying on transfer of measurements from the scan or radiograph [90]. Parallax errors and disorientation of the landmarks in situ could have the potential to bias the incisions in the incorrect location. However, in the planning of a PRESS all the variables and precautions are realized and accounted for, with appropriate adjustments to the dimensions of the lid. If the preliminary impression for the STL is captured correctly, with the proper stretching/thinning of the alveolar mucosa, the final stent will be virtually "bone borne," thereby eliminating any parallax error during the outlining stage. One final advantage of the piezosurgical technique is the ability to modify the angle or level of the root-end resection intra-operatively to address a dentinal defect, fracture, or other unforeseen anomaly without compromising the integrity of the remaining window. With other guided techniques, the surgeon is resigned to a surgical high-speed handpiece for the revision, with all its associated drawbacks of visibility and length control.

In challenging clinical scenarios, especially posterior surgical sites with thick cortical plates, the use of 3D precision is planned, and printed guides simplify site location and definition. Coupled with piezosurgical instruments for acquisition and root-end revision, the bony lid technique allows for unhindered operational visibility without sacrificing post-operative protection and regeneration. The selective nature of the instrument for hard tissues instills a level of confidence in those instances where sensitive structures border the site, and the skill set for proficiency is easily acquired. The outcomes observed in the private practice setting are increased patient comfort post-operatively, accelerated regeneration timetables, and increase in the confidence level of the surgeon.

References

1. Kim S, Kratchman S. Modern endodontic surgery concepts and practice: a review. J Endod. 2006;32(7):601–23.
2. Setzer FC, et al. Outcome of endodontic surgery: a meta-analysis of the literature–Part 2: comparison of endodontic microsurgical techniques with and without the use of higher magnification. J Endod. 2012;38(1):1–10.
3. Setzer FC, et al. Outcome of endodontic surgery: a meta-analysis of the literature–part 1: comparison of traditional root-end surgery and endodontic microsurgery. J Endod. 2010;36(11):1757–65.
4. Farman AG, Scarfe WC. 3 D X-ray: an update. Inside Dentistry. 2007;3(6):70–4.
5. Durack C, Patel S. The use of cone beam computed tomography in the management of dens invaginatus affecting a strategic tooth in a patient affected by hypodontia: a case report. Int Endod J. 2011;44(5):474–83.
6. Vizzotto MB, et al. CBCT for the assessment of second mesiobuccal (MB2) canals in maxillary molar teeth: effect of voxel size and presence of root filling. Int Endod J. 2013;46(9):870–6.

7. Venskutonis T, et al. The importance of cone-beam computed tomography in the management of endodontic problems: a review of the literature. J Endod. 2014;40(12):1895–901.
8. Tang L, et al. Detection of vertical root fracture using cone beam computed tomography: report of two cases. Dent Traumatol. 2011;27(6):484–8.
9. Schryvers A, et al. Endodontic management of a maxillary first molar with two palatal roots: a case report. Aust Endod J. 2019;45(3):420–5.
10. Bornstein MM, et al. Comparison of periapical radiography and limited cone-beam computed tomography in mandibular molars for analysis of anatomical landmarks before apical surgery. J Endod. 2011;37(2):151–7.
11. Braut V, et al. Thickness of the anterior maxillary facial bone wall-a retrospective radiographic study using cone beam computed tomography. Int J Periodontics Restorative Dent. 2011;31(2):125–31.
12. Zahedi S, Mostafavi M, Lotfirikan N. Anatomic study of mandibular posterior teeth using cone-beam computed tomography for endodontic surgery. J Endod. 2018;44(5):738–43.
13. Lavasani SA, et al. Cone-beam computed tomography: anatomic analysis of maxillary posterior teeth-impact on endodontic microsurgery. J Endod. 2016;42(6):890–5.
14. Yeung AWK, et al. Frequency, location, and association with dental pathology of mucous retention cysts in the maxillary sinus. A radiographic study using cone beam computed tomography (CBCT). Clin Oral Investig. 2018;22(3):1175–83.
15. Suter VG, et al. Radiographic volume analysis as a novel tool to determine nasopalatine duct cyst dimensions and its association with presenting symptoms and postoperative complications. Clin Oral Investig. 2015;19(7):1611–8.
16. Schneider AC, et al. Characteristics and dimensions of the sinus membrane in patients referred for single-implant treatment in the posterior maxilla: a cone beam computed tomographic analysis. Int J Oral Maxillofac Implants. 2013;28(2):587–96.
17. Bornstein MM, et al. Characteristics and dimensions of the Schneiderian membrane and apical bone in maxillary molars referred for apical surgery: a comparative radiographic analysis using limited cone beam computed tomography. J Endod. 2012;38(1):51–7.
18. Ducommun J, et al. Distances of root apices to adjacent anatomical structures in the anterior maxilla: an analysis using cone beam computed tomography. Clin Oral Investig. 2019;23(5):2253–63.
19. von Arx T, et al. Perforation of the maxillary sinus floor during apical surgery of maxillary molars: a retrospective analysis using cone beam computed tomography. Aust Endod J. 2020;46(2):176–83.
20. von Arx T, et al. Radiographic study of the mandibular retromolar canal: an anatomic structure with clinical importance. J Endod. 2011;37(12):1630–5.
21. Ugur Aydin Z, Goller Bulut D. Relationship between the anatomic structures and mandibular posterior teeth for endodontic surgery in a Turkish population: a cone-beam computed tomographic analysis. Clin Oral Investig. 2019;23(9):3637–44.
22. Koivisto T, et al. Mandibular Canal location: cone-beam computed tomography examination. J Endod. 2016;42(7):1018–21.
23. Katakami K, et al. Characteristics of accessory mental foramina observed on limited cone-beam computed tomography images. J Endod. 2008;34(12):1441–5.
24. Kalender A, et al. Cone-beam computed tomography analysis of the vestibular surgical pathway to the palatine root of the maxillary first molar. Eur J Dent. 2013;7(1):35–40.
25. Danesh-Sani SA, et al. Radiographic evaluation of maxillary sinus Lateral Wall and posterior superior alveolar artery anatomy: a cone-beam computed tomographic study. Clin Implant Dent Relat Res. 2017;19(1):151–60.
26. Panjnoush M, Rabiee ZS, Kheirandish Y. Assessment of location and anatomical characteristics of mental foramen, anterior loop and mandibular Incisive Canal using cone beam computed tomography. J Dent (Tehran). 2016;13(2):126–32.
27. Creasy JE, Mines P, Sweet M. Surgical trends among endodontists: the results of a web-based survey. J Endod. 2009;35(1):30–4.
28. Khoury F, Hensher R. The bony lid approach for the apical root resection of lower molars. Int J Oral Maxillofac Surg. 1987;16(2):166–70.

29. Lasaridis N, Zouloumis L, Antoniadis K. Bony lid approach for apicoectomy of mandibular molars. Aust Dent J. 1991;36(5):366–8.
30. Khoury F. The bony lid approach in pre-implant and implant surgery: a prospective study. Eur J Oral Implantol. 2013;6(4):375–84.
31. Lindorf HH. Bone flap closure following opening of the maxillary antrum. Dtsch Zahnarztl Z. 1974;29(Jul):587–90.
32. Lindorf HH. Animal studies on osteoplastic maxillary sinus surgery (bone lid method). Dtsch Z Mund Kiefer Gesichtschir. 1983;7:378–83.
33. Khoury F. Surgical procedures and long-term results of preimplantation surgery. Quintessence Dent Implantol. 1995;2:225–35.
34. Eggers G, et al. Piezosurgery: an ultrasound device for cutting bone and its use and limitations in maxillofacial surgery. Br J Oral Maxillofac Surg. 2004;42(5):451–3.
35. Gonzalez-Garcia A, et al. Ultrasonic osteotomy in oral surgery and implantology. Oral Surg Oral Med Oral Pathol Oral Radiol Endod. 2009;108(3):360–7.
36. Beziat JL, et al. Ultrasonic osteotomy as a new technique in craniomaxillofacial surgery. Int J Oral Maxillofac Surg. 2007;36(6):493–500.
37. Gleizal A, et al. Piezoelectric osteotomy: a new technique for bone surgery-advantages in craniofacial surgery. Childs Nerv Syst. 2007;23(5):509–13.
38. Degerliyurt K, et al. Bone lid technique with piezosurgery to preserve inferior alveolar nerve. Oral Surg Oral Med Oral Pathol Oral Radiol Endod. 2009;108(6):e1–5.
39. Magrin GL, et al. Piezosurgery in bone augmentation procedures previous to dental implant surgery: a review of the literature. Open Dent J. 2015;9:426–30.
40. Schaeren S, et al. Assessment of nerve damage using a novel ultrasonic device for bone cutting. J Oral Maxillofac Surg. 2008;66(3):593–6.
41. Wallace SS, et al. Schneiderian membrane perforation rate during sinus elevation using piezosurgery: clinical results of 100 consecutive cases. Int J Periodontics Restorative Dent. 2007;27(5):413–9.
42. Gomez G, et al. Effects of piezoelectric units on pacemaker function: an in vitro study. J Endod. 2013;39(10):1296–9.
43. Schlee M, et al. Piezosurgery: basics and possibilities. Implant Dent. 2006;15(4):334–40.
44. Maurer P, et al. Micromorphometrical analysis of conventional osteotomy techniques and ultrasonic osteotomy at the rabbit skull. Clin Oral Implants Res. 2008;19(6):570–5.
45. Patel S, et al. Cone beam computed tomography in endodontics–a review. Int Endod J. 2015;48(1):3–15.
46. Mayo CV Jr, et al. Accuracy of Presurgical limited field of view cone-beam computed tomography in predicting intraoperative buccal cortical bone. J Endod. 2020;46(2):169–177 e1.
47. Low KM, et al. Comparison of periapical radiography and limited cone-beam tomography in posterior maxillary teeth referred for apical surgery. J Endod. 2008;34(5):557–62.
48. Wang X, et al. Relationship between the mental foramen, Mandibular Canal, and the surgical access line of the mandibular posterior teeth: a cone-beam computed tomographic analysis. J Endod. 2017;43(8):1262–6.
49. Krennmair S, et al. Risk factor analysis affecting sinus membrane perforation during lateral window maxillary sinus elevation surgery. Int J Oral Maxillofac Implants. 2020;35(4):789–98.
50. Sivolella S, et al. The bone lid technique in oral surgery: a case series study. Int J Oral Maxillofac Surg. 2017;46(11):1490–6.
51. Skoglund A, Persson G. A follow-up study of apicoectomized teeth with total loss of the buccal bone plate. Oral Surg Oral Med Oral Pathol. 1985;59(1):78–81.
52. Horton JE, Tarpley TM Jr, Wood LD. The healing of surgical defects in alveolar bone produced with ultrasonic instrumentation, chisel, and rotary bur. Oral Surg Oral Med Oral Pathol. 1975;39(4):536–46.
53. Horton JE, Tarpley TM Jr, Jacoway JR. Clinical applications of ultrasonic instrumentation in the surgical removal of bone. Oral Surg Oral Med Oral Pathol. 1981;51(3):236–42.
54. Stubinger S, et al. Intraoral piezosurgery: preliminary results of a new technique. J Oral Maxillofac Surg. 2005;63(9):1283–7.

55. Kotrikova B, et al. Piezosurgery–a new safe technique in cranial osteoplasty? Int J Oral Maxillofac Surg. 2006;35(5):461–5.
56. Happe A. Use of a piezoelectric surgical device to harvest bone grafts from the mandibular ramus: report of 40 cases. Int J Periodontics Restorative Dent. 2007;27(3):241–9.
57. Sakkas N, et al. Transposition of the mental nerve by piezosurgery followed by postoperative neurosensory control: a case report. Br J Oral Maxillofac Surg. 2008;46(4):270–1.
58. Sivolella S, et al. Retrieval of blade implants with piezosurgery: two clinical cases. Minerva Stomatol. 2007;56(1–2):53–61.
59. Wang N, et al. Treatment outcome in endodontics-the Toronto study. Phases I and II: apical surgery. J Endod. 2004;30(11):751–61.
60. Barone C, et al. Treatment outcome in endodontics: the Toronto study–phases 3, 4, and 5: apical surgery. J Endod. 2010;36(1):28–35.
61. von Arx T, Jensen SS, Hanni S. Clinical and radiographic assessment of various predictors for healing outcome 1 year after periapical surgery. J Endod. 2007;33(2):123–8.
62. Lustmann J, Friedman S, Shaharabany V. Relation of pre- and intraoperative factors to prognosis of posterior apical surgery. J Endod. 1991;17(5):239–41.
63. von Arx T, Hanni S, Jensen SS. Correlation of bone defect dimensions with healing outcome one year after apical surgery. J Endod. 2007;33(9):1044–8.
64. Misch CM. Maxillary autogenous bone grafting. Dent Clin N Am. 2011;55(4):697–713.
65. Pradel W, Eckelt U, Lauer G. Bone regeneration after enucleation of mandibular cysts: comparing autogenous grafts from tissue-engineered bone and iliac bone. Oral Surg Oral Med Oral Pathol Oral Radiol Endod. 2006;101(3):285–90.
66. Arabiun H, et al. Effects of different storage media, temperature, and time on osteoblast preservation in autogenous bone grafts: a Histomorphometrical analysis. J Dent (Shiraz). 2020;21(3):225–33.
67. Dechichi P, et al. Histomorphometric analysis of rabbit calvarial bone: storage in saline solution versus storage in platelet-poor plasma. Int J Oral Maxillofac Implants. 2007;22(6):905–10.
68. Laursen M, et al. Optimal handling of fresh cancellous bone graft: different peroperative storing techniques evaluated by in vitro osteoblast-like cell metabolism. Acta Orthop Scand. 2003;74(4):490–6.
69. Rocha FS, et al. Effect of different storage media on the regenerative potential of autogenous bone grafts: a histomorphometrical analysis in rabbits. J Oral Implantol. 2013;39(6):635–42.
70. Kamijou T, Ozawa H. Effects of osteocytes on osteoinduction in the autogenous rib graft in the rat mandible, vol. 15. Bone; 1994. p. 629–37.
71. Gu G, Peng Z, Hentunen TA, Vaananen HK. Death of osteocytes turns off the inhibition of osteoclasts and triggers local bone resorption. Biochem Biophys Res Commun. 2005;335:1095–101.
72. Mouraret S, et al. Cell viability after osteotomy and bone harvesting: comparison of piezoelectric surgery and conventional bur. Int J Oral Maxillofac Surg. 2014;43(8):966–71.
73. Schweiberer L, et al. Revascularization of the tibia after conservative and surgical fracture fixation. Hefte Unfallheilkd. 1974;119:18–26.
74. Laird WR, Walmsley AD. Ultrasound in dentistry. Part 1–Biophysical interactions. J Dent. 1991;19(1):14–7.
75. Stubinger S, et al. Ultrasonic bone cutting in oral surgery: a review of 60 cases. Ultraschall Med. 2008;29(1):66–71.
76. Torrella F, et al. Ultrasonic ostectomy for the surgical approach of the maxillary sinus: a technical note. Int J Oral Maxillofac Implants. 1998;13(5):697–700.
77. Gruber RM, et al. Ultrasonic surgery–an alternative way in orthognathic surgery of the mandible. A pilot study. Int J Oral Maxillofac Surg. 2005;34(6):590–3.
78. Gonzalez-Garcia A, et al. Piezoelectric bone surgery applied in alveolar distraction osteogenesis: a technical note. Int J Oral Maxillofac Implants. 2007;22(6):1012–6.
79. Vercellotti T. Technological characteristics and clinical indications of piezoelectric bone surgery. Minerva Stomatol. 2004;53(5):207–14.

80. Schaller BJ, et al. Piezoelectric bone surgery: a revolutionary technique for minimally invasive surgery in cranial base and spinal surgery? Technical note. Neurosurgery. 2005;57(4 Suppl):E410. discussion E410
81. Budd JC, Gekelman D, White JM. Temperature rise of the post and on the root surface during ultrasonic post removal. Int Endod J. 2005;38(10):705–11.
82. Robiony M, et al. Piezoelectric bone cutting in multipiece maxillary osteotomies. J Oral Maxillofac Surg. 2004;62(6):759–61.
83. Strbac GD, et al. Guided modern endodontic surgery: a novel approach for guided osteotomy and root resection. J Endod. 2017;43(3):496–501.
84. Giacomino CM, Ray JJ, Wealleans JA. Targeted endodontic microsurgery: a novel approach to anatomically challenging scenarios using 3-dimensional-printed guides and trephine burs-a report of 3 cases. J Endod. 2018;44(4):671–7.
85. Ahn SY, et al. Computer-aided design/computer-aided manufacturing-guided endodontic surgery: guided osteotomy and apex localization in a mandibular molar with a thick buccal bone plate. J Endod. 2018;44(4):665–70.
86. Benjamin G, et al. Preserving the neurovascular bundle in targeted endodontic microsurgery: a case series. J Endod. 2021;47(3):509–19.
87. Khambay BS, Walmsley AD. Investigations into the use of an ultrasonic chisel to cut bone. Part 2: cutting ability. J Dent. 2000;28(1):39–44.
88. Leclercq P, Zenati C, Dohan DM. Ultrasonic bone cut part 2: state-of-the-art specific clinical applications. J Oral Maxillofac Surg. 2008;66(1):183–8.
89. Popowicz W, Palatynska-Ulatowska A, Kohli MR. Targeted endodontic microsurgery: computed tomography-based guided stent approach with platelet-rich fibrin graft: a report of 2 cases. J Endod. 2019;45(12):1535–42.
90. Fan Y, et al. A novel prefabricated grid for guided endodontic microsurgery. J Endod. 2019;45(5):606–10.

The Use of Cone Beam Computed Tomography in Dynamic Navigation

9

Paula Villa-Machado

Abstract

With the emergence of 3D imaging technology today, it is possible to know the anatomy of the teeth and surrounding structures in detail that allows for more accurate diagnosis and less invasive treatment. Computer-aided static and dynamic navigation techniques have been introduced along with the evolution of imaging in dentistry, which, in turn, means better planning and execution of complex procedures, such as locating and negotiating obliterated canals, fiber post removal, and endodontic microsurgery, in a more predictable and less invasive way.

9.1 Introduction

The use of cone beam computed tomography (CBCT) has had a significant impact on endodontics, especially when diagnosing and planning complex cases [1–3]. It has also had a significant influence on the decision-making process regarding endodontic retreatment, dental trauma [4, 5], endodontic microsurgery (EMS), and diagnosis and treatment of root resorptions [6, 7]. It promotes greater confidence and reduces clinician stress when dealing with difficult cases [4, 8, 9].

Combining CBCT data with other technologies has facilitated the development of computer-guided procedures that have turned out to be clinically useful when facing difficult scenarios such as locating obliterated canals, endodontic retreatment, or EMS [10]. Such techniques could be either computer-aided static (C-ASN) or dynamic navigation techniques (C-ADN) [11].

P. Villa-Machado (✉)
Universidad of Antioquia, Medellín, Colombia
e-mail: paula.villa@udea.edu.co

M. I. Fayad, B. R. Johnson (eds.), *3D Imaging in Endodontics*,
https://doi.org/10.1007/978-3-031-32755-1_9

C-ASN techniques need computer-aided design (CAD) and computer-aided manufacturing (CAM) of surgical templates, whereas C-ADN techniques have an optical triangulation tracking system that uses stereoscopic motion-tracking cameras to guide the drilling process in real time as it is monitored on a video screen [12].

9.2 Computer-Aided Dynamic Navigation (C-ADN)

For over 50 years, C-ADN systems, also called computer-assisted surgery, computer-integrated surgery, computer-aided surgery, image-guided surgery, or navigated surgery, have assisted abdominal, head and neck, orthopedic, and ear, nose, and throat (ENT) surgeons locate lesions. In neurosurgery, this technology has allowed surgeons to locate intracranial lesions and develop atraumatic surgical techniques that contribute to the reduction of mortality and morbidity of those interventions [13]. In dentistry, C-ADN has been mainly used to guide dental implant placement [14] as well as in cranio-maxillofacial surgery [15], nonsurgical endodontics, and endodontic microsurgery [16].

This system, which allows us to monitor instrument movement in real time over the CBCT, consists of a moving base that contains a computer with planning/guidance software. It also has a sensor for optical tracking (e.g., MicronTracker stereoscopic camera), a tracer tool, an optically marked handpiece attachment (drill tag), and an optically marked patient jaw attachment (head-tracker for maxillary teeth or jaw-tracker for mandibular teeth) (Fig. 9.1).

Trace registration is the first step after uploading the Digital Imaging and Communications in Medicine (DICOM) files onto the software. For this, three to six hard-tissue anatomical points of reference (teeth) are chosen and marked on the CBCT in order to set the landmarks that are turned into a virtual cloud of points that will match the CBCT by using the tracer tool. This allows the software to track the patient's location. Finally, it will be necessary to verify the registration accuracy (Fig. 9.2).

Next, the handpiece and instrument to be used (i.e., drill, trephine, ultrasonic tip, or piezosurgery saw) must be calibrated (Fig. 9.3). The system offers real-time monitoring of instrument position in the axial, sagittal, and coronal planes of the CBCT. A virtual guide may be planned to indicate the desired path to get to the target (i.e., root canal), but this procedure can also be carried out without this guide by constantly monitoring tool position and displacement [17, 18] (Fig. 9.4).

In vitro studies have demonstrated that the C-ADN system is useful for locating canals [18] and its accuracy is similar to C-ASN [11]. The results that have been observed when using C-ADN have shown less linear deviation and less loss of dentine as compared to freehand access cavity preparation, giving the opportunity to perform less invasive access cavities in a shorter period of time [19–23].

Clinical application of the C-ADN system in endodontics has been considered of great help not only when treating teeth with pulp canal obliteration (PCO) [17] but also during retreatment procedures [24, 25] and endodontic microsurgery (EMS) [26–28].

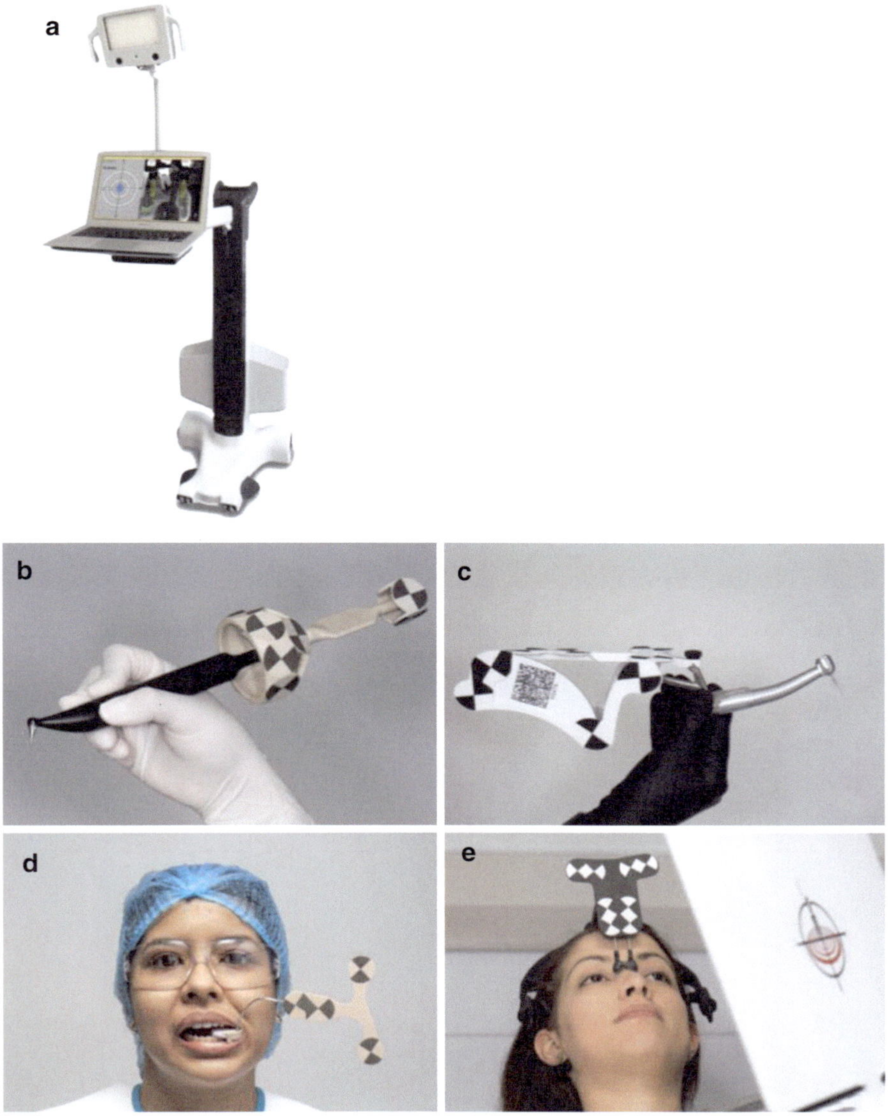

Fig. 9.1 Computer-aided dynamic navigation system Navident® (Claronav, Canada): computer with a planning/guidance software and sensor for optical tracking (**a**), tracer tool (**b**), drill tag (**c**), jaw-tracker (**d**), and head-tracker (**e**)

Some advantages of C-ADN systems are as follows: planning is simple and fast, the entire procedure can be done in a single appointment, it is possible to verify the accuracy in real time during the procedure, irrigation is easy to accommodate, and a large interocclusal space to place templates is not necessary [28]. Some

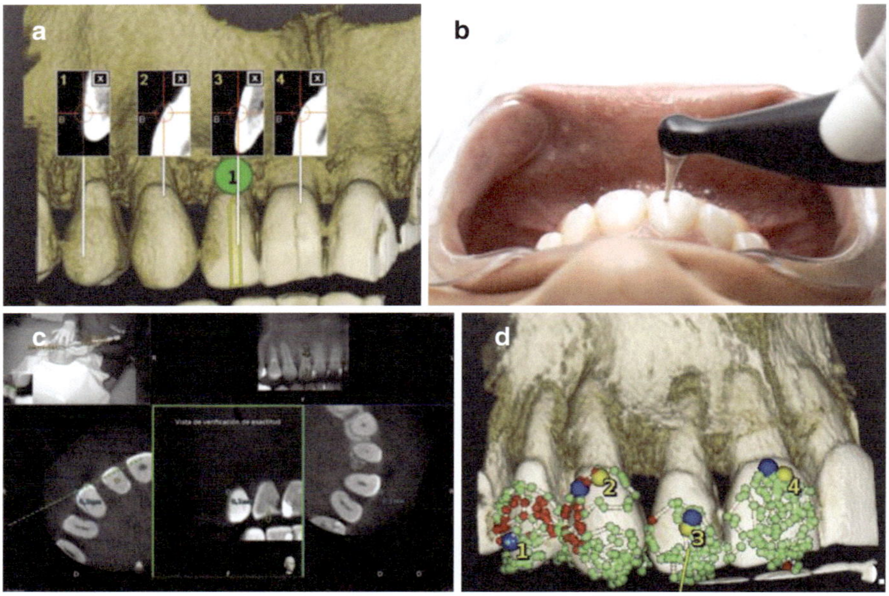

Fig. 9.2 Trace registration process: first, reference points are selected and marked on the CBCT (**a**); then, the tracer tool is placed over these points and displaced along the structures (**b**). In the final step, accuracy is checked (**c**), and the result will be the virtual cloud of points which matches the CBCT (**d**)

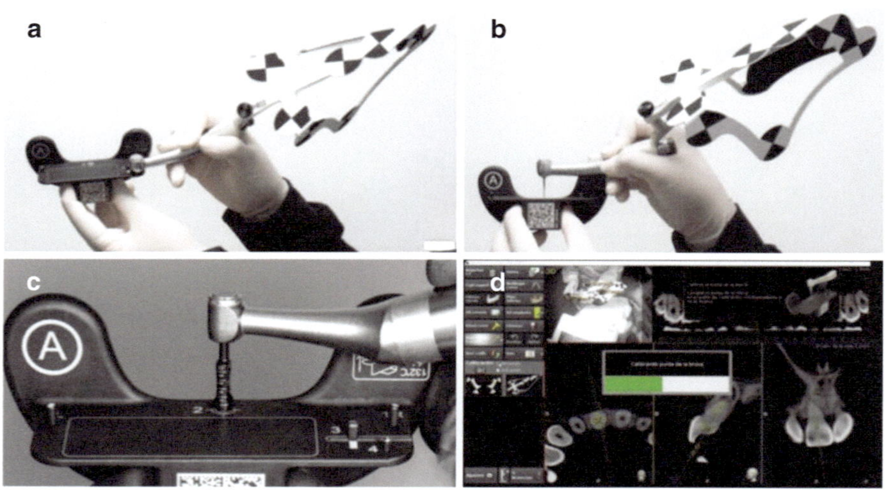

Fig. 9.3 The handpiece with the drill tag attached and the system calibrator are used for calibrating its axis (**a**); after that, every instrument must be calibrated immediately before its use (**b**, **c**). For this, the clinician holds the handpiece over the calibrator right in front of the C-ADN system camera so that the calibrator and drill tag are detected (**d**). The calibrator can also be used for calibrating drills, trephines, ultrasonic tips, or piezosurgery saws

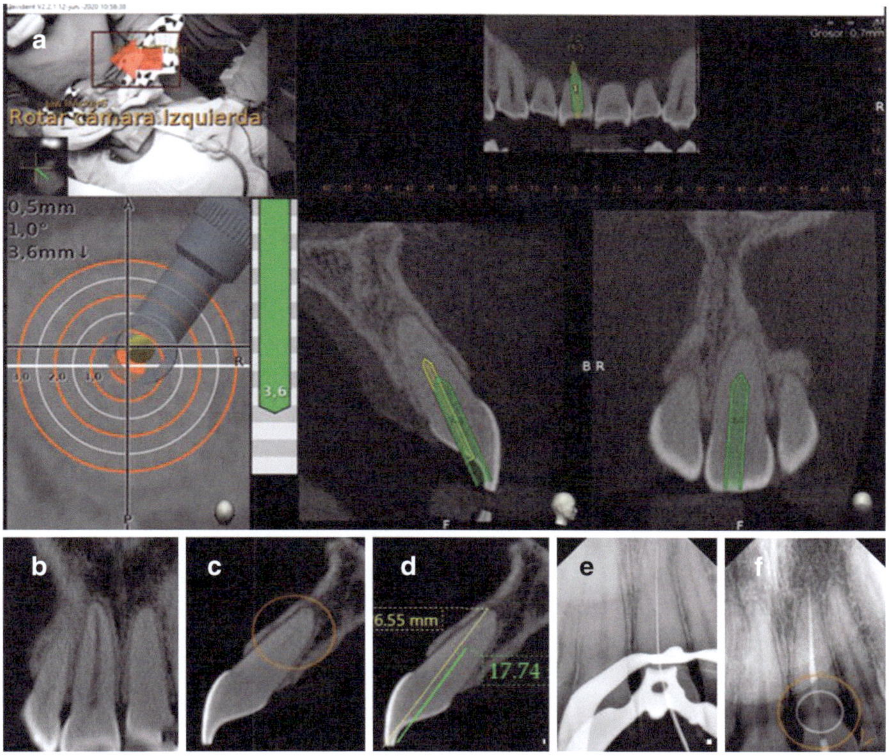

Fig. 9.4 Root canal treatment of maxillary left central incisor with PCO using C-ADN system. Distance from the instrument tip to the center of the virtual guide, angular deviation, and the depth of cut can be monitored in real time during the whole process (**a**). Analysis of the CBCT prior to treatment establishes the distance to reach the partially obliterated canal (**b**–**d**). The result was endodontic treatment through a conservative access cavity (**e**, **f**)

disadvantages of this system could be the cost and the strict training that is required before it can be used [12].

9.2.1 Clinical Applications of C-ADN System in Endodontics

9.2.1.1 Root Canal Treatment

PCO might be a consequence of multiple factors, such as dental trauma, tooth decay, previous pulpotomy, extensive restorations, maxillofacial surgery, and orthodontics, or the result of dentin deposition throughout life in elderly patients. Clinically, these teeth present discoloration, and radiographically, the pulp chamber and part or all of the root canal space are obliterated. Endodontic treatment of teeth with PCO is often not necessary unless internal bleaching is required or when there is presence of an apical lesion, which happens in 7 to 27% of the cases [29].

Root canal treatment of teeth with PCO is quite challenging since there is the possibility of iatrogenic damage during the access cavity preparation. C-ADN systems allow us to set a virtual guide to get to the root canal (Fig. 9.4). They have become a useful tool for locating obliterated canals, and some authors have demonstrated higher accuracy as compared to the freehand approach. In addition, preparations are more conservative and take less time [20]. A C-ADN system is an accurate approach for locating narrow canals [30], no matter the clinician's experience. However, this technique has a learning curve, and a significant amount of training is necessary prior to use [31].

One of the limitations of C-ASN is the necessary interocclusal space for placing the template, leaving room for the use of the handpiece with long drills. In that regard, the C-ADN system is more practical for posterior teeth given that no template must be placed before use, which makes the guided endodontic procedure more practical in posterior teeth. Additionally, it is possible to use any type of bur and not exclusively the systems designed for guided treatments [28] (Fig. 9.5).

9.2.1.2 Endodontic Retreatment

Endodontic treatment is highly predictable; however, some circumstances such as persistent or secondary intraradicular infection might lead to failure, and a revision may be indicated. Failure is determined by the presence of symptoms and clinical or radiographic signs related to infection [32].

One of the biggest challenges faced during endodontic retreatment is the presence of fiber intraradicular posts. Fiber posts have a modulus of elasticity and color similar to dentin. These posts are usually bonded to the dentin, and the most appropriate way to remove them is grinding the post with burs or an ultrasonic tip. This approach may lead to procedural errors such as weakening of the tooth due to excessive dentin removal, ledge formation due to axis post deviation with removal instruments, and microcrack formation or root fracture. Freehand removal of fiber post requires magnification and ultrasound and is time-consuming, and experience is needed [24].

Several authors have shown the usefulness of C-ASN for guiding fiber post removal procedures [33, 34] even in posterior teeth [35]; however, the disadvantages are the same that the system has when accessing teeth with PCO.

The use of C-ADN also seems to be beneficial in removing fiber posts. It is safe and fast and offers the same advantages that it has for endodontic access to teeth with PCO [24].

9.2.1.3 Endodontic Microsurgery

With the use of current techniques, EMS has become a highly predictable procedure with a high success rate [36, 37]. EMS may be the treatment of choice when initial nonsurgical root canal treatment has failed and orthograde retreatment is impractical or unlikely to result in a favorable outcome.

In order to perform this procedure, reflecting a soft tissue flap and accessing the root apex through the cortical bone are necessary so that root-end resection, root-end cavity preparation, and root-end filling can be done.

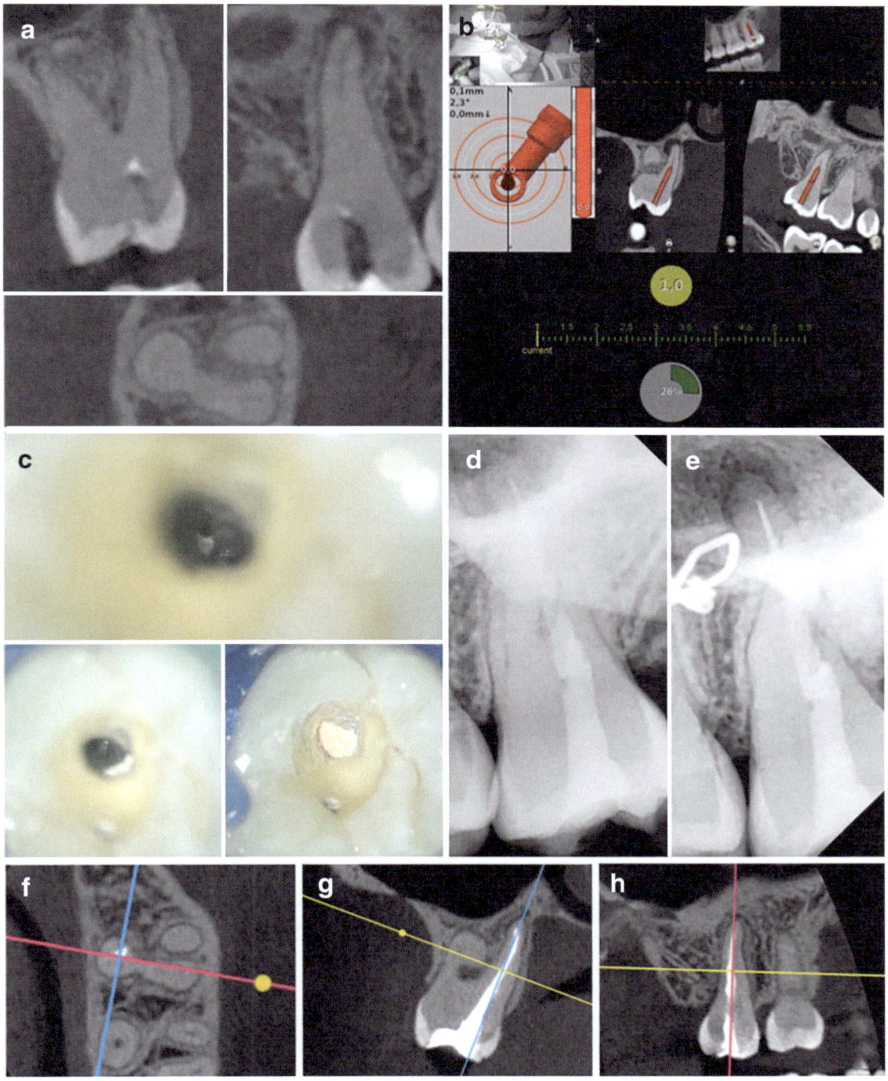

Fig. 9.5 CBCT of maxillary left second molar with evidence of complete PCO of the buccal root canals and obliteration of the palatal root canal extending to the apical third, with apical periodontitis (**a**). The access is planned using the C-ADN system (**b**) and could be performed despite the limited interocclusal space (**d–e**). 6-months follow-up CBCT shows complete healing of palatal apical periodontitis (**f–h**)

Access might be complex when the cortical bone is not fenestrated or when the root to be treated is located close to anatomical structures such as the maxillary sinus, mandibular canal, or mental foramen.

The use of CBCT has had a positive impact on EMS given that it allows an accurate identification of the location and size of the lesion as well as the number of roots involved and cortical bone thickness [38, 39].

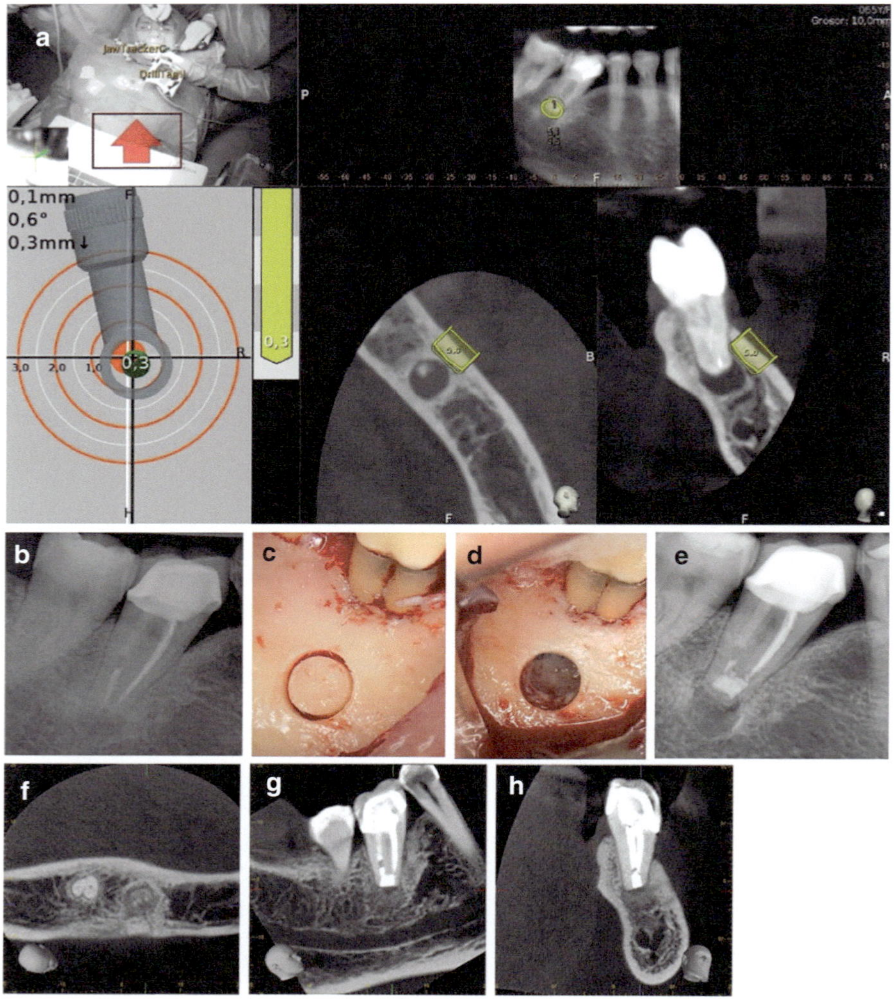

Fig. 9.6 Endodontic microsurgery of mandibular right second molar. The osteotomy is made with a 5.0 mm diameter trephine following the planned virtual guide with C- ADN system (**a**). Pre and post-surgical periapical radiographs (**b**, **e**) show the treatment of the apical third of the roots through a minimally invasive bone cavity (**c**, **d**). 6-months follow-up CBCT reveals healing in progress with adequate reintegration of the bone lid (**f**–**h**)

C-ADN systems may be used during EMS to monitor the movement and cutting of the instruments in real time as the osteotomy and root-end resection are performed, thus allowing for a safer and less invasive procedure [40, 41], even when performed by non-experienced clinicians [42]. The necessary instruments are the same ones regularly used in EMS (i.e., surgical burs, piezosurgery saws, or trephine burs), and the procedure can be planned with the software and performed without a previously designed guide but with constant supervision of instrument movement as it is being used (Fig. 9.6).

9.3 Conclusion

CBCT usage along with C-ADN systems facilitates the performance of complex endodontic procedures in a predictable way due to the possibility of creating a virtual access guide to the target area, allowing conservative cutting and preservation of anatomical structures.

References

1. Bhatt M, Coil J, Chehroudi B, Esteves A, Aleksejuniene J, MacDonald D. Clinical decision-making and importance of the AAE/AAOMR position statement for CBCT examination in endodontic cases. Int Endod J. 2021 Jan;54(1):26–37.
2. Rodríguez G, Patel S, Durán-Sindreu F, Roig M, Abella F. Influence of cone-beam computed tomography on endodontic retreatment strategies among general dental practitioners and endodontists. J Endod. 2017 Sep;43(9):1433–7.
3. Rodríguez G, Abella F, Durán-Sindreu F, Patel S, Roig M. Influence of cone-beam computed tomography in clinical decision making among specialists. J Endod. 2017 Feb;43(2):194–9.
4. Luz LB, Vizzotto MB, Xavier PNI, Vianna-Wanzeler AM, Dias da Silveira HL, Montagner F. The impact of cone-beam computed tomography on diagnostic thinking, treatment option, and confidence in dental trauma cases: a before and after study. J Endod. 2022 Mar;48(3):320–8.
5. Mota de Almeida FJ, Hassan D, Nasir Abdulrahman G, Brundin M, Romani VN. CBCT influences endodontic therapeutic decision-making in immature traumatized teeth with suspected pulp necrosis: a before-after study. Dentomaxillofac Radiol. 2021;50(8):20200594.
6. Rodríguez Mazón M, Garcia-Font M, Doria G, Durán-Sindreu F, Abella F. Influence of cone-beam computed tomography in clinical decision-making among different specialists in external cervical resorption lesions: a before-after study. J Endod. 2022 Jun 8;S0099-2399(22):00407–1.
7. Kakavetsos VD, Markou ME, Tzanetakis GN. Assessment of cone-beam computed tomographic referral reasons and the impact of cone-beam computed tomographic evaluation on decision treatment planning procedure in endodontics. J Endod. 2020 Oct;46(10):1414–9.
8. Viana Wanzeler AM, Montagner F, Vieira HT, Dias da Silveira HL, Arús NA, Vizzotto MB. Can cone-beam computed tomography change Endodontists' level of confidence in diagnosis and treatment planning? A before and after study. J Endod. 2020 Feb;46(2):283–8.
9. Patel S, Brown J, Semper M, Abella F, Mannocci F. European Society of Endodontology position statement: use of cone beam computed tomography in endodontics: European Society of Endodontology (ESE) developed by. Int Endod J. 2019 Dec;52(12):1675–8.
10. Moreno-Rabié C, Torres A, Lambrechts P, Jacobs R. Clinical applications, accuracy and limitations of guided endodontics: a systematic review. Int Endod J. 2020 Feb;53(2):214–31.
11. Zubizarreta-Macho Á, Muñoz AP, Deglow ER, Agustín-Panadero R, Álvarez JM. Accuracy of computer-aided dynamic navigation compared to computer-aided static procedure for endodontic access cavities: an in vitro study. J Clin Med. 2020 Jan 2;9(1):129.
12. Connert T, Weiger R, Krastl G. Present status and future directions–guided endodontics. Int Endod J. 2022 Jan 25;55:995.
13. Grunert P, Darabi K, Espinosa J, Filippi R. Computer-aided navigation in neurosurgery. Neurosurg Rev. 2003;26(2):73–99.
14. Pellegrino G, Ferri A, Del Fabbro M, Prati C, Gandolfi MG, Marchetti C. Dynamic navigation in implant dentistry: a systematic review and meta-analysis. Int J Oral Maxillofac Implants. 2021 Sep-Oct;36(5):e121–40.
15. Zhang W, Wang X, Zhang J, Shen G. Application of preoperative registration and automatic tracking technique for image-guided maxillofacial surgery. Comput Assist Surg (Abingdon). 2016 Dec;21(1):137–42.

16. Vasudevan A, Santosh SS, Selvakumar RJ, Sampath DT, Natanasabapathy V. Dynamic navigation in guided endodontics–a systematic review. Eur Endod J. 2022 Jun;7(2):81–91. https://doi.org/10.14744/eej.2022.96168.
17. Villa-Machado PA, Restrepo-Restrepo FA, Sousa-Dias H, Tobón-Arroyave SI. Application of computer-assisted dynamic navigation in complex root canal treatments: report of two cases of calcified canals. Aust Endod J. 2022 Apr;48(1):187–96.
18. Chong BS, Dhesi M, Makdissi J. Computer-aided dynamic navigation: a novel method for guided endodontics. Quintessence Int. 2019;50:196–202.
19. Connert T, Leontiev W, Dagassan-Berndt D, Kühl S, ElAyouti A, Krug R, Krastl G, Weiger R. Real-time guided endodontics with a miniaturized dynamic navigation system versus conventional freehand endodontic access cavity preparation: substance loss and procedure time. J Endod. 2021 Oct;47(10):1651–6.
20. Gambarini G, Galli M, Morese A, Stefanelli LV, Abduljabbar F, Giovarruscio M, Di Nardo D, Seracchiani M, Testarelli L. Precision of dynamic navigation to perform endodontic ultraconservative access cavities: a preliminary in vitro analysis. J Endod. 2020 Sep;46(9):1286–90.
21. Dianat O, Gupta S, Price JB, Mostoufi B. Guided endodontic access in a maxillary molar using a dynamic navigation system. J Endod. 2021 Apr;47(4):658–62.
22. Jain SD, Carrico CK, Bermanis I. 3-dimensional accuracy of dynamic navigation Technology in Locating Calcified Canals. J Endod. 2020 Jun;46(6):839–45.
23. Jain SD, Saunders MW, Carrico CK, Jadhav A, Deeb JG, Myers GL. Dynamically navigated versus freehand access cavity preparation: a comparative study on substance loss using simulated calcified canals. J Endod. 2020 Nov;46(11):1745–51.
24. Janabi A, Tordik PA, Griffin IL, Mostoufi B, Price JB, Chand P, Martinho FC. Accuracy and efficiency of 3-dimensional dynamic navigation system for removal of fiber post from root canal-treated teeth. J Endod. 2021 Sep;47(9):1453–60.
25. Bardales-Alcocer J, Ramírez-Salomón M, Vega-Lizama E, López-Villanueva M, Alvarado Cárdenas G, Serota KS, Ramírez-Wong J. Endodontic retreatment using dynamic navigation: a case report. J Endod. 2021 Jun;47(6):1007–13.
26. Lu YJ, Chiu LH, Tsai LY, Fang CY. Dynamic navigation optimizes endodontic microsurgery in an anatomically challenging area. J Dent Sci. 2022 Jan;17(1):580–2.
27. Gambarini G, Galli M, Stefanelli LV, Di Nardo D, Morese A, Seracchiani M, De Angelis F, Di Carlo S, Testarelli L. Endodontic microsurgery using dynamic navigation system: a case report. J Endod. 2019 Nov;45(11):1397–1402.e6.
28. Dianat O, Nosrat A, Mostoufi B, Price JB, Gupta S, Martinho FC. Accuracy and efficiency of guided root-end resection using a dynamic navigation system: a human cadaver study. Int Endod J. 2021 May;54(5):793–801.
29. McCabe PS, Dummer PM. Pulp canal obliteration: an endodontic diagnosis and treatment challenge. Int Endod J. 2012;45:177–97.
30. Zubizarreta-Macho Á, Valle Castaño S, Montiel-Company JM, Mena-Álvarez J. Effect of computer-aided navigation techniques on the accuracy of endodontic access cavities: a systematic review and meta-analysis. Biology (Basel). 2021;10(3):212.
31. Torres A, Boelen GJ, Lambrechts P, Pedano MS, Jacobs R. Dynamic navigation: a laboratory study on the accuracy and potential use of guided root canal treatment. Int Endod J. 2021 Sep;54(9):1659–67.
32. Siqueira JF Jr. Aetiology of root canal treatment failure: why well-treated teeth can fail. Int Endod J. 2001 Jan;34(1):1–10.
33. Perez C, Sayeh A, Etienne O, Gros CI, Mark A, Couvrechel C, Meyer F. Microguided endodontics: accuracy evaluation for access through intraroot fibre-post. Aust Endod J. 2021 Dec;47(3):592–8.
34. Cho C, Jo HJ, Ha JH. Fiber-reinforced composite post removal using guided endodontics: a case report. Restor Dent Endod. 2021;46(4):e50.
35. Perez C, Finelle G, Couvrechel C. Optimisation of a guided endodontics protocol for removal of fibre-reinforced posts. Aust Endod J. 2020 Apr;46(1):107–14.

36. Tsesis I, Rosen E, Taschieri S, Telishevsky Strauss Y, Ceresoli V, Del Fabbro M. Outcomes of surgical endodontic treatment performed by a modern technique: an updated meta-analysis of the literature. J Endod. 2013 Mar;39(3):332–9.
37. Setzer FC, Kohli MR, Shah SB, Karabucak B, Kim S. Outcome of endodontic surgery: a meta-analysis of the literature–Part 2: comparison of endodontic microsurgical techniques with and without the use of higher magnification. J Endod. 2012 Jan;38(1):1–10.
38. Mayo CV Jr, Replogle KJ, Marshall JG, Best AM, Sehgal HS, Sousa Melo SL, Sedgley CM. Accuracy of Presurgical limited field of view cone-beam computed tomography in predicting intraoperative buccal cortical bone. J Endod. 2020 Feb;46(2):169–177.e1.
39. Kopacz M, Neal JJ, Suffridge C, Webb TD, Mathys J, Brooks D, Ringler G. A clinical evaluation of cone-beam computed tomography: implications for endodontic microsurgery. J Endod. 2021 Jun;47(6):895–901.
40. Aldahmash SA, Price JB, Mostoufi B, Griffin IL, Dianat O, Tordik PA, Martinho FC. Real-time 3-dimensional dynamic navigation system in endodontic microsurgery: a cadaver study. J Endod. 2022 Jul;48(7):922–9.
41. Fu W, Chen C, Bian Z, Meng L. Endodontic microsurgery of posterior teeth with the assistance of dynamic navigation technology: a report of three cases. J Endod. 2022;48(7):943–50. https://doi.org/10.1016/j.joen.2022.03.010. Epub 2022 Apr 6
42. Martinho FC, Aldahmash SA, Cahill TY, Gupta S, Dianat O, Behzad M, Price JB, Griffin I, Tordik PA. Comparison of the accuracy and efficiency of a 3D dynamic navigation system for osteotomy root-end resection performed by novice and experienced endodontists. J Endod. 2022 Jul 12;S0099-2399(22):00464–2.

Utilization of Cone Beam Computed Tomography in Diagnosis and Treatment of Traumatic Injuries

10

Adham A. Azim

Abstract

Traumatic dental injuries can often result in immediate complications in the form of tooth fracture and mobility, as well as later complications in the form of pulp necrosis and root resorption. Proper diagnosis and management of traumatic injuries is key for the long-term survivability of the tooth. It also provides the patients with the expected outcome and possible needs for intervention in the future. In this chapter, we go through the different types of traumatic injuries that can be encountered in the dental practice, the best management approaches, and how to utilize CBCT to better improve the diagnosis and treatment planning.

10.1 General Considerations

Traumatic injuries to the head can often be accompanied by intra-oral injuries in the form of soft tissue lacerations, dental fractures, and/or alveolar fractures. A thorough examination is essential to ensure a proper diagnosis is reached before intervention. Endodontists are likely not to be the first providers for a dental injury as patients may opt to present to their primary dentist, an emergency clinic, or a trauma center to manage their immediate injury. In the event of needing to manage a dental trauma, clinicians should be aware that more severe injuries to the brain or other body organs can be associated with these dental traumas. Ruling out more severe injuries should be the dentist's priority.

The first step when managing traumatic injuries to the head is to examine the patient's mental status by asking them a few questions, such as their name, age, and the current date and location. Cognitive functions are also important to assess. The

A. A. Azim (✉)
University of the Pacific, Arthur A Dugoni, School of Dentistry, San Francisco, CA, USA
e-mail: aazim@PACIFIC.EDU

M. I. Fayad, B. R. Johnson (eds.), *3D Imaging in Endodontics*,
https://doi.org/10.1007/978-3-031-32755-1_10

patient should have a good recollection of what happened from the time of the injury till presenting to the dentist. Reporting of loss of consciousness, dizziness, or headache may indicate a brain injury. Since some of these traumas may occur to minors, the treating doctor should try to hear from the patient directly without interference from their accompanying parent/guardian. If the patient fails to recollect what happened or feels disoriented, this may indicate that their mental status is impaired. In that case, the doctor should postpone dental treatment and refer the patient to a hospital for a thorough medical evaluation. If the patient can answer these questions and shows normal cognitive functions, the dentists can proceed to address the patient's dental needs.

Examination for traumatic injuries should start with an extra-oral evaluation of the soft tissue to rule out any lacerations. Since traumatic injuries are likely to occur on the streets or open fields, a tetanus shot should be considered in case of significant cuts or abrasions on the face and/or body. Extra-oral evaluation should also include skeletal structures to rule out any fractures. This can be established through palpation and observing any mobility or deviation of the facial skeleton.

10.1.1 Dental Examination

Evaluation of the teeth and the supporting dental structures will provide the necessary information to assess the type of injury and the best treatment approach. This can be achieved through clinical and radiographic examination to determine the degree of injury as well as the stage of root development. Dental traumas can present similar clinical findings, such as fractures, mobility, and displacement. Radiographic presentation, however, makes the diagnosis more definitive in determining the nature of the trauma and the best possible treatment approach.

Historically, two-dimensional imaging, such as periapical radiographs, has often been used as the radiographic method of choice to interpret the extent of the traumatic injury. It, however, lacks accuracy due to the superimposition of the various anatomical structures within the dental field [1]. For example, an alveolar fracture on a periapical radiograph can easily be misdiagnosed as a horizontal root fracture and, accordingly, managed differently (Fig. 10.1). Due to these limitations, cone beam computed tomography (CBCT) has been recommended as the imaging modality of choice to assess traumatic injuries by the American Association of Endodontists and the American Association of Oral and Maxillofacial Radiologists [2]. CBCT usage should not be limited to the initial diagnosis of dentoalveolar injuries but also during the follow-up of these injuries. Traumatic injuries may often suffer from secondary root resorption [3], particularly during the first year, which can be missed on the traditional periapical radiograph [4]. A pre-operative CBCT scan can serve as a baseline following trauma to monitor any radiographic changes moving forward. It's without a doubt that pre-operative and follow-up CBCT scans can be considered the "best practice" in managing of traumatic dental injuries.

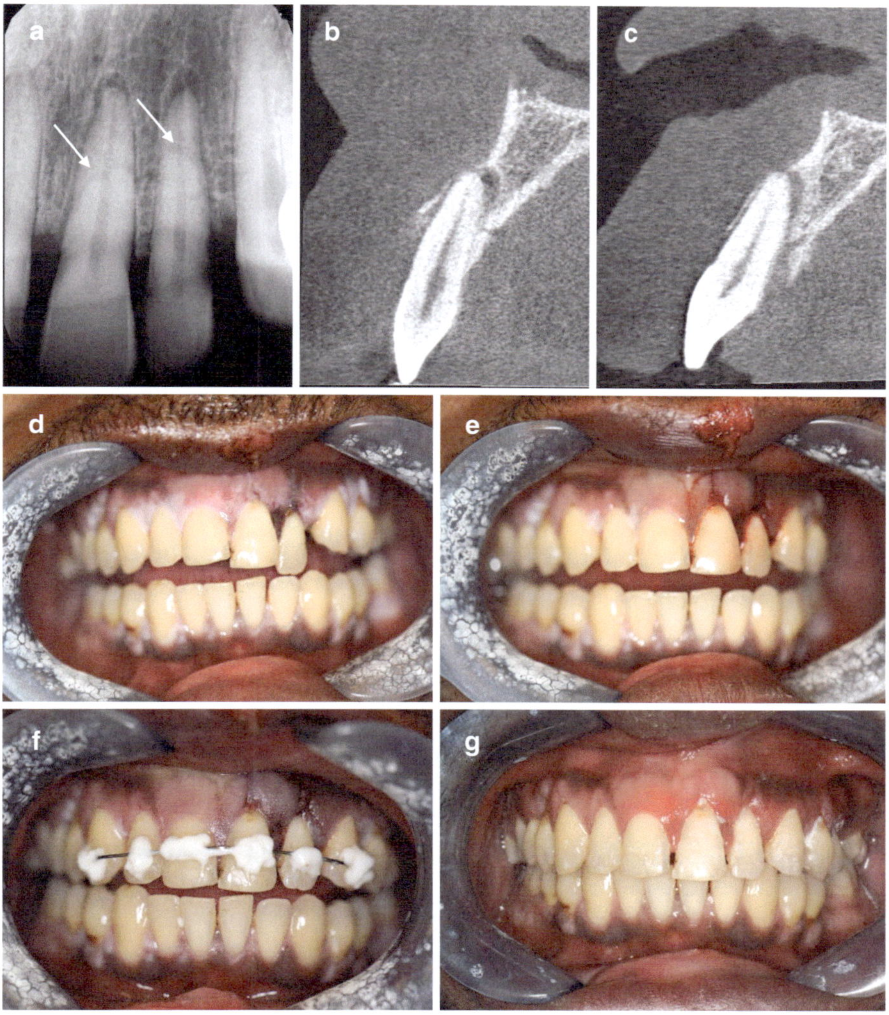

Fig. 10.1 A case of alveolar fracture secondary to a dental trauma misdiagnosed as "horizontal root fracture". (**a**) periapical radiograph suggest oblique fracture at the middle third of the central and lateral incisors (arrows) and was deemed to have poor prognosis due to extensive mobility on both teeth. (**b** & **c**) A Sagittal view of the lateral incisor (**b**) and the central incisor (**c**) showing no signs of horizontal root fracture and evidence of alveolar fracture and luxation injury to both teeth. (**d**-**g**) clinical pictures at different stages of the treatment (**d**) pre-operative € following repositioning of the teeth (**f**) following splinting (**g**) 1 month follow up with no signs of mobility on both teeth

10.2 Type of Traumatic Injuries

10.2.1 Tooth Fracture

10.2.1.1 Crown Fractures

Crown fractures can generally be divided into two categories: uncomplicated and complicated.

Uncomplicated crown fractures refer to a fractured crown that did not include the root canal space and management of these fractures is limited to direct or indirect restoration to restore the aesthetic and functional elements of the tooth. Complicated crown fractures, on the other hand, refer to fractures that include the pulp, which may require some sort of pulpal intervention in the form of direct pulp capping, pulpotomy, or a full root canal treatment depending on the extent of the fracture and the restorative needs of the tooth [5] (Fig. 10.2).

Generally, complicated crown fractures are not associated with high bacterial loads. For these reasons, even when the pulp has been exposed in the oral cavity for a day or two, removal of the coronal pulp followed by placing an appropriate pulp capping material, such as Biodentine, has a high success rate [6]. Once crown fractures extend below the CEJ, it is referred to as a "crown-root fractures." The fractures can be more complicated as the extent of root involvement can be challenging to assess. A CBCT scan can help determine the extent of root involvement and the restorability of the tooth (Fig. 10.3).

10.2.1.2 Root Fracture

Traumatic injuries to the dentoalveolar structure can also result in root fractures. These fractures are relatively rare. Root fractures secondary to trauma tend to run horizontally or obliquely along the root surface and can be associated with displacement of the coronal portion of the tooth. The apical segment, on the other hand, is usually not displaced and maintains vital tissue. The prognosis of horizontal root fractures depends primarily on the position of the fracture within the root (coronal, middle, or apical) and the degree of displacement [7, 8]. A CBCT scan can assist in proper assessment of the level of the fracture and, accordingly, better predict the treatment outcome. The prognosis is worse as the fracture becomes more coronal and associated with a higher degree of displacement. Treatment of horizontal root fracture often involves repositioning the displaced coronal segment followed by splinting the tooth between 4 and 6 weeks. This time can be extended if the location of the fracture is more coronally [8]. Endodontic treatment should be initiated on the coronal segment of the tooth within 10 days following the trauma to minimize infection and further bone loss. For the best clinical outcome, the apical segment should be left untreated as it maintains vital pulp tissue [9]. If an apical infection is evident radiographically, surgical removal of the apical segment should be attempted for the best outcome [9]. The healing of horizontal root fracture can take one of four possibilities [10] (Fig. 10.4):

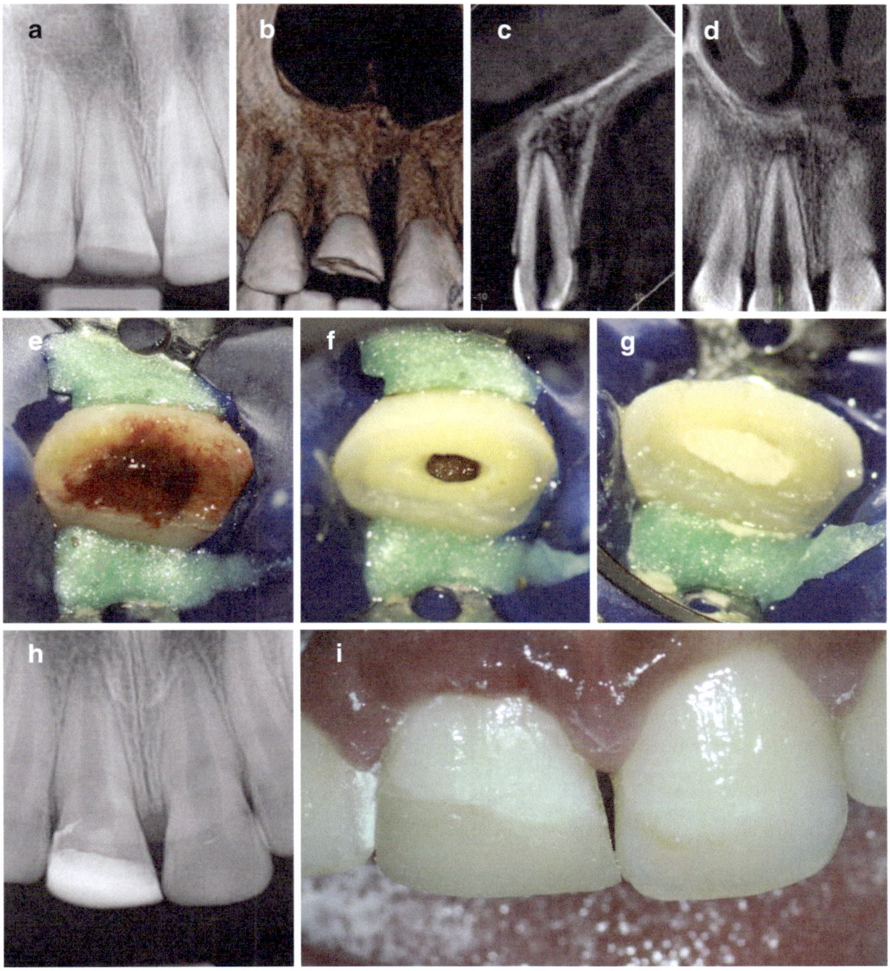

Fig. 10.2 Complicated crown fracture of a maxillary central incisor. (**a**) Periapical radiograph showing crown fracture of a maxillary central incisor. (**b-d**) CBCT images confirming no other injuries to the tooth or the supporting structure. (**e-f**) Exposed pulp chamber following pulpotomy (**e**) hemostasis (**f**) and placement of pulp capping material (**g**). (**h**) post-operative radiograph (**i**) post-operative clinical picture following restoration. UB PG Endo: Dr. Faranak Mahjour

1. Healing with calcified tissue (bone)
2. Healing with bone and connective tissue
3. Healing with connective tissue only

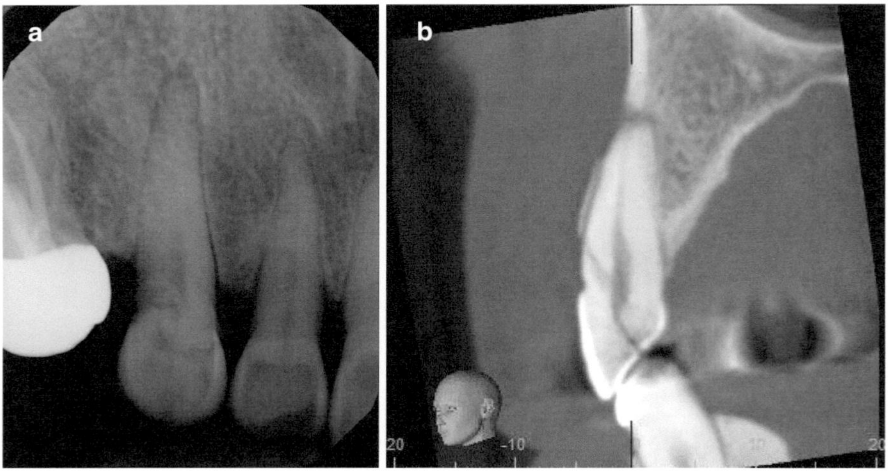

Fig. 10.3 Crown-Root fracture only illustrated through CBCT images. (**a**) Periapical radiograph showing no evidence of fracture (**b**) CBCT showing the extent of the fracture from the crown to the root surface

4. No healing (inflammatory)
    a. *Concussion*: this type of injury implies that the tooth has not been displaced and has no mobility.
    b. *Subluxation*: this type of injury implies that the tooth has no displacement but has increased mobility and sensitivity to percussion.

Management

For concussion and subluxation injuries, no intervention is needed to stabilize the teeth. Clinicians, however, should be aware that pulp canal obliteration or pulp necrosis can be a sequel to these types of injuries [11, 12] (Fig. 10.5). In addition, the neural responses of the pulp can be impaired for up to 1 year, and thus, the results of the pulpal sensibility tests (cold and EPT) can be inaccurate [13, 14]. Only laser Doppler and pulse oximetry tests can provide a more accurate diagnosis of these conditions [14]. Clinicians should constantly monitor these cases to ensure that the pup maintains vitality, with no signs of apical disease or root resorption. In cases of immature teeth, continuous root formation would be an indication that the tooth still maintains a vital pulp.

If clinical evidence is present that the tooth has lost its vitality, such as tooth discoloration and the presence of apical disease or clinical symptoms, endodontic intervention should be initiated in the form of root canal treatment for fully formed roots, and apexification or regenerative endodontic treatment for immature teeth.

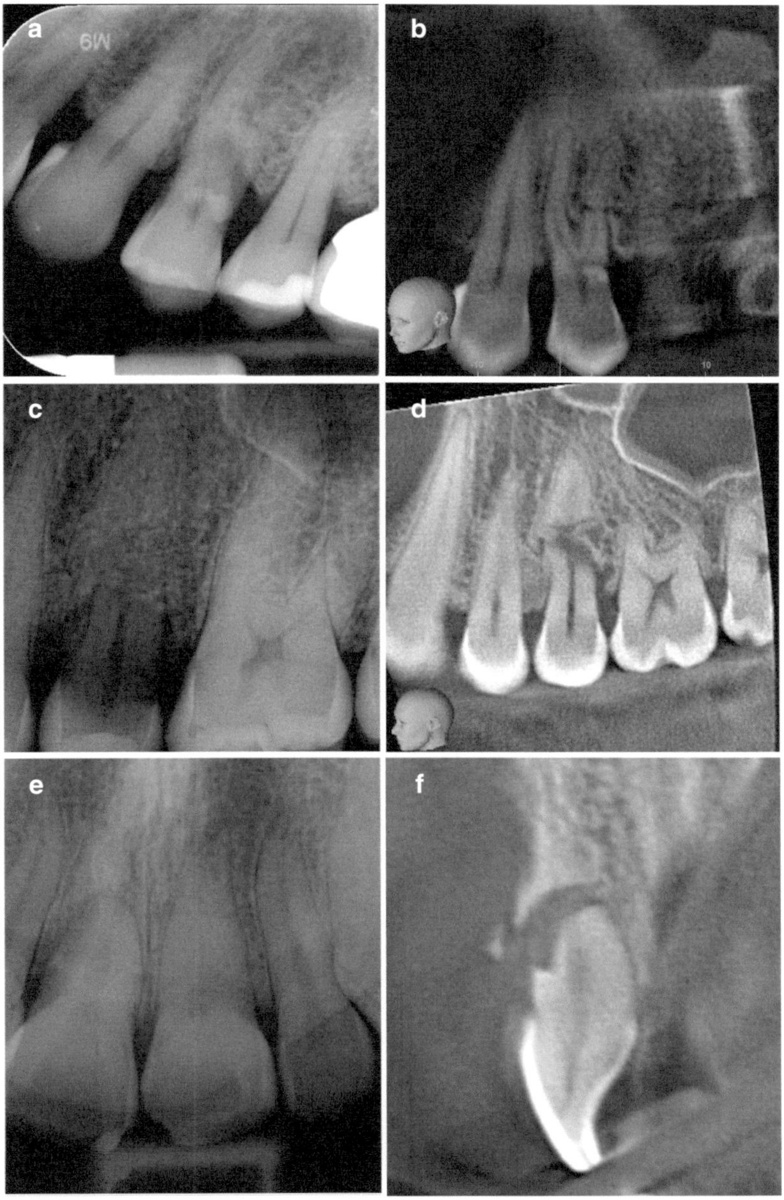

Fig. 10.4 Different types of horizontal root fracture with different forms of healing well illustrated using CBCT scans. (**a**) A periapical radiograph of a maxillary left 1st premolar without clear evidence of fracture (**b**) A CBCT image of the same tooth showing horizontal root fracture of the DB root with evidence of bony healing. (**c**) A periapical radiograph of a maxillary left 2nd premolar without clear evidence of fracture (**d**) A CBCT image of the same tooth showing horizontal root fracture of the the root with evidence of bone and connective tissue healing. (**e**) A Periapical radiograph of a maxillary central incisor with some evidence of horizontal root fracture: (**f**) A CBCT image of the same tooth showing complete separation of the two segements with no evididence of healing

10.2.2 Luxation Injuries

Luxation injuries are the most common type of dental trauma. They can be classified as:

(i) *Extrusive luxation:* In this type of injury, the tooth has been partially displaced along the long axis of the socket without being entirely removed from the oral cavity. In these cases, the tooth will be mobile and potentially lose its vitality [15] (Fig. 10.6).

(ii) *Intrusive luxation:* In these types of injuries, the tooth becomes apically positioned into the socket. This movement is likely to cause severe damage to the periodontal ligament (PDL) as it gets stripped off the root surface from the intrusion. Management of intrusive injuries relies primarily on the degree of intrusion of the stage of root development. In teeth with incomplete root formation (open apex), spontaneous re-eruption may occur and can represent the most conservative approach to avoid further periodontal damage and has been associated with the lowest risk for developing replacement resorption as well as pulp necrosis [16, 17]. For teeth with complete root formation in patients between the age of 12 and 17, a spontaneous eruption can still occur, however; the patients must be monitored very carefully [18]. Surgical or orthodontic extrusion can be attempted on adult patients (>17 years old) together with root canal treatment, as pulp necrosis is inevitable [18] (Fig. 10.7). This aims to avoid external inflammatory root resorption. If the endodontic disease is contained, replacement resorption (ankylosis) is very likely due to the extensive PDL damage secondary to the injury.

(iii) *Lateral luxation:* This type of injury implies that the tooth has been displaced from its original place in a buccal, lingual, mesial, or distal location. Accordingly, the tooth can potentially be in hyper-occlusion. Following lateral luxation injuries, the tooth could be completely stable and locked in its new position and thus missed by the treating doctor, especially if the patient has not experienced any changes in their occlusion. A CBCT image of these cases would illustrate tipping of the root in one direction and the presence of a radiolucency in the opposite direction. This radiolucency is not an apical disease but rather the space created following tooth movement. Management of these cases would include repositioning of the tooth in its original position and splinting in place [15].

10.2.3 Avulsion

This type of injury implies the complete separation of the tooth from its socket because of the trauma. Avulsed teeth are likely to suffer from damage to the pulp and the PDL. The degree of damage depends on the extra-oral dry time as well as the stage of root development. In permanent teeth with closed apex, pulp necrosis following avulsion is expected, and initiating root canal treatment is always

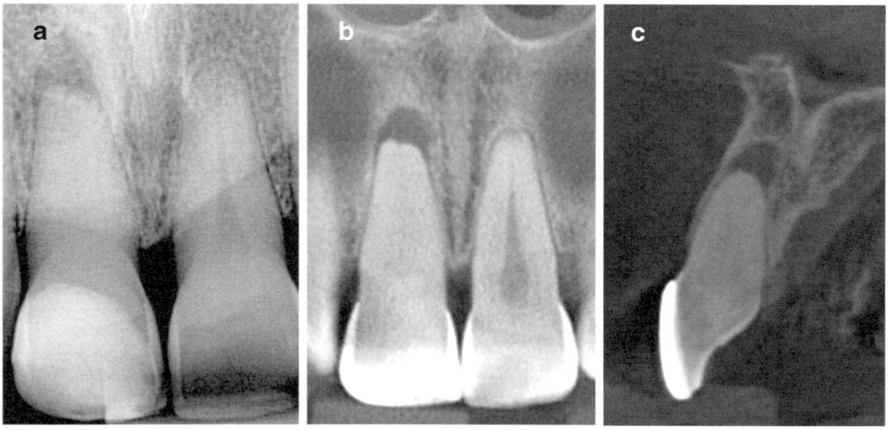

Fig. 10.5 Pulp canal obliteration followed by pulpal necrosis of a maxillary central incisor with a history of a concussion injury and uncomplicated crown fracture. (**a**) Pre-operative PA (**a**) and CBCT coronal view (**b**) and sagittal view (**c**) showing completely calcified canal that was later associated with pulp necrosis and apical periodontitis

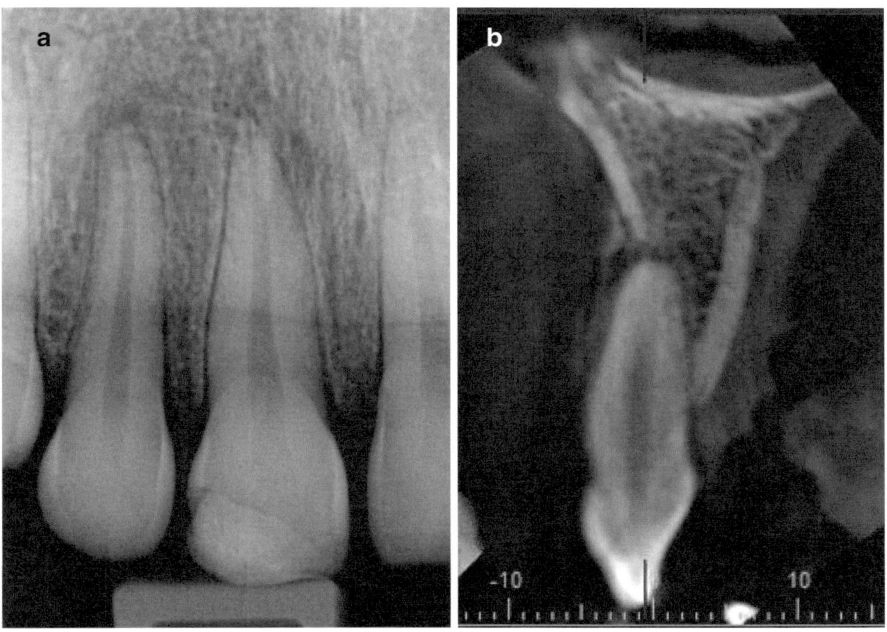

Fig. 10.6 Extrusive luxation of a maxillary lateral incisor shown on periapical radiographs (**a**) and CBCT sagittal view (**b**)

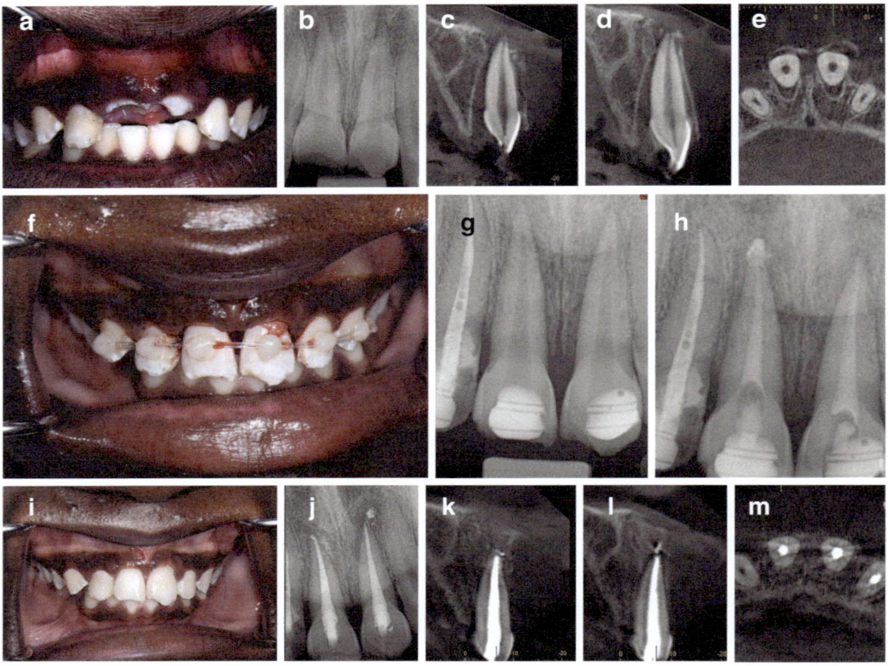

Fig. 10.7 Management of intruded central incisors using surgical extrusion. (**a-e**) Pre-operative condition showing clinical picture (**a**) and periapical radiograph (**b**) of intruded maxillary central incisors. CBCT Sagittal (**c** & **d**) and axial (**e**) views showing intruded central incisors associated with buccal plate fracture. (**f-h**) 2 weeks follow up following surgical repositioning of the maxillary central incisors and initiating root canal treatment. (**i–n**) 3 months follow up showing normal position of the central incisors with healed soft tissue (**i**) and completed root canal treatment (**j**). CBCT Sagittal (**k** & **m**) and axial (**m**) views showing signs of bone healing around the UB PG Endo: Dr. Ibrahim Alaugaily

recommended. Teeth with open apex, however, may revascularize following avulsion injuries [19, 20], and thus, the tooth should be monitored at regular intervals (3, 6, and 12 months following replantation) for any signs of continuing root maturation and apical closure. If regular evaluation showed no signs of root development, absence of vitality, or presence of periapical infection, endodontic treatment in the form of root canal treatment, apexification, or regenerative endodontic should be initiated.

The prognosis of avulsed teeth with complete root formation depends primarily on how soon the tooth can be replanted into its socket. Immediate replantation at the sight of injury following rinsing the tooth with water to remove gross contaminants results in the best outcome and should be encouraged. This will reduce the chances of PDL damage and secondary root resorption [21]. Following replantation, teeth should be splinted with a flexible splint for 2 weeks after confirming that the tooth is properly positioned, and root canal treatment should be initiated within 2 weeks

[22]. If immediate replantation is not feasible, the management protocol may differ depending on the extra-oral dry time. In these cases, the tooth should be stored in a media, such as milk, saline, or saliva, and brought to the office as soon as possible. The best storage medium is Hanks' balanced solution, which can allow the PDL to survive up to 2 days. However, it may not always be available compared to the other mediums mentioned [23]. Keeping the tooth dry should be avoided, and similarly, storing the tooth in water, to avoid damage to the PDL cells [23].

When the patient arrives at the dental office, the tooth should be placed in hanks' balance solution or sterile isotonic saline, and the patient should be assessed for any injuries. A CBCT should be considered to ensure that the trauma did not impact any other teeth through subluxation or luxation (Fig. 10.8). The avulsed site should also be examined to rule out alveolar fracture [22].

(a) *Extra Oral time less than 60 mins*

In cases where the extra-oral time is less than 60 mins, the root surface should be rinsed using isotonic sterile saline to remove any contaminants. The socket should also be examined, and any clot formed should be removed gently without excessive scraping of the socket walls. The crown of the tooth would then be grasped, and the

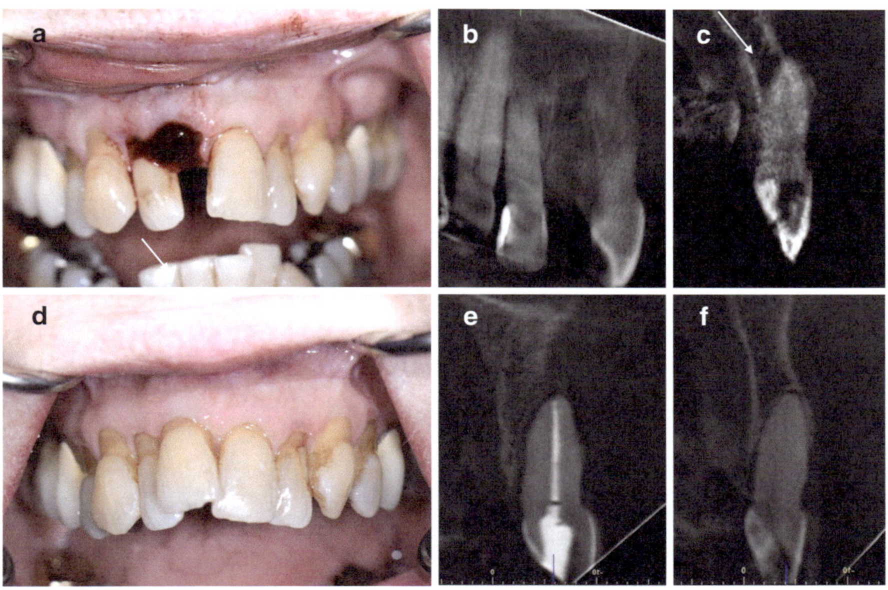

Fig. 10.8 Management of a traumatic injury associated with avulsion and lateral luxation. (**a-c**) preparative clinical pictures (**a**) and CBCT coronal and sagittal view (**b** & **c**) of avulsed central incisor and lateral luxation of the lateral incisor. Arrow pointing to a low-density area created lingual to the luxated tooth. (**d-f**) 1 month follow up showing intra-oral clinical images (**d**) and reimplantation and root canal treatment of the central incisor and repositioned lateral incisor

tooth replanted with minimal pressure until it is fully seated. The tooth would then be stabilized in place using a flexible splint for at least 2 weeks.

(b) *Extra Oral time more than 60 mins*

If the extra-oral time is more than 60 mins, the PDL is not expected to survive the injury. Root canal treatment can be completed extra-orally before replantation and splinting. In the most recent guidelines by the International Association of Dental Traumatology [22], root canal treatment can be initiated within 2 weeks following splinting. Replacement root resorption (ankylosis) is expected to occur in these cases [22, 24]. Dipping the tooth in florid before replantation and treating the root surface with growth factors have been proposed to potentially slow down the resorption process and favor periodontal healing [25, 26]. However, there is currently no consensus on their usage in the management of avulsed teeth [22].

Following replantation and splinting of the avulsed tooth, antibiotics should be recommended. A tetanus shot or a booster should also be considered since avulsed teeth are likely to be in contact with soil or dirt [22]. The patient should keep the site clean and have good oral hygiene while maintaining a soft diet. The splint can be removed 2–4 weeks following avulsion, and the tooth should be monitored at 3 months, 6 months, and 1 year for any signs of root resorption.

References

1. Scarfe WC, Levin MD, Gane D, Farman AG. Use of cone beam computed tomography in endodontics. Int J Dent. 2009;2009:634567.
2. AAE and AAOMR Joint Position Statement. Use of cone beam computed tomography in endodontics 2015 update. J Endod. 2015;41:1393–6.
3. Berude JA, Hicks ML, Sauber JJ, Li SH. Resorption after physiological and rigid splinting of replanted permanent incisors in monkeys. J Endod. 1988;14:592–600.
4. Patel K, Mannocci F, Patel S. The assessment and management of external cervical resorption with periapical radiographs and cone-beam computed tomography: a clinical study. J Endod. 2016;42:1435–40.
5. Aggarwal V, Logani A, Shah N. Complicated crown fractures–management and treatment options. Int Endod J. 2009;42:740–53.
6. Donnelly A, Foschi F, McCabe P, Duncan HF. Pulpotomy for treatment of complicated crown fractures in permanent teeth: a systematic review. Int Endod J. 2022;55:290–311.
7. Andreasen JO, Andreasen FM, Mejare I, Cvek M. Healing of 400 intra-alveolar root fractures. 1. Effect of pre-injury and injury factors such as sex, age, stage of root development, fracture type, location of fracture and severity of dislocation, vol. 20. Dent Traumatol; 2004. p. 192–202.
8. Andreasen JO, Andreasen FM, Mejare I, Cvek M. Healing of 400 intra-alveolar root fractures. 2. Effect of treatment factors such as treatment delay, repositioning, splinting type and period and antibiotics. Dent Traumatol. 2004;20:203–11.
9. Cvek M, Mejare I, Andreasen JO. Conservative endodontic treatment of teeth fractured in the middle or apical part of the root. Dent Traumatol. 2004;20:261–9.
10. Cvek M, Andreasen JO, Borum MK. Healing of 208 intra-alveolar root fractures in patients aged 7-17 years. Dent Traumatol. 2001;17:53–62.

11. Holcomb JB, Gregory WB Jr. Calcific metamorphosis of the pulp: its incidence and treatment. Oral Surg Oral Med Oral Pathol. 1967;24:825–30.
12. Andreasen FM, Pedersen BV. Prognosis of luxated permanent teeth–the development of pulp necrosis. Endod Dent Traumatol. 1985;1:207–20.
13. Bastos JV, Goulart EM, de Souza Cortes MI. Pulpal response to sensibility tests after traumatic dental injuries in permanent teeth. Dent Traumatol. 2014;30:188–92.
14. Ahn SY, Kim D, Park SH. Long-term prognosis of pulpal status of traumatized teeth exhibiting contradictory results between pulp sensibility test and ultrasound Doppler Flowmetry: a retrospective study. J Endod. 2018;44:395–404.
15. Diangelis AJ, Andreasen JO, Ebeleseder KA, Kenny DJ, Trope M, Sigurdsson A, et al. Guidelines for the management of traumatic dental injuries: 1. Fractures and luxations of permanent teeth. Pediatr Dent. 2017;39:401–11.
16. Tsilingaridis G, Malmgren B, Andreasen JO, Wigen TI, Maseng Aas AL, Malmgren O. Scandinavian multicenter study on the treatment of 168 patients with 230 intruded permanent teeth–a retrospective cohort study. Dent Traumatol. 2016;32:353–60.
17. Andreasen JO, Bakland LK, Andreasen FM. Traumatic intrusion of permanent teeth. Part 2. A clinical study of the effect of preinjury and injury factors, such as sex, age, stage of root development, tooth location, and extent of injury including number of intruded teeth on 140 intruded permanent teeth. Dent Traumatol. 2006;22:90–8.
18. Andreasen JO, Bakland LK, Andreasen FM. Traumatic intrusion of permanent teeth. Part 3. A clinical study of the effect of treatment variables such as treatment delay, method of repositioning, type of splint, length of splinting and antibiotics on 140 teeth. Dent Traumatol. 2006;22:99–111.
19. Andreasen JO, Borum MK, Jacobsen HL, Andreasen FM. Replantation of 400 avulsed permanent incisors. 1. Diagnosis of healing complications. Endod Dent Traumatol. 1995;11:51–8.
20. Andreasen JO, Borum MK, Jacobsen HL, Andreasen FM. Replantation of 400 avulsed permanent incisors. 2. Factors related to pulpal healing. Endod Dent Traumatol. 1995;11:59–68.
21. Andreasen JO, Borum MK, Jacobsen HL, Andreasen FM. Replantation of 400 avulsed permanent incisors. 4. Factors related to periodontal ligament healing. Endod Dent Traumatol. 1995;11:76–89.
22. Fouad AF, Abbott PV, Tsilingaridis G, Cohenca N, Lauridsen E, Bourguignon C, et al. International association of dental traumatology guidelines for the management of traumatic dental injuries: 2. Avulsion of permanent teeth. Dent Traumatol. 2020;36:331–42.
23. Udoye CI, Jafarzadeh H, Abbott PV. Transport media for avulsed teeth: a review. Aust Endod J. 2012;38:129–36.
24. Souza BDM, Dutra KL, Kuntze MM, Bortoluzzi EA, Flores-Mir C, Reyes-Carmona J, et al. Incidence of root resorption after the replantation of avulsed teeth: a meta-analysis. J Endod. 2018;44:1216–27.
25. Iqbal MK, Bamaas N. Effect of enamel matrix derivative (EMDOGAIN) upon periodontal healing after replantation of permanent incisors in beagle dogs. Dent Traumatol. 2001;17:36–45.
26. Shulman LB, Gedalia I, Feingold RM. Fluoride concentration in root surfaces and alveolar bone of fluoride-immersed monkey incisors three weeks after replantation. J Dent Res. 1973;52:1314–6.

Root Resorption

11

Peng-Hui Teng and Shanon Patel

Abstract

Root resorption is the loss of dental hard tissue due to the action of clastic cells. In permanent dentition, root resorption is pathological in nature. Root resorption can be classified into internal or external root resorption based on the location of the resorptive lesion. Root resorption may be challenging to be accurately diagnosed and managed. Periapical radiographs are commonly used to identify root resorption. However, periapical radiographs are not reliable in detecting early root resorption or the resorptive lesions on buccal/lingual surfaces. CBCT aids in the detection, assessment and management of root resorption in all planes. In this chapter, periapical and CBCT radiographic features of different types of root resorption will be discussed. Clinical cases will be presented to demonstrate the importance of CBCT in diagnosing and managing root resorption.

11.1 Introduction

Root resorption (RR) is the irreversible loss of mineralized cementum or dentine due to osteoclastic/odontoclastic activity [1]. It can occur in deciduous or permanent dentition. RR in primary dentition is desirable as it helps to exfoliate the deciduous teeth for the eruption of permanent dentition. However, RR in permanent dentition is typically *pathological* and undesirable. RR may be self-limiting, but it can also be sustained by pulp infection and/or pressure and continue to progress. This will cause continued hard tissue destruction and may eventually make the affected tooth unsalvageable.

RR can be classified into internal root resorption (IRR) and external root resorption based on the location of the resorptive lesion; IRR affects the inner wall of the

P.-H. Teng (✉) · S. Patel
Faculty of Dentistry, Oral & Craniofacial Sciences, King's College London, London, UK

M. I. Fayad, B. R. Johnson (eds.), *3D Imaging in Endodontics*,
https://doi.org/10.1007/978-3-031-32755-1_11

root canal, while external RR occurs on the external root surface. Both internal and external RR can be further subclassified based on the pathogenesis [1].

Internal root resorption

- Internal inflammatory root resorption
- Internal replacement resorption

External root resorption

- External surface resorption (ESR)
- External inflammatory root resorption (EIR)
- External replacement resorption (ERR)
- External cervical resorption (ECR)
- Transient apical breakdown (TAB)

The key for the successful management of RR relies on early detection and accurate diagnosis. RR is often asymptomatic during early stage and can only be detected through radiographic examination. Periapical radiographs (PR) are commonly used in endodontic cases for diagnosis and management. However, PR are two-dimensional images which cannot reliably identify resorptive lesions on buccal/lingual/palatal (approximal surfaces), and they are also less accurate in detecting small lesions [2]. Cone beam computed tomography (CBCT) has been increasingly popular in the detection of RR as many studies have demonstrated the excellent accuracy of CBCT in various types of RR [3–5].

11.2 Internal Root Resorption

IRR is initiated within the root canal and can be categorized into two main types based on their pathogenesis: *inflammatory* which consists of granulation tissue only and *replacement* which consists of a combination of granulation tissue and bone-like tissue. Both types of IRR share similar clinical findings. Depending on the extent of IRR lesions and the pulp status, teeth affected by IRR may present symptoms and signs of acute pulpitis and apical periodontitis. IRR can also be asymptomatic and is detected as incidental finding during radiographic examination. Hence, the radiographic examination is important for the diagnosis and subsequent management of IRR. Due to their rarity, transient IRR such as internal tunnel root and internal surface root resorption will not be discussed in this chapter.

Historically, IRR has been described as a symmetrical oval or round-shaped radiolucency on periapical radiograph (PR) within the root canal as the root canal wall balloons out [6]. Patel has reported that there is no ‘classic’ radiographic appearance of IRR [1, 7]. In general, inflammatory IRR presents as a uniformly oval or circular-shaped radiolucency and typically has smooth and well-defined margin (Fig. 11.1), whereas replacement IRR is described as radiolucency with cloudy or mottled appearance (Fig. 11.2) due to the deposition of bone-like tissue within the

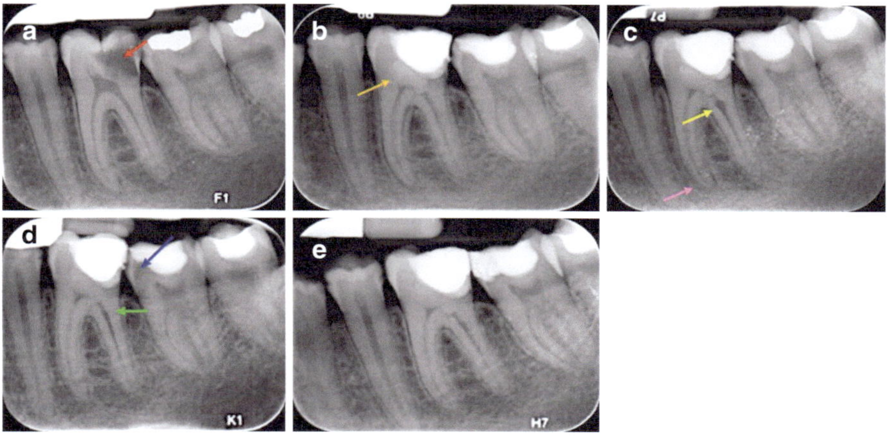

Fig. 11.1 Internal inflammatory resorption following pulpotomy. An 18-year-old male patient with an extensive carious lesion on the left mandibular first molar with symptoms of irreversible pulpitis (**a**) preoperative periapical radiograph showing the deep carious lesion (red arrow), (**b**) a Biodentine pulpotomy (orange arrow) was carried out, (**c**) a 3-month review confirmed that the tooth was asymptomatic; however, the radiographic examination revealed internal inflammatory root resorption (yellow arrow) on the distal canal, diffuse calcification on the mesial canals and apical widening of the periodontal ligament on the mesial root (pink arrow). After discussing the treatment options, as they were asymptomatic, the patient decided to have their tooth reviewed on a periodic basis. (**d**) A 15-month review revealed that the tooth was asymptomatic and there were no signs of endodontic or periodontal disease associated with the tooth; radiographic assessment confirmed that the internal inflammatory resorption has spontaneously resolved and may have become internal replacement resorption (green arrow) but did reveal secondary caries in the left mandibular second molar (blue arrow) which was restored during (**e**) 24-month review. (From Patel S, Saberi N, Pimental T & Teng P-H. (2022) Present status and future directions: Root resorption. *International Endodontic Journal*, 55(Suppl. 4), 892–921)

resorptive lesions [1, 7, 8]. The margin of replacement IRR is usually poorly defined. IRR lesions may be centric or eccentric.

IRR may be misdiagnosed for external cervical resorption (ECR) as they share similar radiographic features on PR [9]. Although parallax technique can be used to differentiate between these two RR, the limitation of PR in multi-rooted teeth remains a challenge for accurately diagnosing IRR or ECR [7]. For example, the IRR in one root canal of a molar can be superimposed to another unaffected root canal, thus being misdiagnosed as ECR. PR is also unable to detect root canal perforation in IRR cases. Root canal perforation may drastically change the management of the IRR [10], i.e. the treatment approach (nonsurgical or surgical) and the choice of obturation materials (*gutta-percha* or hydraulic calcium silicate material).

CBCT is able to provide accurate information about the nature, location and extent of IRR. CBCT can also accurately detect the presence of root canal perforation in IRR cases. These factors may influence the management of IRR. Studies have shown that CBCT has higher specificity, sensitivity and overall accuracy in

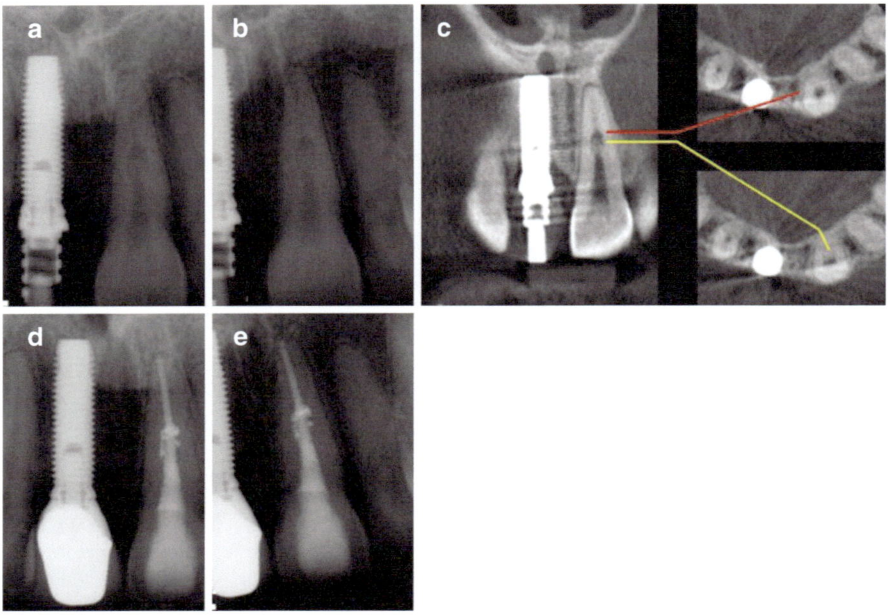

Fig. 11.2 Internal replacement resorption. (**a**, **b**) Periapical radiographs of a maxillary left central incisor with radiographic signs of IRR; note the symmetrical nature of the defect, which remains centred with the parallax view, and the radio-opaque nature of its coronal aspect. This patient sustained a dental traumatic injury 9 years previously. (**c**) CBCT slices through the same tooth reveal a calcified tissue in the coronal part of the lesion. (**d**, **e**) Obturated tooth and a 2-year review radiograph demonstrating the irregular borders of the defect that have been obturated with thermoplasticized gutta-percha. (From Patel S, Ricucci D, Durak C, Tay F. Internal root resorption: a review. *Journal of Endodontics* 2010; 36: 1107–1121)

diagnosing IRR [11, 12], as well as distinguishing IRR from ECR [4, 13], when compared to PR.

11.3 External Root Resorption

11.3.1 External Surface Resorption (ESR)

ESR is a pressure-induced resorption at the external aspect of the root. It is typically non-infective and self-limiting. Pressure exerted by orthodontic treatment, impacted teeth, tumours and cysts have been reported to be the cause of ESR [1, 14–16]. ESR is usually asymptomatic, and the affected teeth usually respond normally to pulp sensibility testing. Hence, the diagnosis is solely dependent on radiographic examination. Orthodontically treated teeth with ESR may have blunted or flattened root apices and may appear shorter than the unaffected teeth on PR (Fig. 11.3). Teeth adjacent to impacted teeth, tumours or cysts may have saucer-shaped or

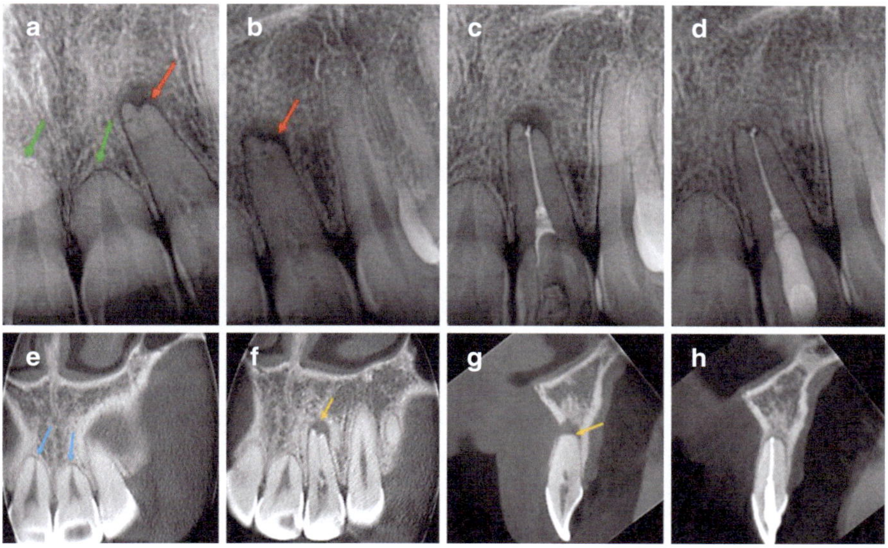

Fig. 11.3 External surface resorption and external inflammatory resorption following childhood dental trauma and orthodontic treatment. Periapical radiographs showing (**a**) external surface resorption (green arrows) on both maxillary central incisors and (**b**) external inflammatory resorption (red arrows) on maxillary left lateral incisor. Note that the roots of central incisors appear blunt and shorter. The external inflammatory resorption in the left lateral incisor was associated with periapical radiolucency. (**c**) Immediate postoperative radiograph in the left lateral incisor. (**d**) One-year follow-up radiograph revealed complete resolution of periapical radiolucency in the lateral incisor, and the external inflammatory resorption has stopped progressing. (**e**, **f**) Coronal CBCT images showing the true nature of the external surface resorption (blue arrows) and external inflammatory resorption (orange arrows) on these teeth. Sagittal CBCT slices show (**g**) the perforation of buccal cortical plate by periapical radiolucency on the maxillary left lateral incisor and (**h**) complete resolution of the periapical radiolucency during 1-year follow-up

irregular-shaped excavation on the root [17, 18]. The periodontal ligament space (PDL) is absent during active resorption and re-establishes once the ESR is stable [1]. The radiographic appearances of ESR on CBCT are similar to PR. However, CBCT can reveal the true extent and the exact position of the resorptive defect. Studies have shown that the use of CBCT increases the detection of ESR [19, 20]. CBCT examination is often taken prior to the treatment planning and management of impacted teeth, tumours or cyst.

11.3.2 External Cervical Resorption (ECR)

ECR mainly affects the cervical region of the tooth, but it can spread to middle and apical third of the root in advanced stage. ECR begins with the damage to the unmineralized cementum and exposure of the underlying dentine to the osteoclastic cells (initiation phase). The osteoclastic cells resorb the dentine and form a fibrovascular lesion (resorption phase). At a later stage, the fibrovascular lesion becomes calcified with bone-like metaplastic tissue as a part of reparative process (reparative phase) [21]. The exact aetiology of ECR is not known. Studies have suggested several predisposing factors that are commonly associated with ECR, i.e. orthodontic treatment, previous history of dental traumatic injuries (DTI), parafunctional habits, viral infection, intracoronal bleaching, etc. [22–24].

The clinical features of ECR are variable and dependent on the nature and extent of the lesions [25]. It is difficult to diagnose ECR clinically as they are often asymptomatic at early stage. In addition, ECR could be misdiagnosed as caries. Therefore, radiographic examination is vital in the diagnosis and management of ECR.

There is no 'classic' radiographic feature for ECR; it may present as a radiolucency in resorptive phase or may take mottled or cloudy appearance in reparative phase due to the deposition of calcified tissue into the lesions [25]. The margin of ECR lesions may be clearly defined or irregular. The root canal outline should be intact and traceable as long as the ECR lesion has not perforated the root canal. As mentioned in the IRR section earlier, ECR may be misdiagnosed as IRR, and there are limitations of using parallax technique in differentiating ECR from IRR.

CBCT reveals the exact position, nature, circumferential spread and perforation of the root canal by ECR lesion. Both in vivo and ex vivo studies have shown significantly higher sensitivity, specificity and overall accuracy with CBCT for the detection of ECR when compared to PR [3, 13]. CBCT is also a more reliable tool to distinguish between ECR and IRR [4]. ECR does not always present at the cervical region on PR, especially where the portal of entry is located at approximal surfaces or the mass of tissue destruction is distant away from the entry point of osteoclastic cells. This may have a negative impact on the management of ECR as these entry points must be managed to stop the progression of ECR lesion. CBCT images will clearly show these details and aid in the management of ECR. A clinical study by Patel et al. [5] reported that CBCT may significantly influence the assessment and the subsequent management of ECR lesions.

Historically, the Heithersay classification is commonly used to classify ECR lesions [26]. This two-dimensional classification is based solely on periapical radiographic findings and has been reported to have lower accuracy than CBCT for the correct ECR classification [3]. A three-dimensional classification (Fig. 11.4, Patel classification) has been introduced to categorize ECR lesions

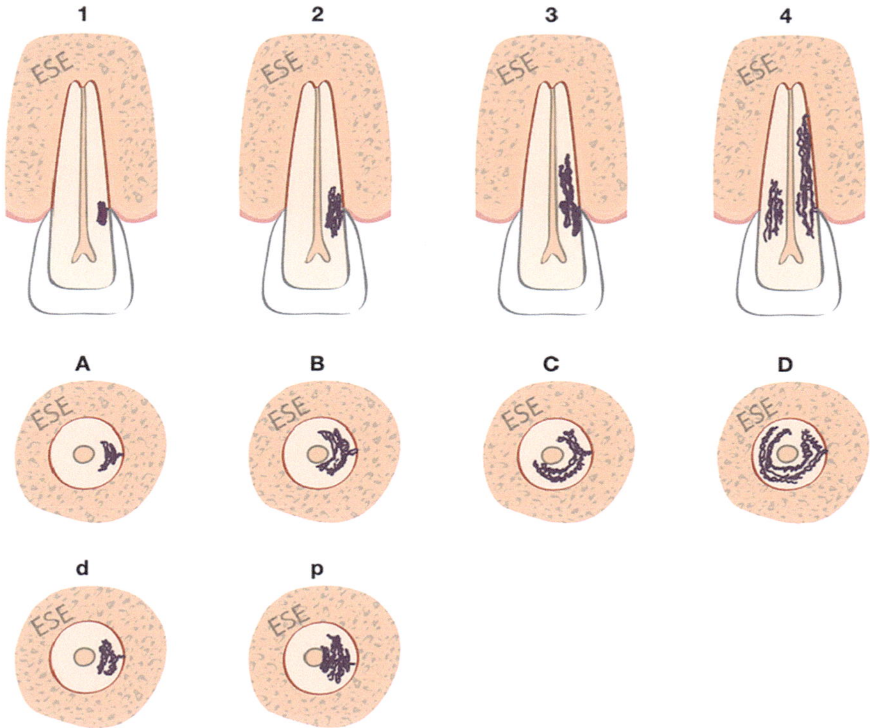

Height	Circumferential spread	Proximity to the root canal
1: At cemento-enamel junction level or coronal to the bone crest (supracrestal)	**A**: ≤90°	**d**: Confined to dentine
2: Extends into coronal third of the root and apical to the bone crest (subcrestal)	**B**: >90° to ≤180°	**p**: Probable/actual pulpal involvement
3: Extends into mid-third of the root	**C**: >180° to ≤270°	
4: Extends into apical third of the root	**D**:>270°	

Fig. 11.4 Patel 3D Classification for external cervical resorption classification. (From Patel S, Krastl G, Weiger R, Lambrechts P, Tjäderhane L, Gambarini G, et al. ESE position statement on root resorption. International Endodontic Journal. 2023;56(7):792–801. https://doi.org/10.1111/iej.13916.)

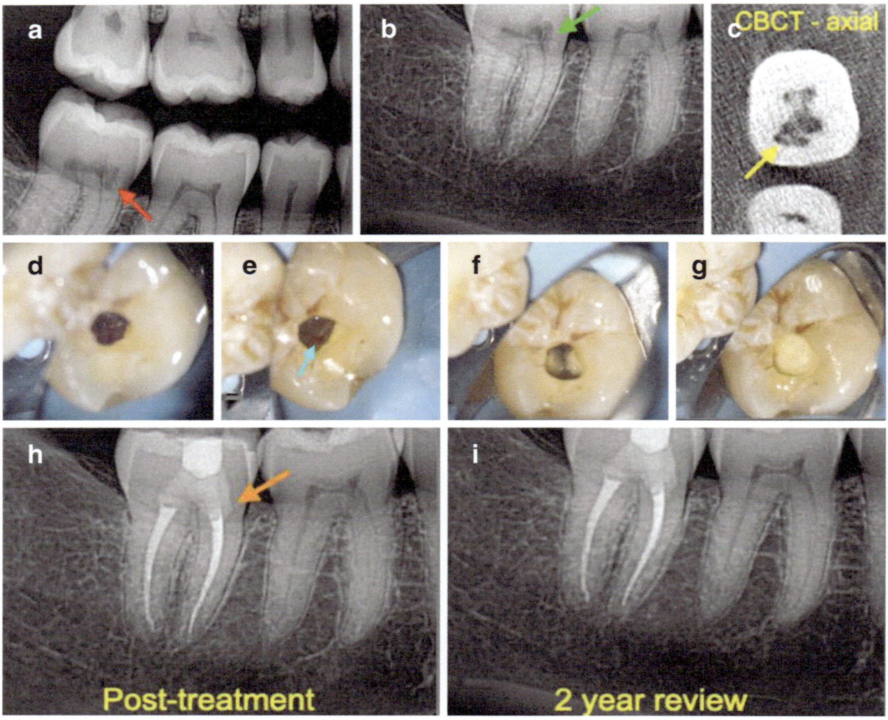

Fig. 11.5 External cervical resorption. (**a**–**c**) Radiographic presentation ECR (Patel 2Ap) on a right mandibular second molar. Endodontic treatment and internal repair (**d**) granulation and pulp tissue access, (**e**) ECR tag resulting in small bleeding point (**f**) access cavity and root canal system prepared (**g**) Biodentine to seal the access cavity (**h**) post-treatment, (**i**) 2-year follow-up. Potential predisposing factor in this case was a previous history of parafunction. (From Patel S, Saberi N, Pimental T & Teng P-H. (2022) Present status and future directions: Root resorption. *International Endodontic Journal*, 55(Suppl. 4), 892–921)

based on both PR and CBCT images [27, 28]. It takes into account the height and circumferential spread of the lesion, as well as its proximity to the root canal (Figs. 11.5 and 11.6). This new classification allows for a better understanding of the true extent of the ECR lesion in all planes and can facilitate the communication between clinicians and has also been shown to be more accurate in classification of the ECR lesion than the Heithersay classification [3]. More accurate treatment options can be recommended for ECR lesions of varying severity under this new classification [29].

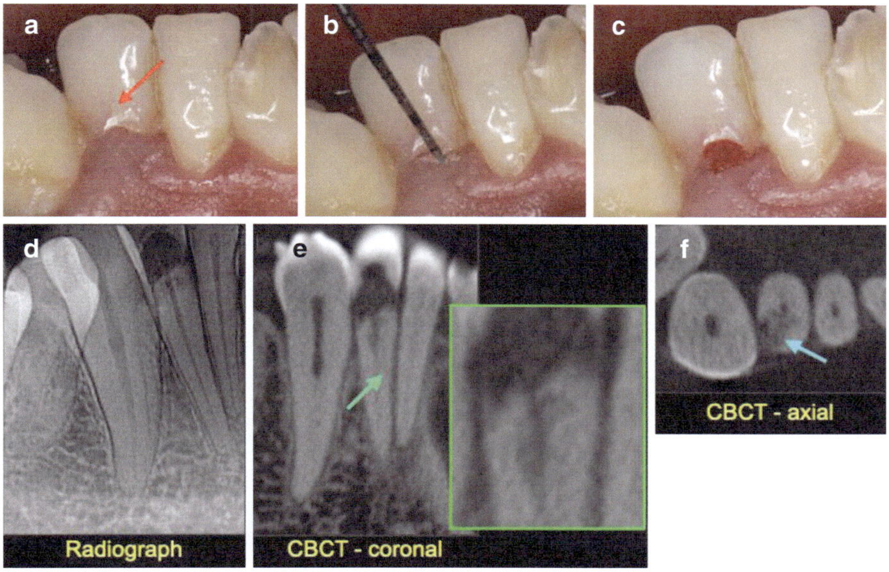

Fig. 11.6 External cervical resorption. (**a**) Subtle pink hue (red arrow) on a right mandibular lateral incisor, (**b**) probing (**c**) resulting in copious bleeding on probing (**d**) well-defined radiolucency (resorptive/destructive phase) appears to show that the ECR is confined to the coronal aspect of the tooth; (**e**) CBCT reveals the ECR extends into the coronal-third of the root (**f**) and nearly up to 180 degrees around the tooth (Patel 2Bp). The potential predisposing factors for this case was cricket ball injury sustained over 20 years ago. (From Patel S, Saberi N, Pimental T & Teng P-H. (2022) Present status and future directions: Root resorption. *International Endodontic Journal*, 55(Suppl. 4), 892–921)

11.3.3 External Inflammatory Resorption (EIR)

EIR is a common finding in majority of the teeth with chronic apical periodontitis [30, 31]. EIR due to solely chronic apical periodontitis is less aggressive and progresses at a slower pace. EIR is also a complication of moderate to severe DTI such as avulsion or luxation. Andreasen and Pedersen [32] reported 38% of intruded teeth has EIR as healing complication. This type of EIR is typically more aggressive in nature and may deteriorate rapidly without treatment.

On PR, EIR caused by solely infected necrotic pulp may present as ragged margin at root end, and the affected root may appear shorter in length. A periapical radiolucency adjacent to the affected root is a common feature. EIR associated with DTI may have ragged crater-shaped indentation along the lateral border of the affected root, loss of PDL space and a periradicular radiolucency on PR (Fig. 11.7). Advanced EIR may perforate root canal wall, but this can only be observed on PR if it involves the mesial/distal (proximal) surface of the root.

The nature and the extent of the EIR can be appreciated better in CBCT. Lesions on approximal surfaces and root canal perforation which were undetected on PR

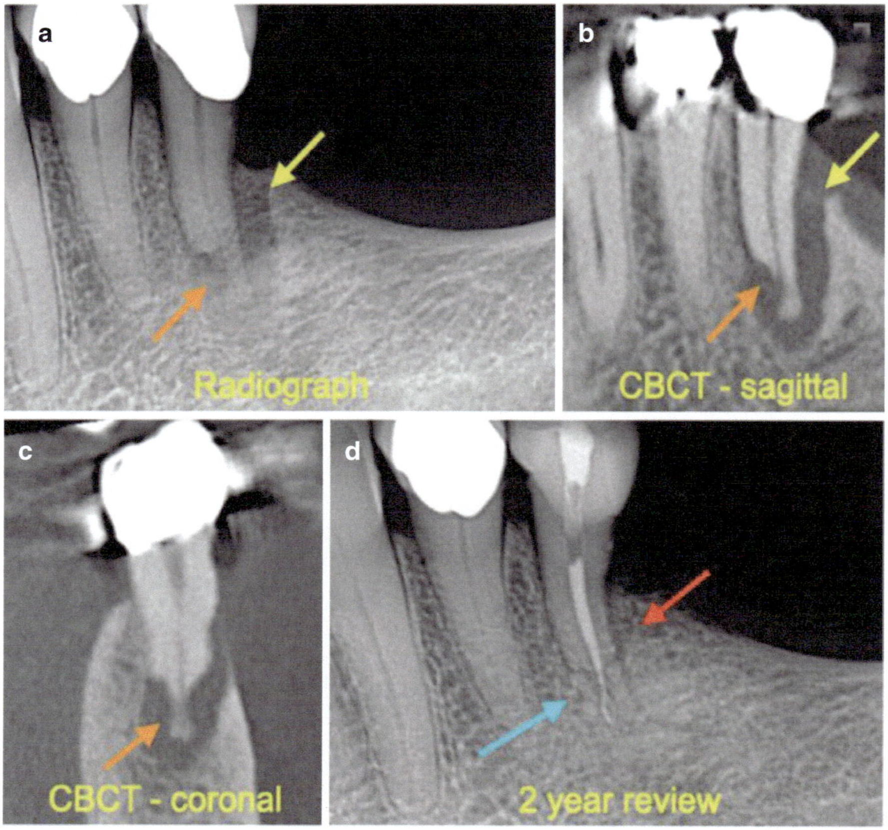

Fig. 11.7 External inflammatory resorption (**a**) A periapical radiograph, (**b**, **c**) sagittal and coronal CBCT scans revealing periradicular bone loss (yellow arrow) and periapical radiolucency associated with external inflammatory resorption (orange arrow) on the apical third of left mandibular second premolar. (**d**) Two-year post-treatment periapical (cyan arrow) and periradicular healing (red arrow). (From Patel S, Saberi N, Pimental T & Teng P-H. (2022) Present status and future directions: Root resorption. *International Endodontic Journal*, 55(Suppl. 4), 892–921)

will be clearly visible on CBCT images. This information aids in planning the root canal treatment of the affected teeth. CBCT has been reported to have higher sensitivity to detect small-simulated EIR compared to PR [33, 34].

11.3.4 External Replacement Resorption (ERR)

ERR is a common complication observed after severe DTI such as intrusion and avulsion [35, 36]. The damaged PDL cells/cementum/dentine are resorbed and replaced with alveolar bone as part of the healing process. Conventional radiographic features of ERR include the absence of PDL space and 'moth-eaten' or irregular appearance on the external root surface [37]. The external root surface will appear to fuse with the surrounding bone tissue. Andersson et al. [38] reported that ERR involving more than 20% of root surface (based on PR) will give rise to the clinical symptoms such as the lack of physiological mobility and/or production of high-pitched metallic sound upon percussion. However, PR are two-dimensional images and can only assess ERR on proximal surfaces. This most probably results in an underestimation of the extent of ERR or even missed ERR on approximal surfaces. CBCT allows reliable detection and assessment of ERR on the approximal root surfaces, as well as the small and early ERR which may be undetected on PR (Fig. 11.8). Early detection of ERR is essential and may help to avoid complications in children or adolescents such as infra-occluded tooth and localized underdevelopment of alveolar ridge.

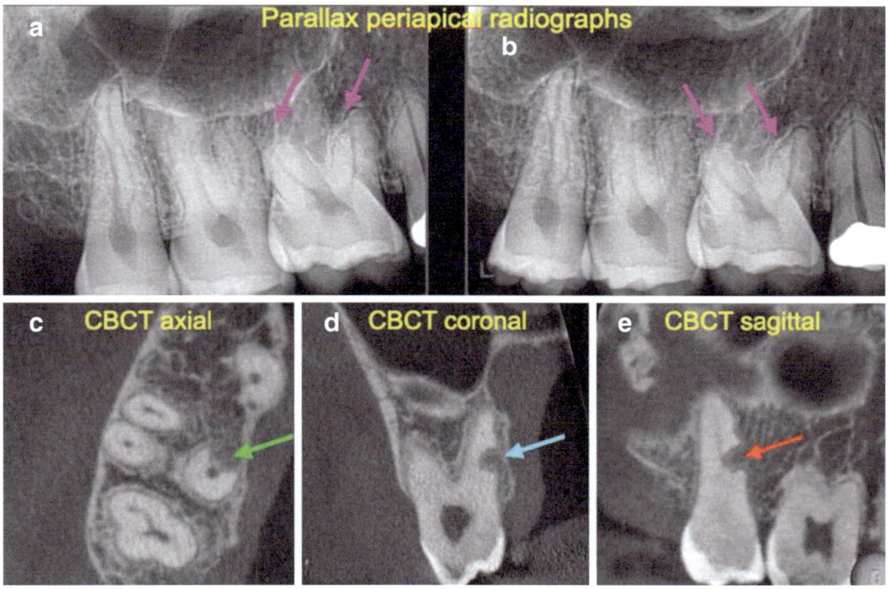

Fig. 11.8 External surface resorption and external replacement resorption. (**a**, **b**) Parallax periapical radiographs of upper right molar region taken to assess the degree of external surface resorption (pink arrow) on the maxillary right first molar after a rapid course of orthodontics, fixed braces were placed from maxillary right first molar to maxillary left first molar. The maxillary left second and third molar were not used for orthodontic anchorage. (**c**–**e**) CBCT slices reveal an unusual presentation of external replacement resorption of the maxillary right second molar, and the orthogonal views reveal the well-defined resorptive defect which is very close proximity to the root canal; no active treatment was advised, instead the patient was advised to attend for annual reviews (watchful waiting), including sensitivity testing and radiographic assessment. Note that the periodontal ligament space is visible confirming that ESR is not active. (From Patel S, Saberi N, Pimental T & Teng P-H. (2022) Present status and future directions: Root resorption. *International Endodontic Journal*, 55(Suppl. 4), 892–921)

11.3.5 Transient Apical Breakdown (TAB)

TAB is a transient resorption of the apical portion of the root after moderate DTI such as extrusion and lateral luxation [39]. Widening of PDL space and blurry or loss of the lamina dura are initial radiographic findings of TAB on PR, and these features usually resolve within 1 year. ESR and pulp canal obliteration (PCO) usually ensue following the resolution of TAB.

Some authors have suggested that TAB is merely a subtle displacement of tooth during luxation injuries and its appearance and disappearance can be caused by inadvertent beam angulation (geometric distortion) when taking periapical radiographs [1, 40]. CBCT is able to overcome the limitations of PR and detect subtle changes in periapical and PDL space to achieve accurate diagnosis in these cases (Fig. 11.9).

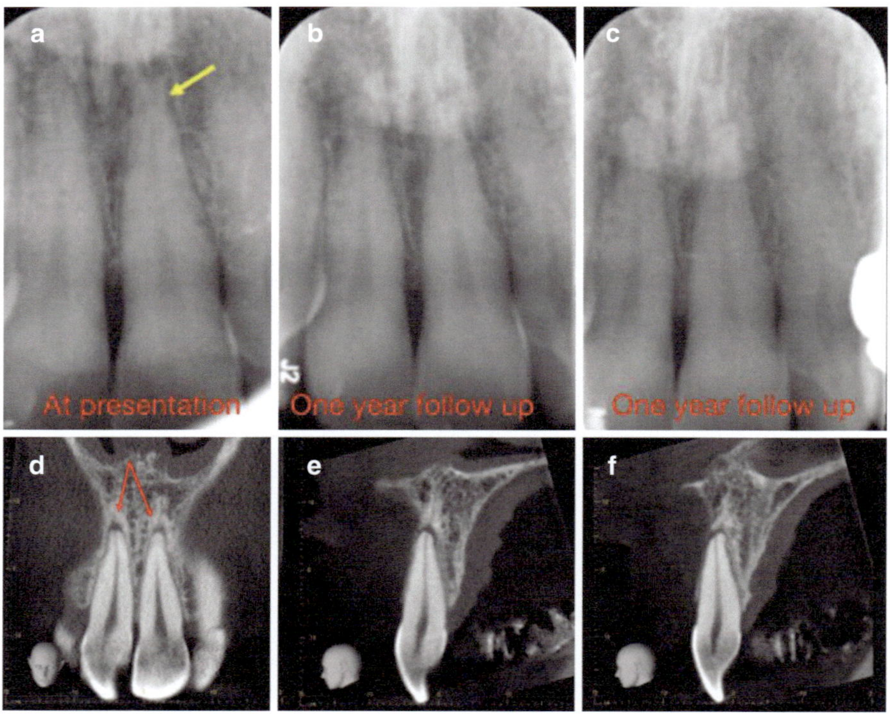

Fig. 11.9 Transient apical breakdown. (**a**) A periapical radiograph revealing widening of the periodontal ligament space and loss of apical lamina dura following subluxation injury to the maxillary anterior teeth (yellow arrow). (**b**) One-year follow-up radiograph demonstrates an improvement, and (**c**) a 10-degree vertical shift eliminates the presence of the lesion altogether, confirming a diagnosis of transient apical breakdown. (**d**–**f**) Coronal and sagittal CBCT slices of the same teeth, however, reveal well-defined periapical radiolucencies associated with the maxillary right and left central incisors (red arrows); therefore, the diagnosis was changed to chronic periapical periodontitis associated with infected necrotic pulp. This case highlights anatomical noise and subtle geometrical distortion associated with conventional radiographs which may be overcome with CBCT. (Patel S, Saberi N (2018) The ins and out of root resorption. *British Dental Journal* **224**, 691–699)

11.4 Conclusion

It is a well-accepted fact that CBCT has a significant higher accuracy and reliability than conventional PR in the assessment, diagnosis and management of various types of RR. A small field of view (FOV) and high-resolution CBCT has been recommended by various position statements in the diagnosis and treatment planning of RR [28, 29, 41, 42].

References

1. Patel S, Saberi N, Pimental T, Teng P-H. Present status and future directions: root resorption. Int Endod J. 2022;55(S4):892–921. https://doi.org/10.1111/iej.13715.
2. Andreasen FM, Sewerin I, Mandel U, Andreasen JO. Radiographic assessment of simulated root resorption cavities. Dent Traumatol. 1987;3(1):21–7. https://doi.org/10.1111/j.1600-9657.1987.tb00167.x.
3. Vaz de Souza D, Schirru E, Mannocci F, Foschi F, Patel S. External cervical resorption: a comparison of the diagnostic efficacy using 2 different cone-beam computed tomographic units and periapical radiographs. J Endod. 2017;43(1):121–5. https://doi.org/10.1016/j.joen.2016.09.008.
4. Kamburoğlu K, Kurşun Ş, Yüksel S, Öztaş B. Observer ability to detect ex vivo simulated internal or external cervical root resorption. J Endod. 2011;37(2):168–75. https://doi.org/10.1016/j.joen.2010.11.002.
5. Patel K, Mannocci F, Patel S. The assessment and management of external cervical resorption with periapical radiographs and cone-beam computed tomography: a clinical study. J Endod. 2016;42(10):1435–40. https://doi.org/10.1016/j.joen.2016.06.014.
6. Gartner AH, Mack T, Somerlott RG, Walsh LC. Differential diagnosis of internal and external root resorption. J Endod. 1976;2(11):329–34. https://doi.org/10.1016/s0099-2399(76)80071-4.
7. Patel S, Ricucci D, Durak C, Tay F. Internal root resorption: a review. J Endod. 2010;36(7):1107–21. https://doi.org/10.1016/j.joen.2010.03.014.
8. Ne RF, Witherspoon DE, Gutmann JL. Tooth resorption. Quintessence Int. 1999;30(1):9–25.
9. Gulabivala K, Searson LJ. Clinical diagnosis of internal resorption: an exception to the rule. Int Endod J. 1995;28(5):255–60. https://doi.org/10.1111/j.1365-2591.1995.tb00310.x.
10. Bhuva B, Barnes JJ, Patel S. The use of limited cone beam computed tomography in the diagnosis and management of a case of perforating internal root resorption. Int Endod J. 2011;44(8):777–86. https://doi.org/10.1111/j.1365-2591.2011.01870.x.
11. Madani Z, Moudi E, Bijani A, Mahmoudi E. Diagnostic accuracy of cone-beam computed tomography and periapical radiography in internal root resorption. Iran Endod J. 2016;11(1):51–6. https://doi.org/10.7508/iej.2016.01.010.
12. Lima TF, Gamba TO, Zaia AA, Soares AJ. Evaluation of cone beam computed tomography and periapical radiography in the diagnosis of root resorption. Aust Dent J. 2016;61(4):425–31. https://doi.org/10.1111/adj.12407.
13. Patel S, Dawood A, Wilson R, Horner K, Mannocci F. The detection and management of root resorption lesions using intraoral radiography and cone beam computed tomography–an in vivo investigation. Int Endod J. 2009;42(9):831–8. https://doi.org/10.1111/j.1365-2591.2009.01592.x.
14. Weltman B, Vig KW, Fields HW, Shanker S, Kaizar EE. Root resorption associated with orthodontic tooth movement: a systematic review. Am J Orthod Dentofacial Orthop. 2010;137(4):462–76.; discussion 12A. https://doi.org/10.1016/j.ajodo.2009.06.021.
15. Teo KW, Shi AH, Teh LY, Lee AMH. External root resorption in common odontogenic cysts and ameloblastomas of the jaw: a retrospective radiographic study in an Asian population. Oral Surg. 2021;14(4):335–41. https://doi.org/10.1111/ors.12628.

16. Matzen LH, Schropp L, Spin-Neto R, Wenzel A. Radiographic signs of pathology determining removal of an impacted mandibular third molar assessed in a panoramic image or CBCT. Dentomaxillofacial Radiol. 2017;46(1):20160330. https://doi.org/10.1259/dmfr.20160330.
17. Durack C, Patel S. Root resorption. In: Patel S, Harvey S, Shemesh H, Durack C, editors. Cone beam computed tomography in endodontics. 1st. ed. Berlin, Germany: Quintessence Publishing Co. Ltd; 2016. p. 119–31.
18. Tronstad L. Root resorption–etiology, terminology and clinical manifestations. Endod Dent Traumatol. 1988;4(6):241–52. https://doi.org/10.1111/j.1600-9657.1988.tb00642.x.
19. Alemam AA, Abu Alhaija ES, Mortaja K, AlTawachi A. Incisor root resorption associated with palatally displaced maxillary canines: analysis and prediction using discriminant function analysis. Am J Orthod Dentofacial Orthop. 2020;157(1):80–90. https://doi.org/10.1016/j.ajodo.2019.08.008.
20. Sondeijker CFW, Lamberts AA, Beckmann SH, Kuitert RB, van Westing K, Persoon S, et al. Development of a clinical practice guideline for orthodontically induced external apical root resorption. Eur J Orthod. 2020;42(2):115–24. https://doi.org/10.1093/ejo/cjz034.
21. Mavridou AM, Hauben E, Wevers M, Schepers E, Bergmans L, Lambrechts P. Understanding external cervical resorption in vital teeth. J Endod. 2016;42(12):1737–51. https://doi.org/10.1016/j.joen.2016.06.007.
22. Mavridou AM, Bergmans L, Barendregt D, Lambrechts P. Descriptive analysis of factors associated with external cervical resorption. J Endod. 2017;43(10):1602–10. https://doi.org/10.1016/j.joen.2017.05.026.
23. Heithersay GS. Invasive cervical resorption: an analysis of potential predisposing factors. Quintessence Int. 1999;30(2):83–95.
24. Friedman S, Rotstein I, Libfeld H, Stabholz A, Heling I. Incidence of external root resorption and esthetic results in 58 bleached pulpless teeth. Endod Dent Traumatol. 1988;4(1):23–6. https://doi.org/10.1111/j.1600-9657.1988.tb00288.x.
25. Patel S, Mavridou AM, Lambrechts P, Saberi N. External cervical resorption-part 1: histopathology, distribution and presentation. Int Endod J. 2018;51(11):1205–23. https://doi.org/10.1111/iej.12942.
26. Heithersay GS. Clinical, radiologic, and histopathologic features of invasive cervical resorption. Quintessence Int. 1999;30(1):27–37.
27. Patel S, Foschi F, Mannocci F, Patel K. External cervical resorption: a three-dimensional classification. Int Endod J. 2018;51(2):206–14. https://doi.org/10.1111/iej.12824.
28. Patel S, Krastl G, Weiger R, Lambrechts P, Tjäderhane L, Gambarini G, et al. ESE position statement on root resorption. International Endodontic Journal. 2023;56(7):792–801. https://doi.org/10.1111/iej.13916.
29. European Society of Endodontology. European Society of Endodontology position statement: external cervical resorption. Int Endod J. 2018;51(12):1323–6. https://doi.org/10.1111/iej.13008.
30. Laux M, Abbott PV, Pajarola G, Nair PN. Apical inflammatory root resorption: a correlative radiographic and histological assessment. Int Endod J. 2000;33(6):483–93. https://doi.org/10.1046/j.1365-2591.2000.00338.x.
31. Vier FV, Figueiredo JA. Prevalence of different periapical lesions associated with human teeth and their correlation with the presence and extension of apical external root resorption. Int Endod J. 2002;35(8):710–9. https://doi.org/10.1046/j.1365-2591.2002.00554.x.
32. Andreasen FM, Pedersen BV. Prognosis of luxated permanent teeth–the development of pulp necrosis. Endod Dent Traumatol. 1985;1(6):207–20. https://doi.org/10.1111/j.1600-9657.1985.tb00583.x.
33. Estrela C, Bueno MR, De Alencar AH, Mattar R, Valladares Neto J, Azevedo BC, et al. Method to evaluate inflammatory root resorption by using cone beam computed tomography. J Endod. 2009;35(11):1491–7. https://doi.org/10.1016/j.joen.2009.08.009.

34. Durack C, Patel S, Davies J, Wilson R, Mannocci F. Diagnostic accuracy of small volume cone beam computed tomography and intraoral periapical radiography for the detection of simulated external inflammatory root resorption. Int Endod J. 2011;44(2):136–47. https://doi.org/10.1111/j.1365-2591.2010.01819.x.
35. Soares AJ, Souza GA, Pereira AC, Vargas-Neto J, Zaia AA, Silva EJ. Frequency of root resorption following trauma to permanent teeth. J Oral Sci. 2015;57(2):73–8. https://doi.org/10.2334/josnusd.57.73.
36. Souza BDM, Dutra KL, Kuntze MM, Bortoluzzi EA, Flores-Mir C, Reyes-Carmona J, et al. Incidence of root resorption after the replantation of avulsed teeth: a meta-analysis. J Endod. 2018;44(8):1216–27. https://doi.org/10.1016/j.joen.2018.03.002.
37. Andreasen JO, Hjørting-Hansen E, Replantation of teeth. I. Radiographic and clinical study of 110 human teeth replanted after accidental loss. Acta Odontol Scand. 1966;24(3):263–86. https://doi.org/10.3109/00016356609028222.
38. Andersson L, Blomlöf L, Lindskog S, Feiglin B, Hammarström L. Tooth ankylosis: clinical, radiographic and histological assessments. Int J Oral Surg. 1984;13(5):423–31. https://doi.org/10.1016/S0300-9785(84)80069-1.
39. Andreasen FM. Transient apical breakdown and its relation to color and sensibility changes after luxation injuries to teeth. Dent Traumatol. 1986;2(1):9–19. https://doi.org/10.1111/j.1600-9657.1986.tb00118.x.
40. Patel S, Saberi N. The ins and outs of root resorption. Br Dent J. 2018;224(9):691–9. https://doi.org/10.1038/sj.bdj.2018.352.
41. American Association of Endodontists/American Academy of Oral & Maxillofacial Radiology. AAE and AAOMR joint position statement: use of cone beam computed tomography in endodontics 2015 update. Oral Surg Oral Med Oral Pathol Oral Radiol. 2015;120(4):508–12. https://doi.org/10.1016/j.oooo.2015.07.033.
42. European Society of Endodontology. European Society of Endodontology position statement: use of cone beam computed tomography in endodontics: European Society of Endodontology (ESE) developed by. Int Endod J. 2019;52(12):1675–8. https://doi.org/10.1111/iej.13187.

MIX
Papier aus verantwortungsvollen Quellen
Paper from responsible sources
FSC® C105338

If you have any concerns about our products,
you can contact us on
ProductSafety@springernature.com

In case Publisher is established outside the EU,
the EU authorized representative is:
Springer Nature Customer Service Center GmbH
Europaplatz 3, 69115 Heidelberg, Germany

Printed by Libri Plureos GmbH
in Hamburg, Germany